Psychopathological Disorders of Childhood

Psychopathological Disorders of Childhood

Edited by

Herbert C. Quay
Temple University

John S. Werry
University of Auckland
School of Medicine

John Wiley & Sons, Inc.
New York • London • Sydney • Toronto

Library of Congress Catalogue Card Number: 76-180273

ISBN 0-471-70249-8

Printed in the United States of America.

10 9 8 7 6 5 4

Contributors

C. Keith Conners
  Director, Child Development Laboratory, Massachusetts General Hospital and
  Associate Professor of Psychiatry, Harvard Medical School
Spencer Gibbins
  Research Associate, Institute for the Study of Mental Retardation, University
  of Michigan
E. Mavis Hetherington
  Professor of Psychology, University of Virginia
Frank M. Hewett
  Professor of Education and Psychiatry, University of California, Los Angeles
Barclay Martin
  Professor of Psychology, University of Wisconsin
K. Daniel O'Leary
  Associate Professor of Psychology, State University of New York, Stony Brook
Herbert C. Quay
  Chairman and Professor, Division of Educational Psychology, Temple University
William C. Rhodes
  Professor of Psychology and Education, University of Michigan
Lee N. Robins
  Professor of Psychiatry, Washington University School of Medicine
Alan O. Ross
  Professor of Psychology, State University of New York, Stony Brook
John S. Werry
  Professor and Head, Department of Psychiatry, University of Auckland School
  of Medicine

Preface

This volume had two main catalysts. Our work in mental health facilities for children in Canada and the United States, revealed that clinical knowledge was used and taught as if its validity and utility had been well examined and documented. Most books for the mental health professional or clinical student are of an anecdotal, how-to-do-it nature. Critical reviews and attitudes aimed at estimating the scientific and practical work of clinical knowledge are few and far between.

The second wellspring of this book was our conviction that clinically derived psychoanalytic theory, which still dominates the clinical scene in North America, had been superseded by new theory, methodology, and technology of treatment derived from behavioral science, particularly the behavioral-social learning approach. This is not meant to denigrate the past role of psycho-dynamic theory and techniques that fifty years ago had been as revolutionary as the behavioral approach seems today. Science progresses by a fickle willingness to jettison theories when they are proven false or superseded by better ways of looking at things. Generally, however, new theories seldom represent dramatic leaps in knowledge but rather the honing, refining, or recasting of old theories so that their heuristic or therapeutic usefulness is enhanced. Thus, in the behavioral approach, one can see traces of psychoanalytic theory—notably in the conceptualization of the learning process. For the psychoanalyst the conceptualization of the learning process is in Freud's pleasure-pain principle, but for the behavior modifier it is Thorndike's law of effect, both of which are essentially similar. The basic differences in the behavioral-social learning approach are in its emphasis on empiricism, pragmatism, and a rejection of the unconscious as a useful hypothetical construct.

This latter is often misinterpreted to mean that behaviorally oriented clinicians and researchers are not interested or reject the inner processes of thinking and feeling. This is not true; simply, primary emphasis is given to phenomena that can be objectified, or to their immediate derivates, intervening variables instead of more remote hypothetical constructs. In this respect, Freud's development of the technique of free association was an attempt to objectify intervening variables—the verbalizations of the patient were presumed to be the observable measurable indicators of the unconscious conflict. The failure of psychoanalytic theory to realize its scientific potential was as much the result of the failure of Freud and its other protagonists to apply rigorously the methodology of scientific investigation to these observable phenomena and to the definition of intervening variables as it was of any inherent nonfalsifiability of the theory.

Although the enthusiasm for the behavioral approach is clear in most of this book (especially Chapters Six, Seven, and Ten), certain notes of caution must be sounded.

The first concerns the theory *qua* theory. No one (hopefully) would ever claim that modern behaviorism is a comprehensive theory of human behavior. Its strength lies less in discovering the nature of man than in the development of a technology (behavior therapy or behavior modification) of changing certain aspects of human behavior and of measuring whether this has been achieved. The functional relationships between stimulus and response or response and reinforcement on which the technology depends are less invariant and less predictable the more complex the behavior and the intervening variables become. Behaviorists need to turn their attention to internal behaviors if the technology is to advance.

The second area for caution lies in certain aspects of the developing technology. Professional and popular acceptance of a clinical technology, such as happened to psychoanalysis and which is now occurring to behavior modification, almost inevitably leads to loss of self-criticism. Behavioral technologies have generally reflected their experimental origins, but there are increasing signs that polemical dispute and dogma are taking the place of empirical demonstration. The criticism has often been made that behaviorists are not treating the "underlying cause." Although such a medical or disease concept of behavioral deviance has not yet been shown to be valid since predicted outcomes such as symptom substitution apparently do not occur, the question of dealing with classes or responses instead of with individual responses or symptoms, which is one of the keys to more efficient treatment, has received less attention than it merits. Although the efficiency of behavior modification looks more promising than intensive individual psychotherapy (see Chapters Five, Seven, and Nine) in its shortness and its ability to use untrained persons including parents as agents of behavior change, the goals of psychotherapy were always more ambitious—fundamental and durable personality change. When behaviorists attack such complex problems as teaching autistic children language or academic skills (see Chapters Five and Seven), the same need for prolonged individual attention characteristic of psychoanalytic approaches is apparent. Furthermore the results, although dramatic and worthwhile, are still quite limited. For example, autistic children seldom seem to develop more than a parrotlike use of language and their repertoire of social behaviors remains quite limited.

There are other areas in the technology that need study. The problems of generalization of effect from the therapeutic situation to the broader social context is perhaps less of a problem than it is with office-centered play or psychotherapies, since the behaviorist usually carries out his treatment (with children) in the environment in which the problem behavior occurs and by the expectation that generalization to environment in which reinforcers are contingent on quite different behavior will occur spontaneously.

Despite these weaknesses we believe that if the behavioral approach adheres to its empirical beginnings and can continue to attract sensitive and ingenious clinicians as well as theoreticians, some of these problems can and will be solved.

Herbert C. Quay
John S. Werry

Orientation and Organization

Our original goal was to cover as completely as possible the whole do-main of clinical knowledge in the form of a unified critical review culminating in pointers for profitable lines of future investigation. This would have neces-sitated our becoming authors and spending two or three years doing little else. In addition, the literature had become so vast and in certain areas so special-ized that the common tactic of multiple authorship had to be used. This has resulted in a certain inevitable unevenness in style and content, but this should present no major handicap. It will be obvious that, with few exceptions, the contributors have been chosen for the compatibility of their outlook with ours, which is less rigidly behaviorial than it is an assumption of the usefulness of the scientific method in studying and treating the psychopathological disorders of childhood.

Chapter One introduces some of the problems and proposed solutions in the classification of deviant behaviors in children. Its major task, however, is to establish a framework for understanding and studying deviant behavior in terms of the basic patterns of aggression, withdrawal, and immaturity that have so consistently emerged from multivariate statistical analyses of children's behavior problems. However, this conception is relatively new to the field and has not been the basis for most theory and research. It is most clearly reflected in the later chapter on parental behavior.

The implications and problems associated with the dimensional approach for assessment and subsequent treatment are also discussed in Chapter Six. In many ways, Chapter One is a highly personal chapter. The author has been deeply involved in the multivariate study of children's psychopathology and the relationships of the patterns of deviant behaviors to both behavior change and education for over 15 years.

In contrast to the fact that much of Chapter One is based on statistical and experimental studies, the next three chapters are based on more clinical studies found generally in the medical and psychiatric literature. Chapters

Eight and Eleven also rely to a considerable degree on the medical-psychiatric literature.

Chapter Ten, on community organization and planning, approaches the field from a broader perspective and presents a conception which is of very recent origin, at least in its relevance to current programming for the deviant child. Since it is a new and emerging area its data base is limited. A historical perspective is also provided in this chapter.

Our original conception included three chapters that do not appear. We had thought that the institutional treatment of the deviant child was a domain of concern requiring separate treatment. Although this is perhaps true, the paucity of empirical literature, the inability to define the milieu therapy as independent from drug, play, behavior, or educational therapy, and the failure to define criteria for success convinced us that there was little merit in attempting to include a separate chapter at this time.

A chapter devoted to verbal and play psychotherapy with children may seem conspicuous by its absence. While an explication of psychotherapeutic techniques and the psychodynamic theories on which they are based would have been possible, the lack of empirical research in the various techniques and their lack of proven effectiveness would have made such a chapter unlike the research reviews that constitute the main emphasis of this book.

Finally, Rema Lapouse, who was one of the most distinguished epidemiologists of children's psychopathological disorders fell ill and subsequently died before she could get beyond the initial sketches of her chapters on epidemiology. It was impossible to do more than allude to the methods, problems, and results in any of the first four chapters or in the brief section of Chapter Eleven devoted to incidence.

During the writing and editing of this book one of us (H.C.Q.) was on the faculty of the University of Illinois as well as in his present position at Temple University. The other (J.S.W.) was also on the faculty of the University of Illinois, and was the Director of the Institute of Juvenile Research prior to returning to his native New Zealand to assume his current position. The preparation of Chapters Two, Three, and Four was supported in part by U. S. Public Health Service Grant MHO7346 from the National Institute of Mental Health and by the Medical Research Council of New Zealand.

H.C.Q.
J.S.W.

Contents

Psychopathological Disorders of Childhood

Chapter One

Patterns of Aggression, Withdrawal, and Immaturity

Herbert C. Quay

The Meaning of Classification

Progress in scientific understanding in many fields has frequently been closely associated with the scientists' ability to describe and classify entities or events into categories. In the field of abnormal psychology understanding has also followed description, particularly when the observed behavioral phenomena have been shown to have a physiological basis. For example, the constellation of behavioral and physical phenomena called general paresis was first described and then its relationship to the syphilis spirochete was discovered. Since such direct cause-and-effect relationships are few and far between in the behavioral realm, it is fortunate that the value of classification in the field of behavior disorders is not limited to relationships between disorder and etiology.

As Lorr (1961) has pointed out, there have been two competing points of view in regard to categories of behavior disorder. The older "class-model" holds that all or nearly all symptoms must be present before the disorder can be considered present. The disorder is either present or absent; it cannot vary in amount. This view also holds that disorders are mutually exclusive; a person cannot be both psychopathic and neurotic. On the other hand, the more recent "quantitative model" conceives of the disorder as a group of symptoms, with the number of symptoms present being the measure of the intensity of the disorder. This model assumes that the symptoms form a dimension of disorder and that all individuals have a place on this dimension, i.e., all persons possess the disorder to a greater or lesser degree. This model also recognizes that since the dimensions are independent, an individual *can* be both neurotic and psychopathic. Further discussion of theories, models, and problems in classification may be found in Eysenck (1961), Eron (1966), and Costello (1970).

Whatever the model, the rationale for any system of classifying psychopathological disorders of children is that the assignment of a child to a category or categories permits useful statements about the child based on his membership in that category. When a child is labeled as having a certain kind of disorder, this label should imply further information about him. For example, such a designation might allow statements or predictions about his relationships with his parents, his school performance, his likelihood of responding to a particular type of treatment, or his future behavior. But before such statements based on category membership can be made, a number of conditions must be met. The first step must be to demonstrate that the category or dimension of disorder actually exists. Is there, in fact, a constellation of behaviors, observable with regularity in one or more situations, that defines the disorder? This is a crucial question, and much of the research discussed in this chapter is directed toward answering it.

After it has been determined that patterns of deviant behavior occur with regularity, the second step is to demonstrate that children can reliably be placed somewhere on the continuum of characteristics defining one or more of the patterns. Obviously, a child cannot be assigned to one pattern by one clinician and to another pattern by a second clinician. Neither can he be extremely high on the continuum today and extremely low tomorrow. A lack of reliability and stability have plagued the use of categories derived from the class model currently employed in the field of adult behavior disorders.

Finally, the relationships between the patterns of deviant behavior and their psychological antecedents and consequences must be demonstrated. The meaningfulness of any pattern depends on those relationships that can be demonstrated in differential etiologies, differential responses to treatment procedures, and differential outcomes. Many of the later chapters of this book are devoted to a review of such relationships as they now exist.

As simple as these requirements may seem, they have rarely been met, even in the field of adult disorders where a "standard" system of categories of behavior disorder is in widespread usage. In a discussion of research on the extent of agreement between clinicians on diagnoses, Zubin (1967, p. 383) points out that "the degree of overall agreement between different observers is too low for individual diagnosis." Reviewing studies on the consistency of diagnosis over time, Zubin also concludes that "for the specific categories, with the exception of several of the organic, the consistency of diagnosis is for the most part low" (p. 386). Also, Costello (1970), reviewing all the problems associated with the current classification system, concludes that a continuation of reliance on psychiatric diagnostic categories of the traditional kind is unwarranted and may be a disservice to both psychiatry and the psychiatric patient. Such conclusions leave clinically derived classification systems stemming from the class model open to serious criticism.

Although no less than 24 different systems of classification have been proposed for children's behavior disorders (Group for the Advancement of Psychiatry, 1966; pp. 297–322), no reliability studies of diagnostic classification have been reported. The absence of such studies is no doubt partly a result of the fact that none of these proposed systems has been widely adopted. As Zubin (1967, p. 400) has succinctly stated in referring to childhood disorders, "the state of diagnostic procedure is even more incoherent in this field than in the adult field." In fact, reports of diagnostic practices in psychiatric clinics (Rosen, Bahn, & Kramer, 1964) indicate that about 70% of children are classified under the rubric of "adjustment reaction." This is a broad category implying little more than the fact that the child has some behavior problem.

To better understand the current state of affairs and to set the stage for the discussion of more recent attempts to solve the problem of classification, we must return to a consideration of the older class model of categories of deviant behaviors. This model has been closely associated with a particular approach to the development of diagnostic categories generally referred to as the clinical method. This method, the traditional one in psychiatry and abnormal psychology, essentially relies on observations made by clinical workers of their patients. Clinicians may come together to discuss their impressions and to try to arrive at consensus, but quantitative statistical methods are not utilized. A fairly close look at this method in action can serve to point up some deficiencies and can permit some corrections to be suggested.

The most recent attempt to develop a comprehensive classification system for psychopathological disorders in childhood is that by the Group of Advancement of Psychiatry (1966). This system resulted from the collaborative efforts of a group of experienced child psychiatrists who worked as a committee. The result of their deliberation is a classification involving ten major headings under which may be found a variety of subtypes. Each of these subtypes is described in terms of symptoms and psychodynamics. Anxious personality, for example, is described as follows:

These children are chronically tense and apprehensive over new situations, often related to their extraordinarily vivid fantasies. They usually perceive the environment as threatening, however, and are not aware of and do not exhibit crippling anxieties, as do those with anxiety neurosis. Marked inhibitions or serious constriction of the total personality are not present, and they are often able to deal adequately with new situations after initial anxiety, in contrast to children with developmental deviations, who do not have stage-appropriate social capacities available (p. 241).

In setting forth Anxious Personality as a category of disorder certain assumptions have been implicitly made. It is first assumed that there is, in fact, a disorder composed of the symptoms and dynamics used to describe Anxious Personality. It has been presumed that these symptoms and dynamics actually occur together; that they form a homogeneous cluster of characteristics which define the disorder. But to what extent do these symptoms actually occur together? What is the correlation between the presence of "chronically tense and apprehensive" and "perception of the environment as threatening?" Does the pattern of intercorrelations between these and other symptoms and dynamics show that they do form a homogeneous cluster of characteristics? Despite the wealth of clinical observation that may go into the makeup of a classification system, the degree of interrelatedness of the characteristics said to comprise a category cannot simply be assumed. The question is really a statistical one and can be answered only by the application of appropriate statistical procedures to data collected under appropriate conditions.

It has also been assumed that clinicians will be able to make reliable judgments about whether a child manifests the symptoms and dynamics of the category. However, the extent to which clinicians can agree on whether a child "perceives the environment as threatening" or has "extraordinarily vivid fantasies" is problematical. It is well known that judgments requiring a high degree of inference are made much less reliably than those made on the basis of observable behavior. When symptoms and other diagnostic indicators are not described in terms of overt behavior, there is less likelihood of agreement among clinicians as to their presence or absence.

The uses to which the proposed classification is to be put must now be considered. At this point the utility of the proposed system can be judged only on the basis of internal consistency and interjudge reliability criteria. But the ultimate proof of the pudding is in the eating. No amount of internal consistency, harmony with theory, or caveats about relativism and dynamism that the Group for the Advancement of Psychiatry considers important can serve to make useful a descriptive scheme with no predictive or etiological correlates. The report itself indicates an awareness of this problem:

> The ideal scheme of classification would, as has been implied, permit a synthesis of the clinical picture, the psychodynamic and psycho-social factors, "genetic" considerations regarding the level or origin, the major ideological forces, a concise prognosis, and the appropriate method of treatment. The conceptual framework described would nevertheless

permit the conclusion that such a clinical-dynamic-genetic ideological scheme of classification is presently premature if not unrealistic. From the information currently available, only the clinical-descriptive aspects can be dealt with in a classification that is susceptible to the use of statistical methods and can be employed by people from differing schools of thought (Group for the Advancement of Psychiatry, pp. 208–209).

It is clear from the above quotation that the correlates of the categories of this system are currently at the implicit and clinical-observation stage. In view of the newness of the proposed system, this is understandable. However, the system, carrying the prestige of the committee, represents a culmination of efforts utilizing the clinical method. Its usage in child psychiatry is clearly intended by its creators.

Finally, it is clear that the proponents of the proposed classification system view all behavior disorder as disease (p. 181); analogies are drawn between psychological processes and physical illnesses. The extent to which all behavior disorder can be considered to be disease has been the subject of lively debate (see Szasz, 1960 and Ausubel, 1961). Regardless of which point of view is correct about the similarity of behavior disorders to disease, for purposes of developing classifications schemes and for the diagnostic process, the disease assumption has some clear-cut consequences. These consequences are related to both etiology and treatment and will be dealt with in later chapters of this volume.

Multivariate Statistical Approaches to Classification

The newer quantitative view of behavior disorder in children has led to another way of attacking the problem which can obviate many of the difficulties associated with the clinical method. This approach involves isolating patterns of behavior that are statistically interrelated. The approach was first used by Ackerson (1942) and Hewitt and Jenkins (1946), who analyzed case histories of problem children by means of lists of behavior traits. Although their methodology was unsophisticated by today's standards, the findings of Hewitt and Jenkins, the more definitive of the two early investigations, have been generally supported by later research. These investigators began with a pool of 500 case records of children who had been referred to a child guidance clinic for some behavior problem. The investigators rated 45 frequently occurring descriptive phrases about behavior for their presence or absence in each of the case records and then intercorrelated them. An analysis of the pattern of interrelationships among the behavior traits was then performed by visual inspection. The purpose of the analysis was to find which traits occurred together, thus forming clusters or syndromes of deviant behavior. Three primary behavioral syndromes were identified. They were labeled the unsocialized aggressive, the socialized delinquent, and the overinhibited child.

Fifty-two children were thus classified as unsocialized aggressive, 70 as socialized delinquent, and 73 as overinhibited. The number of multiple classifications was small but, as the above figures reveal, only about two-fifths of the 500 children could be designated as representative of any of the three major syndromes. This failure to be able to classify over three-fifths of the sample illustrates a problem that arises when one uses behavior dimensions as if they were personality types. This problem will be discussed in greater detail later. Despite this problem, and Hewitt and Jenkins were successful in establishing that a variety of problem-behavior traits were subsumable under a pattern of behavioral inhibition, anxiety, and withdrawal and two distinct patterns of aggression.

A study by Peterson (1961), which has served as a model for much additional work, is an excellent illustration of a more sophisticated methodology. Peterson began by considering carefully the need for an adequate sampling of the many behaviors of children that could be considered as deviant. This complete sampling was an important step since behavior traits not included obviously could not appear in any syndromes that might be isolated. Over 400 representatively selected case folders from the files of a child guidance clinic were inspected and the referral problems of each child were noted. Eliminating overlap and selecting on the basis of relatively frequent occurrence, 58 items descriptive of deviant behavior were chosen and compiled into a checklist. A sample of 831 grammar school students in kindergarten through sixth grade were then rated by their teachers on this problem checklist. The correlations among all the items were obtained and this matrix of intercorrelations was subjected to further study by means of factor analysis. This statistical technique enables one to isolate clusters of behaviors (or other variables) interrelated among themselves and thus forming an underlying behavioral dimension. A "factor loading" is also obtained for each constituent behavior. This factor loading reveals the extent to which that behavior is related to the underlying dimension. Peterson's results indicated that the interrelations among the 58 items could be resolved into two independent clusters, which he called "Conduct Problem" and "Personality Problem." Thus, Peterson demonstrated that the vast majority of problem behaviors in public school students could be accounted for by two major dimensions: essentially one of aggression and one of withdrawal. Furthermore, each child could be placed somewhere on these two dimensions according to the number of problem behaviors related to the dimension that the child manifests. It is important to note that children differ in quantity but not in quality; the normal and abnormal differ only in degree.

In the building of a classification system, the statistical approach clearly obviates two of the basic weaknesses characteristic of the clinical approach. First, empirical evidence is obtained showing that the dimension exists as an observable constellation of behavior. Second, as will be discussed later in this chapter, the objective nature of most of the constituent behaviors permits considerable reliability of judgment about the degree to which a child manifests the dimension. This approach is not, however, without pitfalls of its own. One criticism, which has been applied to the technique of factor analysis in general, is characterized by the statement: "If something does not go into the analysis, it cannot come out." This simply means that a dimension not represented by its constituent behavior traits in the analysis cannot possibly emerge. Neither can a dimension be identified unless there is an intercorrelation of some subset of behaviors (since this intercorrelated subset in fact constitutes the cluster). Such intercorrelation depends on the sample in which the behaviors are observed.

In the Peterson study, for example, a dimension of behavior that might have been labeled "psychoticism" was not found. There clearly is such a syndrome (see Chapter Five) and its failure to emerge was a function of the fact that there were no behaviors related to it in Peterson's checklist and there were no children manifesting the syndrome in the samples studied. Clearly, Peterson's method did not permit a dimension of psychoticism to emerge in his analysis. But such problems are by no means fatal; deviant behaviors can be selected carefully for inclusiveness, and a variety of samples of children can be systematically studied.

An additional criticism of the factor analytic technique which is sometimes voiced is that the factors which emerge are dimensions of behavior, not types of individuals. As we have already pointed out, Peterson's two dimensions are sets of behaviors that all children possess to varying degrees: A child is rarely "all problem" or "no problem." But there are few, if any, instances of clear-cut types in any other area of human behavior. In the field of childhood psychopathology it is likely that behavior description will have to be in terms of dimensions rather than types. However, children who represent extremes of these dimensions will frequently be found, and it is these children who are often a principal cause for concern.

A somewhat more serious and more complex problem for the establishment of factor analytically based descriptive systems has been the degree to which the method of data collection (e.g., ratings and questionnaires) and the settings in which the data are collected influence the results. Are the behavioral dimensions that result from different methods really the same? This problem of "factor matching," which has occurred in studies of adult personality, has stimulated considerable controversy because it involves using the results of studies which employ different methods (Becker, 1960; Becker, 1961;

Cattell, 1961). Empirical studies of the comparability of factors arising from different methods of assessing children's behavior problems are limited in number (see Chapter Six). Categories arising from the analysis of behavior ratings may or may not be the same as those arising from the analysis of life history data even though they look to be the same. There is always some possibility that the method may produce the result. Peterson (1965) for example, has suggested that the meaning systems of those doing the ratings may be reflected more in factors arising from behavior ratings than in the behavior of those being rated. It is also clear that the situation in which the behavior is observed influences what behavior does, in fact, occur. A thorough discussion of the possible influences of methods and situations is beyond the scope of this chapter (see Chapter Six).

Although it may be necessary to develop a particular method to assess a given behavior dimension as it may be observed by a particular setting (e.g., classroom) this complicates, but in no way invalidates, the meaningfulness of the dimension. It is the relationship of factorially derived dimensions of behavior, however measured, to etiological and treatment variables that give the dimensions psychological relevance.

Finally there are the criticisms leveled by those with strong clinical and dynamic orientations who charge that the statistical approaches result in categories that are oversimplified and lack dynamic quality (e.g., Anthony, 1967; Willer, 1967). These criticisms arise from theoretical predilections and no amount of data appear to be able to dispel them. In return one may only inquire about the value of a system, however complex, dynamic, and theoretically elegant, which does not reflect the actual behavior of children, cannot be reliably applied, and whose only usefulness is in its appeal to the clinician because of its compatibility with his theoretical biases.

Clearly multivariate statistical approaches, although not without some associated difficulties, are currently the methods of choice for classification system construction. A sizable number of such studies have been done using data from many different domains and sampling children in a number of different settings. The results of these studies suggest that there are a number of dimensions of problem behavior which consistently appear regardless of the type of data used or of the sample of children studied.

The remainder of this chapter is devoted to the patterns of aggression, withdrawal, and immaturity that have emerged from these studies in terms of their constituent behaviors, the reliability with which they can be observed, their relationships to age and sex, and their correlates with other psychological variables. Additional data on differential etiology and prognosis will appear in later chapters.

Conduct Disorder

Almost without exception multivariate statistical studies of problem behaviors in children reveal the presence of a pattern involving aggressive behavior, both verbal and physical, associated with poor interpersonal relationships with both adults and peers. This pattern has received a variety of labels: e.g., unsocialized aggressive (Hewitt & Jenkins, 1946); conduct problem (Peterson, 1962; Quay & Quay, 1965); aggressive (Patterson, 1964); unsocialized psychopathic (Quay, 1964a; 1964b); psychopathic delinquency (Peterson, Quay & Cameron, 1959); antisocial aggressiveness and sadistic aggressiveness (Dreger, et al., 1964); and externalizing (Achenbach, 1966). Table 1 presents those characteristics most frequently associated with this dimension.

The behaviors listed in Table 1 have been selected to represent data obtained by direct observations and behavior ratings, by the analysis of data from case records, and by the responses of children and adolescents to questionnaires. In addition, they represent the work of different investigators studying children in a variety of different settings. The list is not meant to be exhaustive, nor is it intended to establish precise comparability between studies. Comparability between studies using similar behavior traits has been established empirically (e.g., Quay, 1964a; Quay & Quay, 1965; Quay, 1966; Brady, 1970; Lessing & Zagorin, 1971). Studies employing different trait lists can only be judged as to comparability in terms of the psychological meaning conveyed by the dimensions that emerge.

The ubiquitous nature of conduct disorder is attested to by its appearance in samples of children in public schools (e.g., Peterson, 1961; Quay & Quay, 1965; Ross, Lacey, & Parton, 1965; Quay, Morse, & Cutler, 1966; Brady, 1970), children referred to child guidance clinics (e.g., Patterson, 1964; Dreger, et al., 1964; Miller, 1967), children in institutions for the delinquent (Quay, 1964a; 1964b), and children in hospitals and institutions for the mentally ill and mentally retarded (Spivack & Spotts, 1965; Achenbach, 1966).

The pattern can be elicited from the observations and behavior ratings of teachers (Peterson, 1962; Brady, 1970), parents (Miller, 1967; Lessing & Zagorin, 1971), guidance clinic staff (Patterson, 1964), and correctional workers (Quay, 1964) by the analysis of case history materials (Hewitt & Jenkins, 1946; Quay, 1964b; Achenbach, 1966) and from the responses of children and adolescents themselves to personality questionnaires (Peterson, Quay, & Tiffany, 1961).

Neither is the dimension limited to the American culture. Studies in Canada (Pimm, Quay, & Werry, 1967) and in Great Britain (Collins, Maxwell, & Cameron, 1962) clearly reveal the presence of this pattern in those cultures.

TABLE 1

Selected Behavior Traits, Life History Characteristics, and Questionnaire
Responses Associated with Conduct Disorder

Behavior Traits	Representative Studies[a]							
Disobedience	1,	4,	6,	8,	9,	15		
Disruptiveness	1,	4,	6,	8,	9,	15		
Fighting	1,	4,	6,	8,	9,	2,	5,	15
Destructiveness	1,	4,	6,	8,	9,	7		
Temper Tantrums	1,	4,	6,	8,	9,	15		
Irresponsibility	1,	4,	6,	8,	9			
Impertinent	1,	4,	6,	8,	9,	3,	7	
Jealous	1,	3,	4,	9				
Shows signs of anger	3,	5						
Acts bossy	5,	7						
Profanity	1,	8,	3,	9				
Attention seeking	1,	3,	4,	6,	7,	8,	9	
Boisterous	1,	4,	6,	7,	8,	9		

Life History Characteristics	Representative Studies[a]			
Assaultive	8,	10,	11,	12
Defies authority	8,	10,	11,	12
Inadequate guilt feelings	10,	12		
Irritable	11,	12		
Quarrelsome	8,	11		

Questionnaire Responses	Representative Studies[a]
I do what I want to whether anybody likes it or not	13, 14
It's dumb to trust other people	13, 14
The only way to settle anything is to lick the guy	13, 14
I'm too tough a guy to get along with most kids	13, 14
If you don't have enough to live on, it's okay to steal	13, 14
I go out of my way to meet trouble rather than try to escape it	13, 14

[a] Representative studies are as follows: 1. Peterson (1961), 2. Patterson (1964), 3. Dreger, et al. (1964), 4. Quay (1964), 5. Spivack & Spotts (1965), 6. Quay & Quay (1965), 7. Ross, Lacey, & Parton (1965), 8. Quay (1966), 9. Lessing & Zagorin (1971), 10. Hewitt & Jenkins (1946), 11. Quay (1964a), 12. Achenbach (1966), 13. Peterson, Quay, & Cameron (1959), 14. Peterson, Quay, & Tiffany (1961), and 15. Brady (1970).

The essence of this pattern is an active antisocial aggressiveness almost inevitably resulting in conflict with parents, peers, and social institutions. Children and adolescents extreme on this pattern seem likely to be in such difficulty as to be involved with the courts and institutions for delinquents. More extreme scores on measures of this pattern are, in fact, related to being in legal difficulties (Quay & Peterson, 1964; 1967). Even within a group of offenders more extreme scores are related to disciplinary difficulties during incarceration, assaultive offenses, recidivism, and a failure to adjust in a community work setting (Quay, Peterson, & Consalvi, 1960; Quay & Levinson, 1967; Mack, 1969).

The aggressive, antisocial, conscienceless, impulsive behaviors associated with the conduct disorder pattern make it tempting to either equate this dimension with, or consider it a precursor of, psychopathic personality in adults. In fact, in delinquent groups, where this pattern appears more frequently in extreme form, investigators have sometimes labeled it "psychopathic delinquency." Although the extent to which the extreme of conduct disorder can be considered a precursor of adult psychopathy is problematical, much of the experimental work done on the extreme conduct-disordered child has been guided, at least in part, by theory about adult psychopathy.

Personality Disorder

The second principal pattern of deviant behaviors is as frequent in its appearance as is conduct disorder. It too has received a variety of labels: e.g., overinhibited (Hewitt & Jenkins, 1947), personality problem (Peterson, 1961), disturbed-neurotic (Quay, 1964b), internalizing (Achenbach, 1966), and withdrawn (Patterson, 1964; Ross, Lacey, & Parton, 1965). This pattern also appears in samples of children in public schools, child guidance clinics, psychiatric patients, and juvenile delinquents and may also be extracted from behavior ratings, analysis of life histories, and questionnaires. Personality disorder has also been found in the Canadian and British studies cited earlier. Representative characteristics of personality disorder may be found in Table 2.

These behaviors, attitudes, and feelings clearly involve a different pattern of social interaction than do those comprising conduct disorder; they generally imply withdrawal instead of attack. In marked contrast to the characteristics of conduct disorder are such traits as feelings of distress, fear, anxiety, physical complaints, and open and expressed unhappiness. It is within this pattern that the child who is clinically labeled as an anxiety neurotic or as phobic will be found. Fears, both general and specific are central features of personality disorder.

The impact on the environment of the child who is extreme on the personality disorder dimension will generally be different from that of the conduct-disordered child. His is less aversive to adults and peers and is less likely to excite his environment into action. If anything, he has too little behavior rather

TABLE 2
Selected Behavior Traits, Life History Characteristics, and Questionnaire Responses Associated with Personality Disorder

Behavior Traits	Representative Studies[a]								
Feelings of inferiority	1,			4,	6,	7,		9	
Self-consciousness	1,			4,	6,	7,	8,	9,	15
Social withdrawal	1,	2,	3,	4,	6,	7,	8,		15
Shyness	1,		3,	4,	6,		8,	9,	15
Anxiety	1,	2,		4,			8,		15
Crying	1,						8,	9	
Shyness	1,	2,		4,	6,				15
Hypersensitive	1,			4,		7,	8,	9,	15
Seldom smiles		2							
Chews fingernails		2							
Depression, chronic sadness	1,			4,			8,		15

Life History Characteristics	Representative Studies[a]		
Seclusive	8	10	11
Shy	8	10	11
Sensitive		10	11
Worries		10	11
Timid			11
Has anxiety over own behavior			11

Questionnaire Responses	Representative Studies[a]	
I don't think I'm quite as happy as others seem to be	13,	14
I often feel as though I have done something wrong or wicked	13,	14
I seem to do things I regret more often than most people do	13,	14
I just don't seem to get the breaks other people do	13,	14
People often talk about me behind my back	13,	14
I have more than my share of things to worry about	13	

[a] Representative studies are as follows: 1. Peterson (1961), 2. Patterson (1964), 3. Dreger, et al. (1964), 4. Quay (1964), 5. Spivack & Spotts (1965), 6. Quay & Quay (1965), 7. Ross, Lacey, & Parton (1965), 8. Quay (1966), 9. Lessing & Zagorin (1971), 10. Hewitt & Jenkins (1947), 11. Quay (1964a), 12. Achenbach (1966), 13. Peterson, Quay, & Cameron (1959), 14. Peterson, Quay, & Tiffany (1961), and 15. Brady (1970).

than too much. In fact, avoidance behaviors may be so widespread that the child appears almost behaviorally paralyzed.

It should be recognized, however, that fear, anxiety, and tension, when coupled with impulsiveness and cast into certain environmental circumstances, can result in overt behavioral acts defined as antisocial. The presence of extremes of this pattern in institutions for the delinquent as well as psychiatric clinics amply attests to this. However, when in the correctional (or other) setting the personality disorder behaves differently; he is less aggressive, more accepting of authority, more responsive to attempts to help him to change, and less likely to commit repeated delinquencies (Quay, Peterson, & Consalvi, 1960; Quay & Levinson, 1967).

Immaturity

Although the third major pattern has not been as pervasive and prominent as the previous two patterns, it has nevertheless appeared in a number of studies. It has been labeled, among other things, autism (Peterson, Becker, Shoemaker, Luria, & Hellmer, 1961), immature (Patterson, 1964), inadequacy-immaturity (Quay, 1964), immaturity (Quay & Quay, 1965), social immaturity (Dreger, et al., 1964), and daydreaming-inattentive (Conners, 1969).

As with conduct and personality disorder, immaturity has been found in samples of children and adolescents studied in public schools, child-guidance clinics, and institutions for the delinquent. It has occurred most frequently in behavior ratings, but has also emerged in studies of case histories. It appeared in one analysis of questionnaire items (Peterson, Quay, & Cameron, 1959) but was not replicated in later work (Peterson, Quay, & Tiffany, 1965; Quay & Peterson, 1967). With the notable exception of a study of emotionally disturbed children in special classes (Quay, Morse, & Cutler, 1966), it is generally less prominent than either conduct disorder or personality disorder.

Representative characteristics of the immaturity pattern may be found in Table 3. Since most of the behaviors listed seem appropriate to all children at some stage in their development, this pattern seems to represent a persistence of these behaviors when they are inappropriate to the chronological age of the child and society's expectations of him. At the same time, regression to an earlier form of behavior could also be involved. Again, this pattern occurs in all settings where deviant children are found. It seems especially prominent in public school classes for the emotionally disturbed (Quay, Morse, & Cutler, 1966; McCarthy & Paraskevopoulos, 1969) and the learning disabled (Paraskevopoulos & McCarthy, 1970).

Socialized Delinquency

The characteristics of the three previous patterns may all be said to be clearly maladaptive either from the social or individual viewpoint. Extremes

TABLE 3
Selected Behavior Traits and Life History Characteristics
Associated with Immaturity

Behavior Traits	Representative Studies[a]										
Preoccupation	1				5	6			9	12	
Short attention span	1		3		5	6			9		13
Clumsiness	1		3					8	9		13
Passivity	1	2	3		5	6					13
Daydreaming	1				5	6			9	12	13
Sluggish	1					6			9	12	
Drowsiness	1					6				12	
Prefers younger playmates	1		3	4				8			
Masturbation		2	3								
Giggles		2									
Easily flustered			3								
Chews objects		2					7				
Picked on by others				4							
Plays with toys in class							7				

Life History Characteristics	Representative Studies[a]
Habitually truant from home	10
Unable to cope with a complex world	10
Incompetent, immature	10
Not accepted by delinquent subgroup	10
Engages in furtive stealing	11

[a] Representative studies are as follows: 1. Peterson et al. (1961), 2. Patterson (1964), 3. Quay (1964), 4. Dreger, et al. (1964), 5. Quay & Quay (1965), 6. Quay, Morse, & Cutler (1966), 7. Pimm, Quay, & Werry (1969), 8. Miller (1967), 9. Lessing & Zagorin (1971), 10. Quay (1964a), 11. Quay (1966), 12. Brady (1970), 13. Conners (1969).

of such behaviors are at variance with either the expectations of self, parents, or educational and other social institutions. The child behaving in such a fashion is either a problem to most of society which surrounds him or is a victim of subjectively experienced emotional and social distress. Each of the previous patterns also involves interpersonal alienation with peers, attack in the case of conduct disorder, withdrawal in the case of personality disorder, or lack of engagement in the case of immaturity.

The fourth pattern represents behavior which is neither generally a source of personal distress nor clearly maladaptive when one considers the social conditions under which it seems to arise. Neither does it involve alienation from the peer group. Instead, it encompasses behavioral traits that are acquired in response to environmental circumstances. Both direct reinforcement by peers and modeling of the behavior of adults and peers are likely to influence the learning of these behavioral traits.

First empirically identified in the work of Hewitt & Jenkins (1946), this pattern has usually been labeled socialized or subcultural delinquency. Its emergence has been limited to studies of samples of juvenile delinquents or child guidance clinic cases in metropolitan areas. Because it involves environmental and social factors (e.g., gang activities, delinquent companions) and is comprised of behaviors generally not manifest in institutional settings, it has generally been elicited only from case history and questionnaire data.

Table 4 sets forth salient characteristics of this pattern as they have emerged from a number of studies. In view of the social structure of urban deteriorated areas, these behaviors would not seem obviously maladaptive. At the same time, it must be recognized that many children grow up in slum areas without becoming extreme on the characteristics of this dimension (Reckless, Dinitz, & Kay, 1957). Conditions for the acquisition of the characteristics in-

TABLE 4

Life History Characteristics and Questionnaire Responses Associated
with Socialized Delinquency

Life History Characteristics	Representative Studies[a]		
Has bad companions	1	2	3
Engages in gang activities	1	2	
Engages in cooperative stealing	1	2	3
Habitually truant from school	1	2	
Accepted by delinquent subgroups	1	2	
Stays out late at nights	1	2	
Strong allegiance to selected peers		2	

Questionnaire Responses	Representative Studies[a]
My folks usually blame bad company for the trouble I get into	4
Before I do something, I try to consider how my friends will react to it	4
Most boys stay in school because the law says they have to	4
When a group of boys get together they are bound to get in trouble sooner or later	4
It is very important to have enough friends and social life	4
I have been expelled from school or nearly expelled	4
Sometimes I have stolen things that I didn't really want	4

[a] Representative studies are as follows: 1. Hewitt & Jenkins (1947), 2. Quay (1964b), 3. Quay (1966), 4. Quay & Peterson (1967).

volve parental behaviors as well as more general social-environmental factors (Hewitt & Jenkins, 1947; see also Chapter Two of this volume).

Reliability

The reliability of the measurement of the four patterns is a function of the method used to assess them, the setting in which the data are collected, the skill of the data collectors, and other factors, as well as the objectivity and consistency of the constituent behaviors of the patterns. Peterson (1961) found ratings from two or more teachers to correlate .77 for conduct disorder and .75 for personality disorder on the rating scale used in his study. Quay, Sprague, Shulman, & Miller (1966) found ratings of mothers and fathers to correlate .78 for conduct disorder and .67 for personality disorder in a child guidance clinic sample. Mothers correlated .33 and .41 with teachers for the two patterns; father-teacher correlations were only .23 and .32. Peterson et al. (1961) found interparent ratings to correlate .48 for conduct disorder, .52 for personality disorder, and .62 for immaturity. Interteacher reliabilities were .82, .68, and .74 respectively, while the degree of parent-teacher agreement was predictably less; .41, .24, and .41 for the three dimensions.

Internal consistency reliabilities of .89, .83, and .68 for conduct disorder, personality disorder, and immaturity as these patterns were measured in a sample of over 1000 delinquents by means of ratings by correctional workers were reported by Quay & Parsons (1970).

Test-retest correlations of .75 for conduct disorder, .76 for personality disorder, and .61 for socialized delinquency were obtained on a sample of 65 delinquents over a time interval of three months by use of a questionnaire (Quay & Peterson, 1964). Ross, Lacey, & Parton (1965) report stability correlations which range from .71 to .96 for the various groups involved obtained after a six-month interval. These values may be somewhat high since the same teacher made both ratings.

Results of these studies indicate that the patterns can be measured reasonably reliably in a variety of settings by a variety of techniques and that they are stable over at least brief time intervals.

Independence of the Dimensions

In most studies the statistical methods used to isolate the factors have been those most likely to produce uncorrelated patterns. Even so, these methods cannot guarantee that when a new sample is measured there will not be correlations among the patterns in the scores obtained, i.e., children who show

TABLE 5

Intercorrelations Among Scores on the Four Dimensions

	Personality Disorder		Immaturity	Socialized Delinquency
Conduct Disorder	−41⁵(H)	.18¹(R)	.49²(R)	.08³(H)
	.30⁵(Q)	.33²(R)	−.03³(H)	.05⁵(H)
		−.31³(H)	.59⁴(R)	.02⁵(Q)
		.10⁴(R)	.37⁵(R)	
		.22⁵(R)	.00⁵(H)	
			.73²(R)	−.32³(H)
Personality Disorder			.07³(H)	.05⁵(H)
			.57⁵(R)	.49⁵(Q)
			.37⁵(H)	
Immaturity				− 23³(H)
				− 09⁵(H)

Key: (H) History, (R) Behavior Rating, (Q) Questionnaire. [1] Peterson (1961), [2] Quay (1964a), [3] Quay (1964b), [4] Quay & Quay (1965), [5] Quay (1966).

high scores for one pattern may show high (or low) scores on another. Table 5 provides correlations between scores obtained by groups of children on the four patterns in a number of studies. In general, correlations between the pattern scores are low, although there is variation depending on the method used to obtain the scores and the particular samples and judges (in the case of ratings) employed. The highest correlations among conduct, disorder, personality disorder, and immaturity were obtained in a study of delinquents rated by correctional staff with little training or sophistication in behavior rating procedures (Quay, 1964a). Thus, although certain ways of measuring the patterns may result in scores with varying degrees of correlation (positive and negative), the patterns themselves are adequately independent.

The evidence clearly supports the contention that the four patterns are statistically homogeneous, can be judged reliably, and show reasonable persistence over short time intervals.

Age and Sex Relationships

Studies from which the dimensions have emerged have involved subjects ranging in age from about 4 to about 18. However, only a relatively few have provided data permitting a comparison of scores of children on the dimension either at various age or grade levels or by sex. Peterson (1961) found that boys displayed more conduct disorder than girls throughout the grades kindergarten to sixth. On the personality disorder dimension, however, boys exceeded girls until about the third grade when girls' scores become higher. There were no trends related to grade for either dimension or either sex except for a slight rise in both groups on both dimensions at the fifth and sixth grade level. This finding was interpreted by Peterson as possibly a result of the "early agitation of adolescence and the difficulty this can bring about in our society" (1961, p. 208).

Quay, Sprague, Shulman, & Miller (1966) studied correlates of conduct disorder and personality disorder in a sample of consecutive referrals to a child guidance clinic. The fact that the sample was 81% male attenuated possible correlations between dimension scores and sex. However, conduct disorder scores tended to be correlated with maleness, while personality disorder scores were positively related to being a girl. In this group with an average age of 10.5 years there was some tendency for younger children to receive higher ratings from mothers, fathers, and teachers on conduct problem behaviors. This is, of course, in contrast to Peterson's (1961) data on public school children noted above but consonant with the later findings of Werry & Quay (1971) that there tends to be a decrease in deviant behavior traits from ages 5 to 7.

Spivack and Spotts (1965) found conduct disorder traits to correlate slightly with age in a sample of children ages 6 to 12 but to be unrelated to sex. Traits in their study related to the personality problem dimensions were more frequent in females and decreased with age.

Achenbach's (1966, p. 35) data on sex indicate that of his sample of 600 psychiatric patients, males classified as "externalizers" (conduct disorder) were twice as frequent as females. The reverse was true for "internalizers" (personality disorder). His data on age suggest a tendency for cases of both types to be more prevalent among older (9 to 15) than among younger (4 to 9) children in both sexes.

Ross, Lacey, & Parton (1965) utilized only male subjects but did provide a comparison of scores on the conduct and personality dimensions by grade level. Their data do not suggest the presence of any age trend in their group of public school children. Miller (1967) also failed to find increasing dimension scores with increasing age in a child guidance clinic sample. Neither does the data of Sines, Parker, Sines, & Owen (1969) show consistent age relationships for males in the age range 5 to 16.

In a sample of 1075 institutionalized male delinquents (mean age about 19) correlations of the four patterns with age ranged from .02 to —.26. While 8 of the 10 relationships were negative, suggesting decreasing severity with age in this sample, none of the relationships were large enough to have practical significance (Quay & Parsons, 1970).

The British study of Collins, Maxwell, & Cameron analyzed data obtained for boys and girls separately, thus making comparison on commonly derived dimensions impossible. Although they report similar dimensions for both sexes, some of the constituent items were different as well as the relationships among the dimensions themselves. For example, while the dimensions of conduct disorder ("rebelliousness") and socialized delinquency ("rootlessness") are independent for males, they are positively correlated for girls. It is also of interest to note that in this study of psychiatric clinic cases boys outnumbered girls by more than two to one.

Finally, while the study by Dreger et al. (1964) of children being served in 13 child guidance clinics did not provide an analysis of dimension by age or sex, it is interesting that their sample also contained more than twice as many boys as girls.

At this juncture the evidence for sex differences is very consistent with boys scoring higher on the conduct problem dimension than girls while girls generally obtain higher scores on the personality disorder dimension. It should also be noted that in the studies cited using clinical populations, boys outnumbered females at least two-to-one unless samples were specifically equated for sex. Much less consistent are findings relating problems to age. About the best that can be said on the basis of current evidence is that age trends are probably related to the type of sample studied and the method by which scores on the dimension are obtained if, in fact, age relationships actually exist.

Prevalence

What little empirical research there is on the frequency with which behavior problems are found in the general child population has usually considered deviant behavior traits individually rather than as representatives of the four patterns. Thus, this research indicates something about the frequency with which we may expect to find such traits as loss of temper, crying, fears and worries, thumb-sucking, restlessness, etc. in the general child population but does not indicate what the distribution of scores might be on instruments constructed to measure the four dimensions.

In general, however, such surveys of various samples of children in the general population reveal that deviant behavior traits are more frequent than might be suspected. For example, Lapouse and Monk (1958) interviewed 482 representatively chosen mothers in an urban area relative to the behavior of their children ages 6 to 12. They found that 7 or more fears and worries were present in 43% of the children, nightmares in 28%, overactivity in 49%, restlessness in 30%, nail-biting in 27%, and temper loss at least twice a week in 48%.

Werry and Quay (1971) obtained ratings on the Behavior Problem Check-list (Quay & Peterson, 1967) on 926 boys and 827 girls in kindergarten, first and second grades. The children represented almost the entire population of children in those grades in a midwestern university town. Their data indicate a mean of 11.4 deviant behaviors for boys and a mean of 7.6 for girls (out of a possible 55). On the list, 37 items were significantly more common in boys than in girls. A greater number of symptoms in boys has also been reported by Lapouse & Monk (1964) and Rutter and Graham (1966).

What is clearly revealed by all of these studies is high frequency in the general population of behaviors thought by many clinicians to be indicative of psychopathology. Thus, most deviant children differ from their normal peers in the number instead of in the kind of deviant behaviors. This is clearly the case for the patterns of aggression, withdrawal, and immaturity although perhaps not so well established in the case of childhood psychosis (see Chapter Five).

Correlates of the Dimensions

The relative newness of the factor analytic approach to classification and the even more recent tendency to view (nonpsychotic) behavior problem children within a four-dimensional framework means that experimental and cor-relational studies of children exhibiting these dimensions are relatively few. Most studies of behaviorally disordered or emotionally disturbed children have contrasted children grouped into such gross categories as normal versus dis-turbed, delinquent versus nondelinquent, etc. Results of such studies have not been particularly revealing either in regard to etiology, basic correlates of psychological functioning such as learning and perception, or responses to treatment.

Although limited, available data contrasting children or adolescents se-lected to represent extremes of the dimensions are encouraging in that they demonstrate differences among extremes in the psychological processes that are relevant to both etiology and approaches to behavior change.

Learning and Performance

Much of the experimental investigation of the extremes of conduct dis-order in children and adolescents has arisen from theoretical speculation about psychopathic behavior. Considerable research with adult psychopaths (see Hare, 1970 for a review of much of this literature) has suggested that the psychopath is comparatively slow to acquire conditioned reactions, especially those of avoidance, and may possess a relatively underreactive autonomic nervous system. Quay (1965) has proposed a theory that relates the clinical behavior of the psychopath and many of the experimental findings to a pathological need for stimulation. The essence of the hypothesis is that much of the psychopaths' senseless aggressive and thrill-seeking behavior represents an attempt to relieve a state of effective distress brought about by boredom. The psychopath cannot tolerate boredom (lack of change in quality and quantity of sensory inputs) and thus actively seeks stimulation.

In a study testing an extrapolation of this hypothesis to a group of juvenile delinquents, Orris (1969) predicted that those subjects high on the conduct disorder dimension would show poorer performance on a boring task requiring continuous attention than would a group representing extreme scores on personality disorder. His hypothesis was confirmed with the added observation that the psychopathic boys engaged to a greater degree in boredom-relieving activities such as singing and talking to themselves.

A much more complex inquiry into both conduct disorder and personality disorder in a delinquent population was undertaken by Skrzypek (1969). He contrasted the preference behavior of the two groups for novelty and complexity of stimuli under conditions of both perceptual arousal and perceptual isolation. He also investigated the relative strength of an anxiety component in the two groups. The procedures of the study were too detailed to report here but the results were of considerable interest. On initial testing the conduct disorder group indicated a greater preference for the complex and the novel. In contrast, the personality disorder group preferred the less complex and more mundane. This group was also significantly higher in anxiety; the mean anxiety score for this group was over twice that for the conduct group. Scores on the behavior rating used to measure conduct disorder correlated —.84 with the anxiety measure (The Anxiety Differential, Husek & Alexander, 1963). This finding was in keeping with an earlier study relating anxiety to personality disorder (Quay, Peterson, & Consalvi, 1960). Skrzypek also found that the effect of a brief period of perceptual isolation was to significantly increase preference for novelty and complexity in the conduct disorder group, a substantiation of a derivation from the theory (Quay, 1965) discussed earlier. The arousal experiences served to increase the anxiety of the personality disorder group and to decrease their preference for complexity. The results of this extremely complex experiment serve further to demonstrate differences in psychological processes between the two groups. The results also support a hypothesis that relates extremes of conduct disorder, at least in adolescents, to a need for varied stimulus inputs.

Psychopathic, neurotic, and socialized delinquents were verbally conditioned to dependency and aggressive verbs by Stewart (1970). As predicted from earlier studies (see Hare, 1970), the neurotics and the socialized groups increased the frequency with which they used the reinforced verb while the psychopathic group decreased its use of the reinforced verb. Even though both aggressive and dependent verbs were reinforced the neurotics increased in dependency verbs while the subculturals increased in aggressive verbs. The differences in conditionability among the groups was magnified by the frustration conditions.

Physiological Correlates

An exploration of difference, in autonomic nervous system reactivity among conduct disorder, personality disorder, and socialized delinquent groups was undertaken by Borkovec (1970). Evidence for significantly lowered responsiveness in the conduct group was obtained on the galvanic skin response. Data on heart rate change to stimuli, although not statistically significant, were suggestive of lessened reactivity. The results of this study support the notion that the extreme conduct disorder suffers relatively lower autonomic reactivity, this perhaps being one basis for the stimulation-seeking behavior in this group.

In another study of physiological correlates Müller and Shamsie (1967) studied 78 girls admitted to the adolescent unit of a psychiatric hospital by means of the EEG. Subjects were classified clinically as overinhibited, unsocialized, or socialized according to the criteria suggested by Hewitt & Jenkins (1946). The overinhibited (personality disorder) group manifested more fast activity in the temporal region, a finding which, according to the authors, might be expected in anxious and sensitive individuals and which might also contribute to the inhibition of impulses originating in lower parts of the central nervous system. The unsocialized aggressive (conduct disorder) group exhibited more generalized slow waves interpreted by the authors as related to a lack of inhibition. The socialized group provided records more regular and more normal than either of the other two groups.

Although these results are consonant with expectations based on the behavior of the three groups, as the authors point out, the study did not include a nonproblem control group and results could have been influenced by medication being taken by some, although not all, of the subjects. Nevertheless the study demonstrates the value of considering an abnormal population in terms of empirically derived subgroups.

Other Personality Correlates

The meaningfulness and generality of the dimensions can be enhanced by demonstrating their relationships to other personality variables. The extent to which empirically related personality characteristics fit logically within psychological meaning of the dimensions further confirm the reality and usefulness of the dimensions.

In the context of a study of personality changes over time in a sample of institutionalized delinquents, Hedlund (1970) administered the Sixteen Personality Factor Questionnaire (Cattell & Eber, 1967) to groups identified as psychopathic, neurotic, inadequate-immature, and socialized on the basis of case history, behavior ratings, and a questionnaire (see Quay & Parsons, 1970). This test was developed by factor analytic methods to measure 16 dimensions of more or less normal personality. Only 4 of these factors were significantly different across the 4 delinquent groups. The psychopaths were found to be more happy-go-lucky (as opposed to sober) than either of the other three groups. On a scale measuring "tough-mindedness" they scored higher than immatures, but were not significantly different from the other two groups. On the factor of apprehensiveness the neurotic groups scored highest, but differed significantly only from the psychopaths. On the "tenseness" scale the neurotics were significantly higher than all of the other groups. While these differences are consonant with expectations, a failure to find differences on such factors as emotional stability, assertiveness, venturesomeness, and self-sufficiency did not fit expectations. As Hedlund's data demonstrate, however, the reliability of some of the subscales of the Sixteen Personality Factor Questionnaire is rather poor.

In another study in a correctional setting Smyth & Ingram (1970) compared youthful offenders classified into one of the four patterns in terms of reasons for sick call. Sick-call visits were classified by medical staff as being primarily medical, emotional, or malingering. Although complete staff ignorance of the behavioral classification of Ss could not be maintained, the size of the population and their newness to the institution (which had just opened) reduced possible contamination to a minimum. No differences among the groups were found for the purely medical visits. The neurotic (personality disorder) group had significantly more emotional sick calls; they accounted for two-thirds of the visits judged to be emotional while accounting for less than 25% of the Ss. The conduct disorder group accounted for 39% of visits judged to be malingering while representing only 16% of the samples.

While research is limited, it is clear that reliable selection of groups representing the four patterns of psychopathology leads to the demonstration of meaningful differences among them on a number of psychological and physiological variables. More such research is needed to further extend the meaning and utility of the patterns.

Acquisition of Deviant Behavior

The environmental circumstances in which both traits and patterns of deviant behavior can be acquired and the mechanisms by which acquisition occurs have been widely studied. The sociological literature has emphasized social class (Miller, 1958), deviant social organization (Cohen, 1955), and social inequalities (Cloward & Ohlin, 1960) in the generation of what we have discussed as subcultural delinquency.

The family context as a setting in which deviant behavior is produced has been the subject of a great deal of research. A review of this research with particular reference to the four-dimensional framework developed in this chapter appears in Chapter Two of this volume.

The mechanisms whereby deviant behavior is acquired and maintained have also been extensively studied. Discussions of various learning mechanisms may be found in such sources as Bandura & Walters (1959; 1963) and Ullmann & Krasner (1969).

Although a review of these circumstances and mechanisms is beyond the scope of this chapter, it is obvious that there are environmental circumstances, including both the family and the larger social context in which the child develops, that make the acquisition of one or another of the principal patterns of deviant behavior more probable. The learning mechanisms, such as modeling, parental reinforcement, peer reinforcement, frustration effects, and aversive conditioning, can also be seen to operate within these contexts to influence the acquisition and maintenance of the specific deviant behaviors comprising the four different patterns.

Even though research is extremely limited, the possibility of hereditary predispositional factors cannot be completely ignored (see Chapter Two). Neither can the possible contributions of the various organic factors discussed in Chapter Three be ruled out. In the light of present evidence the view that these four patterns of psychopathology are primarily composed of learned behaviors is clearly the most tenable.

Conclusions

There is now abundant evidence that the application of empirical multivariate statistical techniques has demonstrated that the vast majority of deviant behaviors of children and adolescents (which occur with a frequency high enough to permit such analysis) can be subsumed under four major headings: conduct disorder, personality disorder, immaturity, and socialized delinquency.

The homogeneity of the behaviors comprising the patterns and their relative independence is essentially a by-product of the methods of deriving the patterns themselves. There need be no speculation over the inclusion or exclusion of a given deviant behavior trait within a pattern. It can be determined by statistical means that a behavior either relates to the rest of the behaviors in the pattern and thus belongs, or that it does not correlate with the other behaviors and is not a part of the pattern.

The basic four patterns are also widely replicable. They have been repeatedly found in the range of normal children in the public school as well as those defined as emotionally disturbed or learning disabled, in children served by child guidance clinics, psychiatric hospitals, residential schools, and correctional institutions. Children being served by these various institutions differ in quantity rather than in quality of deviant behavior. This finding serves to provide a common framework for communication about and treatment of behavioral deviance for school, clinic, hospital, and correctional institution. The implications of a common framework for consideration of behavioral deviance for improved service and research are favorable, to say the least.

While the method used to assess the presence or absence of the behavior related to the patterns has some influence, none of the patterns is solely a function of any method (rating, questionnaire, life history analysis) nor of any group of observers.

In addition to homogeneity, independence, and generality, the patterns can also be measured reliably. Judges can agree on the relative positions of groups of children and adolescents on the patterns. The degree to which individuals are judged to possess the behaviors constituting the patterns is also stable over at least brief time intervals.

Finally, while much additional research needs to be done, differences in basic psychological processes and in a variety of social behaviors can be experimentally shown to exist among the patterns. Evidence for the relevance of the basic patterns to both the etiology and treatment of behavior disorder, will be found in later chapters of this volume.

References

Achenbach, T. M. The classification of children's psychiatric symptoms: a factor analytic study. *Psychological Monographs*, 1966, **80**, 6.

Ackerson, L. *Children's behavior problems*. Chicago: The University of Chicago Press, 1942.

Anthony, E. J. Taxonomy is not one man's business. *International Journal of Psychiatry*, 1967, **3**, 173–178.

Ausubel, D. P. Personality disorder is disease. *American Psychologist*, 1961, **16**, 69–74.

Bandura, A., & Walters, R. H. *Adolescent Aggression*. New York: Ronald, 1959.

Bandura, A., & Walters, R. H. *Social learning and personality development*. New York: Holt, Rinehart & Winston, 1963.

Becker, W. C. The matching of behavior rating and questionnaire peronality factors. *Psychological Bulletin*, 1960, **57**, 201–212.

Becker, W. C. Comments on Cattell's paper on "perturbations" in personality structure research. *Psychological Bulletin*, 1961, **58**, 175.

Borkovec, T. D. Autonomic reactivity to sensory stimulation in psychopathic, neurotic and normal juvenile delinquents. *Journal of Consulting and Clinical Psychology*, 1970.

Brady, R. C. Effects of success and failure on impulsivity and distractibility of three types of educationally handicapped children. Unpublished Ph.D. thesis, University of Southern California, 1970.

Cattell, R. B. Theory of situational, instrument, second order, and refraction factors in personality structure research. *Psychological Bulletin*, 1961, **58**, 160–174.

Cattell, R. B., & Eber, H. W. *Interim manual supplement for form E, Sixteen Personality Factor Questionnaire*. Champaign, Ill.: Institute for Personality and Ability Testing, 1967.

Cloward, R., & Ohlin, L. *Delinquency and Opportunity*. Glencoe, Ill.: The Free Press, 1960.

Cohen, A. *Delinquent boys*. Glencoe, Ill.: The Free Press, 1955.

Collins, L. F., Maxwell, A. E., & Cameron, K. A factor analysis of some child psychiatric clinic data. *Journal of Mental Science*, 1962, **108**, 274–285.

Conners, C. K. A teacher rating scale for use in drug studies with children. *American Journal of Psychiatry*, 1969, **126**, 152–156.

Costello, C. G. Classification and psychopathology. In C. G. Costello (Ed.) *Symptoms of Psychopathology*. New York: Wiley, 1970.

Dreger, R. M., Lewis, P. M., Rich, T. A., Miller, K. S., Reid, M. P., Overlade, D. C., Taffel, C., & Flemming, E. L. Behavioral classification project. *Journal of Consulting Psychology*, 1964, **28**, 1–13.

Eron, L. D. *Classification of behavior disorders*. Chicago: Aldine, 1966.

Eysenck, H. J. Classification and the problem of diagnosis. In H. J. Eysenck (Ed.) *Handbook of Abnormal Psychology*. New York: Basic Books, 1961.

Group for the Advancement of Psychiatry. *Psychopathological Disorders in Childhood: Theoretical Considerations and a Proposed Classification*. New York: The Authors, 1966.

Hare, R. D. *Psychopathy: Theory and research*. New York: Wiley, 1970.

Hedlund, C. S. A validational study of a program utilizing a differential treatment approach for the treatment of juvenile delinquency. Unpublished Master's thesis, West Virginia University, 1970.

Hewitt, L. E., & Jenkins, R. L. *Fundamental patterns of maladjustment, the dynamics of their origin*. Springfield: State of Illinois, 1946.

Husek, T., & Alexander, S. The effectiveness of the Anxiety Differential in examination stress situations. *Educational and Psychological Measurement*, 1963, **23**, 309–318.

Lapouse, R., & Monk, M. A. An epidemiologic study of behavior characteristics in children. *American Journal of Public Health*, 1958, **48**, 1134–1144.

Lapouse, R., & Monk, M. A. Behavior deviations in a representative sample of children—variation by sex, age, race, social class and family size. *American Journal of Orthopsychiatry*, 1964, **34**, 436–446.

Lessing, E., & Zagorin, S. Dimensions of psychopathology in middle childhood as evaluated by three symptom checklists. *Educational and Psychological Measurement*, 1971.

Lorr, M. Classification of the behavior disorders. In P. R. Farnsworth, O. McNemar, & Q. McNemar (Eds.) *Annual Review of Psychology*. Palo Alto, Calif.: Annual Reviews, Inc., 1961.

Mack, J. L. Behavior ratings of recidivist and non-recidivist delinquent males. *Psychological Reports*, 1969, **25**, 260.

McCarthy, J. McR., & Paraskevopoulos, J. Behavior pattern of learning disabled, emotionally disturbed, and average children. *Exceptional Children*, 1969, **36**, 69–74.

Miller, L. C. Dimensions of psychopathology in middle childhood. *Psychological Reports*, 1967, **21**, 897–903.

Miller, W. B. Lower class culture on a generating milieu of gang delinquency. *The Journal of Social Issues*, 1958, **14**, 5–19.

Müller, H. F. & Shamsie, S. J. Classification of behavior disorders in adolescents and EEG findings. Paper presented at the 17th Annual Meeting of the Canadian Psychiatric Association, Quebec City, June, 1967.

Orris, J. B. Visual monitoring performance in three subgroups of male delinquents. *Journal of Abnormal Psychology,* 1969, **74**, 227–229.

Paraskevopoulos, J., & McCarthy, J. McR. Behavior patterns of children with special learning disabilities. *Psychology in the Schools,* 1970, **7**, 42–46.

Patterson, G. R. An empirical approach to the classification of disturbed children. *Journal of Clinical Psychology,* 1964, **20**, 326–337.

Peterson, D. R. Behavior problems of middle childhood. *Journal of Consulting Psychology,* 1961, **25**, 205–209.

Peterson, D. R. The scope and generality of verbally defined personality factors. *Psychological Review,* 1965, **72**, 48–59.

Peterson, D. R., Becker, W. C., Shoemaker, D. J., Luria, Z., & Hellmer, L. A. Child behavior problems and parental attitudes, *Child development,* 1961, **32**, 151–162.

Peterson, D. R., Quay, H. C., & Cameron, G. R. Personality and background factors in juvenile delinquency as inferred from questionnaire responses. *Journal of Consulting Psychology,* 1959, **23**, 392–399.

Peterson, D. R., Quay, H. C., & Tiffany, T. C. Personality factors related to juvenile delinquency. *Child Development,* 1961, **32**, 355–372.

Pimm, J. B., Quay, H. C., & Werry, J. S. Dimensions of problem behavior in first grade children. *Psychology in the Schools,* 1967, **4**, 155–157.

Quay, H. C. Personality dimensions in delinquent males as inferred from the factor analysis of behavior ratings. *Journal of Research in Crime and Delinquency,* 1964a, **1**, 33–37.

Quay, H. C. Dimensions of personality in delinquent boys as inferred from the factor analysis of case history data. *Child Development,* 1964b, **35**, 479–484.

Quay, H. C. Psychopathic personality as pathological stimulation-seeking. *American Journal of Psychiatry,* 1965, **122**, 180–183.

Quay, H. C. Personality patterns in preadolescent delinquent boys. *Educational and Psychological Measurement,* 1966, **26**, 99–110.

Quay, H. C., & Levinson, R. B. The prediction of the institutional adjustment of four subgroups of delinquent boys. Unpublished manuscript, 1967.

Quay, H. C., Morse, W. C., & Cutler, R. L. Personality patterns of pupils in special classes for the emotionally disturbed. *Exceptional Children,* 1966, **32**, 297–301.

Quay, H. C., & Parsons, L. B. *The differential behavioral classification of the juvenile offender.* Washington, D. C.: Bureau of Prisons, U. S. Department of Justice. 1970.

Quay, H. C., & Peterson, D. R. The questionnaire measurement of personality dimensions associated with juvenile delinquency. Mimeo., 1964.

Quay, H. C., & Peterson, D. R. Manual for the Behavior Problem Checklist. Mimeo., 1967.

Quay, H. C., Peterson, D. R., & Consalvi, C. The interpretation of three personality factors in juvenile delinquency. *Journal of Consulting Psychology,* 1960, **24**, 555.

Quay, H. C., & Quay, L. C. Behavior problems in early adolescence. *Child Development,* 1965, **36**, 215–220.

Quay, H. C., Sprague, R. L., Shulman, H. S., & Miller, A. L. Some correlates of personality disorder and conduct disorder. *Psychology in the Schools,* 1966, **3,** 44–47.

Reckless, W. C., Dinitz, S., & Kay, B. The self-component in potential delinquency and potential non-delinquency. *American Sociological Review,* 1957, **22,** 566–570.

Rosen, B. M., Bahn, A. K., & Kramer, M. Demographic and diagnostic characteristics of psychiatric outpatient clinics in the United States, 1961, *American Journal of Orthopsychiatry,* 1964, **34,** 455–468.

Ross, A. O., Lacey, H. M., & Parton, D. A. The development of a behavior checklist for boys. *Child Development,* 1965, **36,** 1013–1027.

Rutter, M., & Graham, P. Psychiatric disorder in 10 and 11 year old children. *Proceedings of the Royal Society of Medicine,* 1966, **59,** 382–387.

Sines, J. O., Parker, J. D., Sines, L. K., & Owen, D. R. Identification of clinically relevant dimensions of children's behavior. *Journal of Consulting and Clinical Psychology,* 1969, **33,** 728–734.

Skrzypek, G. J. Effect of perceptual isolation and arousal on anxiety, complexity preference, and novelty preference in psychopathic and neurotic delinquents. *Journal of Abnormal Psychology,* 1969, **74,** 321–329.

Smyth, R. A., & Ingram, G. Relationship between type of offender and reasons for seeking medical care in a correctional setting. *Nursing Research,* 1970, **9,** 456–458.

Spivack, G., & Spotts, J. The Devereux Child Behavior Scale: Symptom behaviors in latency age children. *American Journal of Mental Retardation,* 1965, **69,** 839–853.

Stewart, D. Dependency correlates of psychopathic, neurotic and subcultural delinquents. Unpublished Ph.D. thesis, Temple University, 1970.

Szasz, T. The myth of mental illness. *American Psychologist,* 1960, **15,** 113–118.

Ullmann, L., & Krasner, L. *A psychological approach to abnormal behavior.* Englewood Cliffs, N. J.: Prentice Hall, 1969.

Werry, J. S. & Quay, H. C. The prevalence of behavior symptoms in younger elementary school children. American Journal of Orthopsychiatry, 1971, **41,** 136–143.

Willer, L. H. Compounding the difficulties of classification. *International Journal of Psychiatry,* 1967, **3,** 186–187.

Zubin, J. Classification of the behavior disorders. In P. R. Farnsworth, O. McNemar, & Q. McNemar (Eds.) *Annual Review of Psychology,* Palo Alto, Calif.: Annual Reviews, Inc., 1967.

Chapter Two

Family Interaction and Psychopathology in Children
E. Mavis Hetherington and Barclay Martin

Most theories of child development emphasize the interaction between parent and child as an important factor contributing to the development of personality and psychopathology. Theories vary not so much in emphasizing the importance of this relationship but in the aspects and processes of the relationship that they regard as critical. Psychoanalytic theory has stressed the caretaking functions of the mother as they interact with psychosexual development and the role of parental behavior in the resolution of the Oedipus complex as basic in the development of psychopathology. Behavior theory has focused on the parents as models and as sources of reinforcement which shape normal or deviant behaviors in the child; and role theory has emphasized the critical function of parents in communicating social roles and standards to the child.

Problems in the Study of Parent-Child Interaction

The investigator who is interested in the relationship between family interaction and psychopathology is confronted with a variety of problems in research strategy, conceptualization, and interpretation of findings, which frequently have been inadequately dealt with in past studies.

Criteria for subject selection are often ill-defined and inadequate. Heterogeneous populations, uncontrolled for social status, age, and sex and with a variety of deviant behaviors, are frequently utilized (Frank, 1965; Fontana, 1966). Thus, the literature is replete with studies of family relations of disturbed versus nondisturbed families (Alkire, 1969; Schuham, 1970), or clinic versus nonclinic populations (Becker & Iwakami, 1969; Murrell & Stachowiak, 1967), although few theories of psychopathology would predict the same antecedent familial variables for diverse forms of psychopathology. Other studies define their deviant groups more precisely and differentiate between types of disorder, but lack the nondeviant control groups that are essential to evaluate whether obtained interaction patterns really differ significantly from those of normal families.

Recent emphasis has been placed on the importance of studying the interaction of the entire family unit; however, there are few investigations that include direct measures of paternal behavior. When paternal variables have been assessed, it has usually been indirectly through mothers' or childrens' reports of fathers' characteristics, with the accompanying possible distortions that accrue to such procedures.

Most studies have focused on the mother-child relationship, partly because of the greater accessibility of mothers than fathers as participants in such research and partly for theoretical reasons. Psychoanalytic theory has emphasized the role of maternal caretaking functions in personality development; learning theorists have stressed the importance of the mother-infant relationship as the first sustained social relationship for the child, which will determine his subsequent patterns of responsiveness and adaptability. This is unfortunate since it may well be that fathers are a main source of contingent stimulation in the critical period of infancy. Much of the mother's interaction with the child is focused on routinized caretaking functions, which are less susceptible to modification by the child's responses than are the playful situations in which father and child usually interact. There is some support for this position since research on the effects of caretaking behavior on personality development has in general yielded negative results (Caldwell, 1964); whereas responsivity and stimulation by caretakers have been found to relate to later emotional responses of the child (Schaffer & Emerson, 1964; Moss, 1967).

Problems in Assessment

After the investigator has selected the pathological groups of interest, the major issues that confront him are the choice of family variables and the measurement techniques to be utilized in the study of family interaction.

In the past decade there has been a decrease in the use of retrospective parental reports of general child-rearing attitudes and an increase in direct observations of reports of more specific contemporary parental behaviors. There has also been a marked shift from self-report to observational measures, from inferential to noninferential measures and from interest in content to interest in process in family interaction. Contemporary experimenters often are concerned with the study of contengencies and sequences of behaviors within the interaction instead of the simple recording of frequencies of various responses emitted by family members.

Questionnaires and Interviews

The majority of early child-rearing studies utilized some measure of retrospective report either in the form of a questionnaire or an interview. Such measures were frequently used for gathering information on both child-rearing practices and child behavior, which led to systematic correlated biases on both the independent and dependent variables. The use of such methods has been seriously criticized in terms of reliability, accuracy of recall, and systematic distortion of reports. Yarrow (1963) has commented on the difficulty of the task with which the parent is confronted. The parent is being asked to recall details that have occurred in the past, to rate herself and her child in relation to ambiguously defined referents of child-rearing, and to formulate principles that guide her behavior with her child. In the face of such demands, it is not surprising to find little stability of reports over time (MacFarlane, 1938; Wenar, 1961; Yarrow, Campbell, & Burton, 1968) and distortion in the direction of precocity (MacFarlane, 1938), idealized expectations (Chess, Thomas, Birch, & Hertzig, 1960), and cultural stereotypes (McCord & McCord, 1961).

Studies of agreement between reports of parents, children, and extrafamilial sources of information find only moderate concordance (Becker, 1960; Goddard, Broder, & Wenar, 1961; Haggard, Brekstad, & Skard, 1960; Helper, 1958; Kohn & Carroll, 1960; Lapouse & Monk, 1958; Levitt, 1959; McCord & McCord, 1961). It has been suggested that reports of fathers tend to be more biased by a social desirability response set than those of mothers (Becker, 1960; Eron, Banta, Waller, & Lauchlit, 1961). However, it may well be that children exhibit more conforming behavior in the presence of the father and that such findings reflect valid situational differences in children's behavior instead of response bias. A recent study that involves direct observation of nine- and ten-year-old children interacting separately with their mothers and fathers found less oppositional behavior in the presence of the father than the mother (Martin & Hetherington, 1970). It is interesting to note that when family members know that other members of the family will also be interviewed they give more favorable reports of the behavior of others (Kohn & Carroll, 1960). This finding of shifts in reports parallels Reid's finding (1970) that there are dramatic increases in interobserver reliabilities of ratings when the judges *know* reliability checks are being run.

Systematic reviews of the literature (Becker & Krug, 1965; Yarrow, Campbell, & Burton, 1968) conclude that parent attitude questionnaires are seldom able to predict independently assessed child behavior. Although focusing on specific, contemporary practices rather than broad retrospective attitudes improves the predictive validity of self-report measures (Winder & Rau, 1962; Bell, 1964; Kagan & Moss, 1962), the continued use of such scales, as the sole measure of family relationships, reflects an unfortunate tendency of some experimenters to value ease over validity in assessment.

Direct Observation

In order to circumvent some of the problems inherent in the use of parental reports many experimenters have resorted to the direct observation of parents and children. These range from naturalistic observations in the home to the use of highly structured tasks in the laboratory.

It is obvious that observational data are not necessarily valid. They are valid only to the extent that representative patterns of interaction have not been disrupted or distorted by the observer. The awareness of being observed may result in changes in characteristic modes of interaction. The experimenter must determine what observational situations, conditions, procedures and periods will be least intrusive and will yield stable estimates of interactive measures. Unfortunately, there are few studies that suggest optimum periods and conditions for stabilization of behavior in various observational settings.

Bell (1964) points out that if observational situations are completely unstructured, behavior may tend to accumulate only in categories that are irrelevant to the hypotheses being tested. Thus, structuring situations in order to elicit responses of interest leads to more efficient hypotheses testing. However, it has also been suggested that subjects doing familiar things in familiar situations are less likely to modify their customary interaction patterns than they are in highly structured laboratory situations.

Even with the use of unobtrusive measures and a reasonable period of adaptation the investigator must cope with the problem of situational specificity in family interaction patterns. Situational variables account for much of the behavior emitted in a given setting and there may be little generality of interaction from one situation to another.

Studies suggest that as families are shifted from familiar to unfamiliar settings, from the home to the laboratory, or from unstructured to structured situations there is a tendency for family members to register less negative emotion, exhibit more socially desirable responses, and assume socially prescribed role behavior. O'Rourke (1963) found that with a shift from a laboratory to a home situation there was a change from stereotyped sex role behavior to an increase in expressiveness in the father and instrumentality in the mother. The father exhibited more social-emotional behaviors and the mother more decision making, controlling behaviors. Similarly, mothers are more directive and less passively attentive in the home than in a laboratory playroom situation (Moustakas, Sigel, & Schalock, 1956). Even within a laboratory setting little consistency may be demonstrated from one structured situation to another (Hatfield, Ferguson, & Alpert, 1967).

Although the structure of laboratory interaction situations may facilitate the occurrence of the family behaviors of interest (Bell, 1964), the situational demands may be so powerful that the behavior that is emitted is specific only to that situation. If family interaction is to be understood, an experimental model of representative design of family interaction is advisable. It seems necessary to assess the behavior of families in a variety of situations in order to establish the specificity or generality of patterns of relationships. If the main focus of interest is in family interaction patterns in the home, then the assessment situation should be as similar to the home situation as possible. However, if it is in relatively stable interactions across situations, representative situations should be sampled.

Observational Measures

After the investigator has considered the selection of an appropriate situation in which to observe family interaction he is confronted with the problem of the actual measurement of behavior. Decisions must be made about the methods of recording behavior, the use of global or specific, of inferential or direct measures, and the focus on the assessment of content or process. Behavior may be concurrently rated in the ongoing interaction situation, or multichannel audio tapes or video tapes of the interaction session may be rated at a later time. Observation of ongoing interaction may permit the assessment of more subtle and complex interactional cues, but tapes of the interaction facilitate repeated observations and rechecking in making ratings.

One of the most controversial issues in the measurement of family interaction concerns the use of inferential versus direct measures. It has been argued that global inferential ratings such as warmth, permissiveness, or hostility are more conceptually relevant than narrower behavioral measures such as number of words spoken, or who speaks first or last; and that although reliabilities tend to be lower in the former, it is more than compensated for by the ease of making meaningful statements about these measures in comparison to the latter measures. In contrast, Haley (1964) protests the admission of any inference into the measurement process. In attempting to develop useful measures of the interaction process, Haley assessed the frequency with which a family member spoke after every other family member during the construction of group TAT stories and a discussion of questionnaire items. Although such a measure is completely objective, the experimenter must make inferential statements about the measure in order to contribute to the understanding of inter-actional processes, and it might be questioned whether such a variable has any psychological meaning at all. Two of the most frequently used objective, behavioral sets of measures are those developed to measure conflict and domi-nance in the Revealed Difference Test (Farina, 1960). In the Revealed Differ-ence Test, each member of the family is asked separately how he would handle a series of child-rearing problems if he were alone. The family is then brought together, their various solutions presented, and they are asked to jointly discuss and come to agreement on a mutually compatible solution for dealing with the problems. The indices of dominance are: (1) speaks first, (2) speaks last, (3) passive acceptance of solution, (4) percent of total family speaking time, and (5) yielding from original individual solution to final group decision. Measures of conflict include: (1) frequency of simultaneous speech, (2) interruptions, (3) disagreements and aggressions, (4) failure to reach agreement, and (5) total speaking time. These measures are obviously highly noninferential. On most of the measures, almost perfect interjudge reliabilities (Farina, 1960; Hetherington & Frankie, 1967) are obtained. Many of the measures have been demonstrated to be stable over time (Ferriera & Winter, 1966), and to have adequate split-half reliabilities (Becker & Iwakami, 1969). The problem with such measures lies not with their objectivity and reliability but with the invalidity of grouping and labeling the various measures dominance and con-flict (Beeker & Iwakami, 1969; Hetherington, Stouwie, & Ridberg, 1970). In the above study by Hetherington et al. (1970), who investigated family interaction in nondelinquent and in socialized, neurotic, and psychopathic delinquent adolescents, these measures were factor analyzed. It was found that the measures which were previously assumed to assess dominance were more closely related than the presumed conflict measures. All dominance measures, with the exception of yielding, tended to load on the same factor. The fact that yielding, which measures a change from one position to another, is not cor-related with the other measures suggests that labels other than dominance may be more appropriate for these two factors. Yielding could be measuring lack of control in the decision-making process, a willingness to compromise, or incon-sistency in disciplinary practices. The other "dominance" factor may be mea-suring control of the families' verbal interaction but not of the decision-making process.

The conflict measures showed variations in the clustering of variables within experimental groups and marked differences for boys and girls. For example, it was found that failure to agree was related to daughter's disagree-ments and aggression, interruptions and simultaneous speech with father, but was unrelated to other "conflict measures" in families of boys. Since the families have been specifically instructed to reach agreement, on the basis of face validity, this inability to do so would appear to be a manifestation of conflict. Further support for this position is yielded since failure to agree was more frequent in the delinquent than in the nondelinquent families. The experimenters posit that disagreeing, aggressing, and intervening in the conversation of the nominal head of the household, the father, is sex inappropriate behavior for girls and hence may be a true measure of conflict and maladaptive behavior. This is supported by the finding that these behaviors are more frequent in social and psychopathic delinquent than in nondelinquent girls. In contrast, assertiveness and active participation in family interaction is more congruent with the instrumental male role and may not indicate gross dissension. This is supported not only by the low intercorrelations between failure to agree and other "conflict measures" and more failure to agree in delinquent than nondelinquent families, but also by the finding of more active and aggressive family interchanges by nondelinquent boys.

These findings in conjunction with those of other studies (Becker & Iwakami, 1969; Rohrbaugh, 1966) that find different patterns of intercorrelations on the dominance and conflict measures among children of different ages and different types of pathology suggest that these objective variables may have different meanings and correlates for various populations. The usefulness and validity of such measures can only be determined by examining their correlates within specific populations and situations.

Mishler and Waxler (1968) have advocated use of multiple coding systems on the same data, and Yarrow (1963) has supported convergent validity procedures utilizing a variety of measures as a partial solution to this problem.

Most of the studies of family interaction have yielded separate frequency measures of parent and child behavior recorded while they were interacting. However, investigators are usually actually interested in the etiology, contingencies, and sequencing of these observed behaviors and often generalize to such questions on the basis of inappropriate methodology. Raush (1965) suggests that the study of parent-child interaction must involve the assessment of interchange where the family members influence each other and subject each other to a variety of constraints. Such studies should look sequentially at interchanges involving chains of interpersonal exchanges and should investigate shifts in probabilities of response in one family member as they are related to the specific behavior of others. A recent study (Perry, 1970) performed a sequential analysis of withdrawn and aggressive children's responses to direct blame or lecturing by parents. Following parental blame the rate of avoidance in withdrawn children was high, whereas the rate of avoidance in aggressive children was low. In contrast, parental lecturing led to greater avoidance in aggressive than withdrawn children. There has been growing interest in the use of such sequential analyses techniques in order to assess contingencies within family interaction processes (Raush, 1965; Waxler & Mishler, 1970).

Interpretation of Self-Report and Observational Data

In spite of the fact that studies in socialization are basically correlational, most experimenters have interpreted their findings in terms of the attitudes and behaviors of the parents causing the behaviors in the child. Recent investigators propose a more truly interactional model of family dynamics whereby we study both the effects of parents on each other and their child, and the effects of the child on the parents (Bell, 1968; Moss, 1967). Even infants exert considerable control over the behavior of parents and with age it might be expected that social skills in shaping others' behavior would increase. Bell has argued that upper limit controls such as parental physical punishment could as easily be considered a result as a cause of children's aggression or impulsivity. Similarly, lower limit controls may be stimulated by passivity, inhibition, or lack of competence in the child. The frequently reported rejection by delinquent parents may be a response to the child's antisocial behavior. The intrusiveness of the parents of withdrawn children may be an attempt to elicit behavior from the passive child.

As a corollary to this problem, the investigator of the relationship between family interaction and psychopathology faces the formidable task of estimating how similar the present interaction patterns are to those that preceded the labeling of the child as deviant, of identifying which behaviors in the families of deviant children are a result and which a precursor of the child being labeled deviant. Such problems in interpretation are difficult to deal with except in longitudinal, prospective studies. Although most procedures used to study parent-child relationships present methodological problems, these problems do not seem to be quite as marked in observational as in self-report studies. Therefore the focus of the present chapter will be on results of studies using direct observation.

Heredity and Constitutional Factors in Psychopathology

Although this paper concentrates on the role of family interaction variables in psychopathology, it is important to note that certain physiological or temperamental characteristics in the young child, possibly hereditary in nature, can influence the course of subsequent family interaction. Autonomic nervous system reactivity, sociability, and activity level are likely factors for this role.

Relatively stable individual differences in patterns of autonomic reactivity have been identified (Lacey, 1950; Richmond & Lustman, 1955; Wenger,

Clemens, Coleman, Cullen, & Engel, 1961) and investigators have attempted to relate these autonomic styles to dimensions of personality (Darling, 1940; Eysenck, 1956; Theron, 1948). Comparisons of identical and fraternal twins on various measures of autonomic reactivity have consistently found that identical twins have a greater degree of similarity than do fraternal twins (Jost & Sontag, 1944; Lader & Wing, 1966; Vandenberg, Clark, & Samuels, 1965). An inherited tendency toward unusually strong autonomic reactivity, combined with greater ease of autonomic conditioning, may be associated with susceptibility to the development of facets of personality disorders such as anxiety, phobic and perhaps obsessive-compulsive reactions. In addition, autonomic lability has been found to be associated with conduct disorder characteristics such as impulsivity, lack of self-control, and inability to resist temptation (Grim, Kohlberg, & White, 1968; Boyle, Dykman, & Ackerman, 1965; Lacey & Lacey, 1958; Levy & Lang, 1966; Kagan & Rosman, 1964). However, these findings must be viewed with some caution since several studies have been unable to replicate the relationship between autonomic lability and motoric impulsivity (Docter, Kaswan, & Nakamura, 1964; Williams, Schachter, & Rowe, 1965).

It has been suggested that Eysenck's Neuroticism factor, Cattell's Anxiety Factor, and Bronson's Placidity-Explosiveness dimension are similar personality variables that can be appropriately labeled emotional reactivity (Bronson, 1969). Bronson's longitudinal analysis of orientations in the personality development of children in the Berkeley Guidance Study found that although Placidity-Explosiveness in children is influenced by parental behavior, it is a relatively stable and enduring behavioral characteristic.

Sociability refers to a dimension represented at one end by individuals who are shy, socially fearful, and inhibited, especially with respect to strangers or new situations, and at the other end by individuals who are outgoing, expansive, ebullient, and at ease in most situations. Again studies of twins have found greater concordance between identical than fraternal twins on sociability (Freedman & Keller, 1963; Gottesman, 1962; Gottesman, 1966; Scarr, 1965; Shields, 1962). Bronson (1969) found that her sociability dimension of Emotional Expressiveness-Reserve was even more stable and pervasive than that of Placidity-Explosiveness, and was relatively independent of parental behavior. It seems possible that a tendency to be inhibited, apprehensive, and restrained or outgoing and assertive in social encounters will be differentially related to the development of various types of psychopathology.

Several studies have dealt directly with the role of heredity in personality disorders and have found greater similarity for identical than fraternal twins for presence of neurotic symptoms (Shields, 1954) and diagnosed anxiety reactions (Slater & Shields, 1969).

Research on infant development has suggested a third variable, activity level, which appears to be constitutional or genetic in origin and may affect the development of pathology. Even in neonates marked individual differences in activity level and irritability exist, and these factors remain relatively stable over time. It has been speculated that an extremely motorically active infant is more likely to manifest aggressive behavior in later years, and that high infant activity is a sign of inability to control or limit the effects of internal tension and impulsivity (Escalona & Heider, 1959). Some evidence for a possible relationship between an innate activity factor and assertiveness is suggested since even as neonates boys are more active than girls, boys are more physically aggressive than girls as early as 13 months, and there is a correlation between activity level and aggression. Hamburg and Lunde (1966) point out that differences in activity and assertiveness in males and females may not necessarily be genetic in origin but may result from maternal changes in androgen level during critical periods in human prenatal development, which may result in sensitizing circuits in the central nervous system—mediating aggressive behavior. However, the child's activity level may be only indirectly related to the development of aggressive behavior, since the active infant elicits a wider variety of more intense and frequent patterns of social and sensory stimulation from his caretakers than does the passive infant (Dennis, 1941; Moss, 1967).

Several longitudinal studies have suggested that if hereditary or temperamental predispositions do exist, they are modified by the child's life experience, particularly those associated with early social interactions (Kagan & Moss, 1962; Kris, 1957; MacFarlane, Allen, & Honzik, 1954; Murphy, 1962; Chess, Thomas, & Birch, 1968). The Chess, Thomas, & Birch (1968) study illustrates the interaction between possible genetically produced traits and social learning experiences. In this research, the development of 136 children was followed from birth to ages 6–12 in 85 families. Measures of child behavior and temperament were obtained by parent interviews at 3-month intervals during the first 18 months of life, at 6-month intervals until 5 years, and at yearly intervals thereafter. The interviews emphasized factual descriptions of recent or current behavior. The validity of the interview data was checked by home observations of child behavior on a subsample of families. Other sources of data included school observations, teacher interviews, and standardized psychological tests.

In the course of the study, 42 of the children developed mildly to moderately severe behavior disorders and were seen more intensively by the staff. Thus the study provides an opportunity to examine what kind of temperamental characteristics were present in these children *before* the onset of the behavior disturbances—an unusual circumstance in psychopathology research.

When the children were still less than 2 years of age, the investigators had identified a subgroup of 14 children that they labeled "difficult children." Prominent temperamental characteristics of these children were as follows: (1) biological irregularity, especially with respect to sleep, feeding, and elimination cycles; (2) withdrawal and associated expressions of distress to new stimuli, for example, to the first bath, to new foods, new people, or new places; (3) slow adaptability to change, taking many exposures to new situations before overcoming the initial negative reaction; and (4) a predominance of negative mood, involving a greater readiness to fuss and cry with high intensity. Of these difficult children, 70% subsequently developed behavior disorders. These children comprised 6% (4 cases) of the 66 children who did not develop behavior disturbances and 24% (10 cases) of those who did.

Parent interviews indicated that the parents of the difficult children did not differ from the parent group as a whole in their approach to child care during the early years. However, as the difficult child grew older, disturbances in parent-child interaction emerged in a number of cases that appeared to be reactive to the special characteristics of these children. Many of these college-educated mothers reacted to the troublesome features of the child with self-blame, for example, by interpreting their child's difficult behavior in terms of psychodynamic theories in which the mother's unconscious attitude of rejection must be producing the problem. Other parents interpreted the child's crying and irregularity as being intentionally defiant and reacted punitively. The development of child disturbance is traced in a number of families in a way that highlights the interaction between child predisposition and parent reaction. In fact, the findings would suggest that if hereditary dispositions do exist, either in the form of the temperament traits measured in this study or in the form of autonomic reactivity as discussed previously, the subsequent development of an emotional disorder is largely dependent on social learning experiences.

Classification of Child Psychopathology

As we have seen in Chapter One, no consistent classification and use of diagnostic terminology is found in personality diagnosis in childhood. Since familial correlates of childhood psychoses have been reviewed in Chapter Five, this section will focus on three of the categories of disorders discussed extensively in Chapter One: those problems that lead to disruption and suffering for others (conduct disorders), those disorders that result mostly in discomfort and suffering for the child himself (personality disorder), and those that involve the interaction of psychological factors and physical symptoms (psychosomatic disorders).

Perhaps because of their greater negative social impact more research has focused on conduct disorders, particularly in the form of juvenile delinquency, than on personality disorders.

Conduct Disorders

The following discussion of familial influences on the development of conduct disorders will incorporate studies of both juvenile delinquency and aggressive behavior in the preadolescent child. It seems reasonable to combine investigations of these groups of children for two reasons. First, the family correlates of early antisocial aggression and most forms of delinquency appear to be similar; second, antisocial behavior in childhood is frequently predictive of severe psychiatric disturbances as adolescents and adults. As will be shown in Chapter Ten, young children who exhibit antisocial behaviors such as truancy, stealing, and lying are likely to display these and other deviant characteristics in later life.

Parental Absence and Conduct Disorders

The effects of both maternal absence, with subsequent institutionalization, and paternal absence have been related to conduct disorders in children. The difficulties of differentiating the effects of maternal deprivation from those of institutionalization have been well documented (Yarrow, 1961). Whatever the most salient factors may be, institutionalized children exhibit gross deviations in personality development. Goldfarb (1945) did a comparative analysis of children who had been reared in an institution for the first three years of life and then placed in a foster home and a group who had been reared in a foster home since infancy. Children of four age groups, 3-1/2, 6-1/2, 8-1/2, and 12 years were studied. The institutionalized children were more impulsive and uninhibited, as manifested in temper tantrums, lying, and stealing; they showed more unpredictable cruelty and aggression to peers, adults, and animals; and they made more demands for attention and affection from adults. The author speculates that the lack of feeling and consideration for others demonstrated by these children at all ages is based on the lack of early attachment to a specific caretaker. It is also noted that these children do not show appropriate guilt or anxiety following transgressions or unprovoked demonstrations of hostility. Lack of self-control, unsocialized aggression, inability to form lasting emotional ties and to internalize prohibitions in institutionalized children have also been reported by other investigators (Bowlby, Ainsworth, Boston, & Rosenbluth, 1956; Lowry, 1940).

The effects of partial maternal absence, in the form of working mothers, remains an open question (Hoffman, 1963; Stolz, 1960). There has been some suggestion that maternal employment is more closely related to delinquency in girls than in boys (Nye, 1958), and is found more often when the mother is involved in part-time rather than regular employment (Glueck & Glueck, 1957). However, the results of a variety of studies have not been consistent and they seem to suggest that if family relations are positive and stable, the effects of maternal employment need not be detrimental.

Broken homes have frequently been stressed as an important contributing factor in the development of conduct disorders. Children with conduct disorders more frequently come from homes that have been disrupted by desertion, divorce, death, and absence of the father than do nondeviant children. Even crosscultural studies have found that in societies in which the father's effective presence is minimal, a high rate of theft and personal crime exists (Bacon, Child, & Barry, 1963).

Siegman (1966) found that medical students whose fathers had been absent for at least one year in the preschool period reported more antisocial behavior in childhood than did father-present boys. The Glueck and Glueck (1950) study, which compared 500 delinquents with carefully matched 500 nondelinquents, found that less than one-fourth of the nondeviant group came from father-absent homes, in contrast to over two-fifths in the delinquents. Although McCord, McCord, and Thurber (1962) report no differences in incidence of delinquency between father-present and father-absent boys, the father-absent boys had been involved in more felonies. It has been proposed that lower-class boys from basically feminine controlled homes, particularly those with absent fathers, are demonstrating compensatory masculinity in their frequent antisocial behavior (Biller, 1969).

There is some suggestion that the effects of a broken home are more disruptive if the child is preadolescent when the separation occurs and if the child is a girl. Studies by Toby (1957) and Monahan (1957, 1960) show broken homes to be more frequent among female than male delinquents.

This is congruent with the findings of a recent study (Hetherington & Deur, 1970) which indicates that although there are few gross deviations in personality manifested by preadolescent girls from father-absent homes, following puberty marked disruption in heterosexual behavior occurs. This sexual deviation appears either as severe sexual anxiety, shyness, and discomfort around males or as inappropriately assertive and promiscuous behavior. The former syndrome appears to be more frequent when separation is a result of death and the latter of divorce or desertion.

Monahan (1957, 1960) also found that both male and female delinquents from broken homes show more recidivism than those from intact homes, although there is less overall recidivism among girls.

Further support for the damaging effects of father absence on sexual behavior is found in the work of O'Connor (1964) and West (1967) who report that father absence during childhood is more frequently associated with homosexuality than neurosis in males. Passive or absent fathers and a close relationship with mothers are frequently found in the histories of homosexual males. A similar pattern of paternal absence or inadequacy is reported among female homosexuals.

Peterson and Becker (1965) in their excellent review of family interaction and juvenile delinquency suggest that both the cause of disruption and the conflict preceding separation must be considered in evaluating the effects of broken homes. In general, death of a parent seems less damaging than separation by divorce or separation following a period of strife.

Parental Characteristics and Interactions

A survey of the research literature suggests that deviant parents have deviant children. Social learning theorists have emphasized imitation of an aggressive model as one of the important factors in the development of aggressive behavior in children (Bandura & Walters, 1963; Berkowitz, 1962). Becker, Peterson, Hellmer, Shoemaker, & Quay (1959) reported that parents of children with conduct disorders were maladjusted, inconsistent, arbitrary, and given to explosive expressions of anger. Mothers were often tense and frustrating, and fathers were inadequate and emotionally distant. Kagan (1958) also found that aggressive elementary school boys fantasied their parents as angry individuals.

These findings parallel those of studies of parents of delinquents that show a high incidence of deviant or criminal behavior in families of delinquents. Glueck and Glueck (1950) found that 84% of the delinquents in Massachusetts reformatories had families that included criminals. Shaw and McKay (1942) also reported a high incidence of antisocial behavior in the siblings and parents of delinquents. McCord and McCord (1958) found a criminal father and cold mother was the combination of parental characteristics most likely to lead to delinquency, particularly if the father were also cruel and neglecting. Where mothers were lacking in affection and served as a deviant model, delinquency was also frequent. However, consistent discipline or affection from one parent could partially counteract the effects of a criminal role model.

Unhappy marital relationships and interparental conflict are found in parents of delinquents (Glueck & Glueck, 1950; McCord, McCord, & Gudeman, 1960; Nye, 1958). Such parents are described as indifferent and isolated from each other or as actively quarreling and aggressing against each other. Antagonistic relations between parents are more frequent among families with a delinquent than a neurotic child (Bennett, 1960). Studies involving observations of family interaction in decision-making situations have also found more spontaneous agreement between normal families than families of delinquents (Ferreira & Winter, 1968) and less failure to agree following discussion in parents of nondelinquents (Hetherington, Stouwie, & Ridberg, 1970).

These results are in agreement with those of an experimental study (Hetherington & Frankie, 1965) of identification with the aggressor in preschool children; the study assessed parental conflict, dominance, and warmth in family interaction through a modified revealed difference test and measured the child's imitation of the mother's and father's behavior in a game-playing session. It was found that children imitated a dominant, hostile parent when the home was high in conflict and when both parents were low in warmth. If either interparental conflict was low, or the other parent was warm, the imitation of the hostile dominant parent decreased. Imitation of the aggressor was found to occur more frequently in boys than in girls, and more frequently for boys if the aggressive, dominant model was the father.

Parent-Child Interactions

Although interparental relations are important in the development of deviant behavior in children, a critical factor is also the parents' interactions with their child. Models of parent behavior have frequently emphasized two dimensions: a control dimension ranging from restrictiveness to permissiveness and an affective dimension ranging from warmth to hostility (Schaefer, 1961). In addition, research has focused on characteristics of the specific disciplinary techniques used to direct the child, such as consistency versus inconsistency, and psychological, love-oriented versus power assertive, physical forms of discipline. It is obvious that these dimensions are not independent. Low use of physical punishment and high reasoning has been found to correlate with warmth in both mothers and fathers (Becker, Peterson, Luria, Shoemaker, & Hellmer, 1962). Frequent use of physical punishment also relates to hostile restrictiveness (Becker, et al., 1962) and authoritarianism as reported by parents. Extremes of restrictiveness and permissiveness, hostility and rejection, power assertive forms of discipline such as severe physical punishment, and inconsistency have all been found to be associated with antisocial behavior in children.

Rosenthal, Finkelstein, Ni, and Robertson (1959) analyzed the relationship between maternal behavior and problem behavior in case histories of 450 children seen at the Illinois Institute for Juvenile Research. Maternal punitiveness, inconsistency, overpermissiveness, and conflicting authorities related to conduct disorders. A parallel study on fathers (Rosenthal, Ni, Finkelstein, & Berkwits, 1962) found an association between children's conduct disorders and paternal punitiveness, authoritarian control, neglect, and conflicting authorities.

Physical Punishment and Hostility.   Becker (1964) suggests that because of the close association between use of physical punishment and hostility in parents, it is necessary to evaluate their combined effects on the child. The relationship of physical punishment and hostility with aggressive behavior, and warmth and reasoning with prosocial behavior has been partially supported in studies of both normal and deviant populations. The relationship between rejection or punishment and aggression is perhaps better documented than that between internalized control and warmth (Aronfreed, 1969). Although conclusions drawn from early studies based largely on parental reports of discipline practices have been criticized because of methodological weaknesses and inconsistency of results (Yarrow, Campbell, & Burton, 1968), recent observational studies lend some support to the former relationship (Baumrind, 1967; Hetherington, Stouwie, & Ridberg, 1970).

Studies of delinquents find a high incidence of rejection and hostility, particularly by fathers, in parents of delinquent boys (Andry, 1960; Bandura & Walters, 1959; Glueck & Glueck, 1950; McCord, McCord, & Zola, 1959; Merrill, 1947).

Similar results have been found in studies of aggressive but nondelinquent children. The Sears, Maccoby, and Levin (1957) study, which correlated maternal interview responses about disciplinary practices with maternal reports of the behavior of their five-year-old children, found that reported aggression in boys in the home was positively related to both severity of punishment and permissiveness for aggression. Congruent results were obtained from the Sears, Whiting, Nowlis, and Sears study (1953), which related maternal reports of childrearing with the child's behavior in nursery school. High severity of punishment for aggression was positively correlated with aggression in school for boys, but a curvilinear relationship was found for girls. Extremes of punishment were related to passivity and low assertiveness in daughters.

When Becker et al. (1962) studied the combined effects of hostility and punitiveness of both parents of 5-year-old children with behavior problems, again a differential pattern of relationship between parental punishment and aggression in school for boys and girls was obtained. Linear relations to child aggression in the home were obtained for both boys and girls, and for boys in school. For girls, the effects of moderate parental hostility and punishment was related to aggression in school. However, this relationship was not found at more intense levels of punishment. It might be speculated that the sex appropriateness of aggressive behavior restricts or alters the expression of direct aggression in girls. This is given some support—in a study relating early discipline practices to aggression in 12-year-olds, it was found that punishment of girls was associated with aggression anxiety and prosocial aggression (Sears, 1961).

An alternate explanation in terms of differential treatment of boys and girls is put forward by Bronfenbrenner (1961a, 1961b). Bronfenbrenner related children's reports of parental discipline to teacher's ratings of leadership and responsibility in adolescents. High warmth combined with high control was associated with conforming overinhibited behavior, while lower amounts of control were associated with responsibility and leadership. However, this relationship must be qualified since when warmth was relatively low, high controls were related to more desirable behaviors and low control to lack of self-control and internalization. Thus, with warm parents there is a danger of overcontrolling the child and with cold parents the danger is of underinhibiting the child unless firm controls are utilized. Bronfenbrenner speculates that because girls are more frequently treated with warmth and receive less physical punishment, overcontrol is more common and inhibition occurs more frequently in girls than in boys.

Aronfreed (1969) suggests that the relationship between the warmth-hostility dimension and internalized controls is attributable entirely to studies involving children who have suffered extremes of parental rejection or punishment. In many studies using normal populations, no association has been found between self-control, prosocial behavior, resistance to temptation, and parental nurturance (Grinder, 1962; Heinecke, 1953; Sears, & Rau, Alpert, 1965).

Parental Control. Studies of the effects of parents' control over their child's behavior suggest that either extreme restrictiveness or extreme permissiveness may lead to aggressive or antisocial behavior. McCord, McCord, & Howard (1961) grouped mothers as exerting subnormal, normal, or overcontrol. Mothers using subnormal control were lax, neglecting, and unconcerned. Mothers exerting normal control permitted their child considerable autonomy in some areas but were more directive and controlling in others. Overcontrolling mothers completely structured, directed, and intruded on all aspects of their child's activity. It was found that maternal overcontrol was associated with low aggression in sons, normal control with assertive behavior in sons, and both subnormal and overcontrol with aggressive behavior.

Studies of delinquents (Glueck & Glueck, 1950; McCord, McCord, & Zola, 1959) suggest that an interaction between extremely lax discipline by mothers of delinquents and rigid, overly restrictive discipline by fathers is often present in families of delinquents. A similar pattern of family relations was found in Bandura and Walters' (1959) study of aggressive but nondelinquent adolescents.

In further clarifying the effects of parental control, the importance of studying the interaction between affective behavior and the parental control dimension again is clearly demonstrated in the classic study by Levy (1943) of maternal overprotection in 20 cases selected from the Institute for Child Guidance in New York. Although Levy's mothers were all warm and overprotective, those who were dominant, infantilizing, and restrictive had children who were passive, timid, overconscientious and conforming, and withdrew from social interactions with their peers. In contrast, those mothers who were excessively permissive and indulgent had children who were rebellious, aggressive, disobedient, and uncontrolled in the home.

A recent study (Baumrind, 1967), which utilized both structured observations and interviews, also suggests that impulsive aggressive behavior in preschool children is associated with moderate levels of parental warmth but low maturity demands and control.

The studies of Levy and Baumrind suggest that even with adequate parental warmth some parental control is necessary for the development of self-control in the child. Further support for this is yielded by behavior modification studies, which find that a differential reinforcement program, combined with time-out procedures for antisocial behavior, is more effective in suppressing aggressive or oppositional behavior than is reinforcement alone in both institutionalized adult patients and children (Holz, Azrin, & Allyon, 1963; Bostow & Bailey, 1969; Wahler, 1968).

Consistency. A third attribute of disciplinary practices that has been found to be prevalent in families having children with conduct disorders is inconsistency in discipline. This may be either in the form of interparental inconsistency involving widely disparate disciplinary practices or in intraparental inconsistency characterized by erratic discipline. Baruch and Wilcox (1944) find an association between interparental disagreements over child-rearing practices and interparental tension, and child maladjustment. Read (1945) finds a higher incidence of unfavorable behavior in nursery school children when one parent is restrictive and the other lax. McCord, McCord, & Howard (1961) also report erratic control ranging from extremes of permissiveness and restrictiveness in mothers of aggressive boys.

Studies of delinquents have consistently yielded a finding of more erratic, lax, and inconsistent discipline by parents of delinquents (Andry, 1960; Bandura & Walters, 1959; Burt, 1929; Glueck & Glueck, 1950; McCord, McCord, & Zola, 1959; Merrill, 1947). As was previously noted, maternal laxity combined with paternal severity and restrictiveness is the most common pattern in families of delinquents.

McCord, McCord, & Zola (1959), in one of the few prospective studies of delinquency, report a low incidence of delinquency, even in homes with a criminal parent when the mothers and fathers were consistent in their discipline. The specific form of discipline, whether punitive or love-oriented, did not seem to matter as long as it was applied consistently. In fact, the lowest rates of delinquency were found in homes in which both parents were consistently punitive or love-oriented in their discipline practices. It has been proposed that extremely restrictive, power assertive discipline, particularly in a hostile family atmosphere, leads to frustration of dependency needs and a heightened predisposition to respond aggressively. If the opportunity to express this aggression occurs through inconsistent discipline, laxity in one parent, or active reinforcement for aggressive behavior outside the home, this may increase the probability of antisocial aggressive responses by the child.

Family Interaction and Dimensions of Delinquency

The previously presented studies of juvenile delinquency usually involved a simple comparison of delinquents and nondelinquents and seemed to assume that delinquency is a homogeneous form of psychopathology. However, recent investigations have indicated that delinquency should be viewed as a legal classification involving the performance of antisocial acts, but which subsumes a variety of psychological dimensions with different patterns of behavior and etiology associated with them.

Three main dimensions of delinquency have been identified with great consistency, as we have seen in Chapter One. In review, the first dimension is the unsocialized psychopathic dimension characterized by amorality, hostility toward authority, impulsivity, assaultiveness, and rebelliousness. The second, the neurotic-disturbed dimension, is associated with guilt, low self-esteem, anxiety, withdrawal, and depression. As was indicated in Chapter One, these dimensions derived from studies of delinquents parallel the conduct and personality factors found in the analysis of other deviant populations. The third, the socialized-subcultural dimension, is related to neither a failure to socialize nor gross personality disturbance. It involves the acceptance of social values of a delinquent subgroup, and within these standards social concern, responsibility, and guilt may be manifested.

The few experimenters (Hewitt & Jenkins, 1946; Lewis, 1954) using case history material who attempted to relate parental behavior to these dimensions of problem behavior suggest that the unsocialized psychopathic factor is associated with parental rejection, the neurotic disturbed factor with overcontrol, and the socialized subcultural factor with neglect, permissiveness, and exposure to delinquent norms.

A recent study (Hetherington, Stouwie, & Ridberg, 1970) investigated family interaction in delinquent boys and girls who scored above the mean on one of these dimensions and below on the other two dimensions, and control groups of nondelinquent male and female adolescents. The dimensions of delinquency were measured by a forced-choice questionnaire developed by Quay and Peterson (1964). The parents and adolescent son or daughter participated in a three-way interaction based on a modification of the Revealed Difference Test and the parents also answered the Stanford Parent Questionnaire (Winder & Rau, 1962). Distinctive patterns of family relations could be differentiated for the four groups of families of boys and girls.

In families of boys, on behavioral measures on the Revealed Difference Test, a clear picture emerged of the neurotic delinquent family being dominated by the mother and the social delinquent family being dominated by the father. Although the mother of the neurotic delinquent boy was controlling in decision making, the father did not accept his role passively. He disagreed and aggressed frequently against his wife, and marital conflict was present. The mother's relationship with her son was less strife ridden; although she dominated her son, there was no evidence of conflict between them.

In contrast, the mother of the social delinquent boy was overtly nondominant and frequently passively yielded to her husband's opinions but some passive resistance was suggested since she frequently failed to reach final agreement with her husband. Although the father controlled the verbal interaction in terms of starting and terminating discussions and yielding little in his initial position, the sons were not acquiescent in the decision-making process. They participated actively in the conversation, shifted their opinions less than any other sons, and were often unwilling to compromise with their father's opinions.

The interactions in families with psychopathic sons were not as clearly delineated although the father appeared to dominate. The mother was more active than the social delinquents' mother. The son participated minimally in interaction and decision-making processes, although he did disagree and aggress against his mother frequently and failed to reach final agreement with his father.

The families of nondelinquent boys showed no stable pattern of differential parental dominance; however, significantly more power was exerted by the son than was the case in delinquent families. Findings of other studies using direct behavioral measures have not been altogether consistent with respect to parental dominance patterns in normal families. Consistent with the Hetherington, Stouwie, and Ridberg results, Martin and Hetherington (1970) found in relatively large samples of families with nondeviant male and female children that fathers and mothers were, on the average, about equally dominant. However, Rohrbaugh (1966) and Schuhan (1970) found father dominance and Murrell and Stachowiak (1967) reported mother dominance in normal families. Since these studies varied in age of the subjects and interaction situations utilized, and the number of family members involved in the interaction, it is difficult to evaluate whether these findings represent true differences in dominance in the various populations or whether they should be attributed to procedural variations.

There seems to be little conflict and disagreement between normal parents, but there is considerable activity and conflict between sons and parents. An extremely low rate of final failure to reach agreement in these families may indicate that members feel free to disagree initially but through active discussion are flexible enough to adapt to a mutually acceptable position.

The questionnaire measure suggests that parents of neurotic delinquent sons, like those of the other delinquent groups, reject their children, make high use of deprivation of privileges and physical punishment, and have little confidence in their child's moral development and self-control in the face of temptation. In contrast to the permissiveness of parents of social delinquents, the parents of neurotic and psychopathic delinquents tend to be extremely restrictive in limitations on their sons' activities. One marked difference between the parents of neurotic and psychopathic delinquents lies in their attitudes toward aggression. The former show considerable anxiety about aggression, whereas the latter actively encourage aggression outside of the home, although they do not permit the son to be assertive within the family.

In many ways, the families of social delinquent boys appear more stable than those of the other two delinquent groups. These parents describe their marriages as happy and gratifying and share a common interest in social activities. Their rejection of their son seems to be part of an ambivalent response since they also score high on warmth. The father's emphasis on appropriate sex role behavior, and both parents' stress on conformity and early independence and mastery by the son, suggest that these parents have rather conventional hopes for an appropriately masculine and competent son. In addition, their high anxiety about aggressive behavior and concern with social approval suggest that these parents may be particularly distressed by their son's antisocial activities. It seems possible that the ambivalence may be a response to instead of a cause of their son's delinquent behavior.

The difference between groups on the Revealed Difference Test for girls is not as clear, consistent, or readily interpretable as those for boys. Again, we find marked maternal dominance in mothers of neurotic delinquents and even greater powerlessness and passivity in these fathers. These daughters are unusually passive, speak less than any other daughters, and have little influence in the decision-making process.

In the homes of the psychopathic and social delinquent girls, no clear pattern of parental dominance emerges. Little effective control is exerted by either parent. There is an active pattern of dissent between these daughters and their parents, particularly with the father. In contrast, the nondelinquent daughter seldom intervenes in her father's conversation and is less dominant and assertive than these two groups of delinquent girls. It could be argued that the low activity and dissension in normal girls is sex appropriate, whereas the greater activity and freedom to disagree in normal boys is congruent with the assertive masculine sex role.

The questionnaire measures again show greater rejection by fathers and mothers of neurotic and psychopathic delinquent girls than by parents of nondelinquent girls.

Both parents of the neurotic delinquents try unsuccessfully to rigidly restrict their daughters' activities. In contrast, interparental inconsistency in discipline in found in parents of psychopathic delinquent girls, since their fathers but not their mothers are restrictive.

Again, we find greater acceptance of the child and greater permissiveness by parents of social delinquents than in the other delinquent groups.

As was found in the boys' study, parents of nondelinquents have a happy marriage, are self-confident, and have a high sense of self-esteem. Unlike parents of delinquent girls, they show little concern about sexual anxiety. No differences between groups were obtained on aggression anxiety; in fact, in contrast to mothers of nondelinquent girls, the mothers of delinquent girls actually encourage and reinforce aggression. This differs from the parents of boys where there were no differences between groups on sex anxiety, but parents of neurotic and social male delinquents showed considerable concern about aggression. This could well be associated with the reasons for committal of males and females. Female delinquents are frequently committed for incorrigible sexual behavior, whereas males almost never are. Males are usually committed for aggressive or destructive acts against people or property. Parents may be exhibiting concern on the basis of the past areas of difficulty with their child.

Personality Disorder

Parent Characteristics and Interaction

Statistical surveys have consistently shown that neurotic individuals tend to come from homes in which a higher proportion of parents have neurotic symptoms than in the general population (Bennett, 1960; Jenkins, 1966; Shields & Slater, 1961). And, Liverant (1959) found significantly more deviant Minnesota Multiphasic Personality Inventory profiles in parents of children referred to child guidance clinics than in parents of normal children. These empirical findings, of course, tell us nothing about the relative contribution of heredity and social learning; either, or more likely an interaction between the two, can readily account for the facts.

There is a tendency for married couples to have greater similarity on the presence or absence of neurotic disorder than would be the case if they had been paired without respect to whether one or the other was neurotic (Buck & Ladd, 1965; Pond, Ryle, & Hamilton, 1963). Such a relationship suggests that assortative mating has occurred, that is, neurotic individuals tend to marry other neurotic individuals and nonneurotics marry nonneurotics. Buck and Ladd, however, suggest that in addition to assortative mating there may be a tendency for similarity in "neurotic" status to increase with length of marriage. Such a finding suggests that either a neurotic spouse tends to produce neurotic reactions in a nonneurotic mate or a nonneurotic spouse helps a neurotic mate to overcome the neurotic reaction, or both. The evidence for progressive increase in similarity is not strong, however, and more research is necessary.

Neurotic disorder in one or both parents is likely to be accompanied by marital conflict. In recent years, the marriage relationship has been given central importance by many clinical writers as a focal point from which other neurosis-inducing social interactions derive (for example, Satir, 1964). Cummings, Bayley, and Rie (1966) found that parents of emotionally disturbed or deviant children report more dissatisfaction and conflict with their spouse than do parents of normal children. Gassner and Murray (1969) found direct behavioral measures of interparent conflict to be higher in parents of neurotic than in parents of normal children. Ferreira and Winter (1968) found that in three-way (father-mother-child) interaction, families with a neurotic child exchanged less information, took longer to reach a decision, and spent a greater proportion of time in silence.

There is no empirical research that illustrates the specific mechanisms whereby conflicted marital interaction eventuates in child disturbance. There is, however, ample speculation derived from clinical experience about how this might happen. Some common ideas along these lines are listed below and are presented more in the spirit of plausible hypotheses than substantiated findings.

(1) Simple displacement of anger and aggression from spouse to child may be the most common occurrence. (2) Husband-wife antagonism, although originally stemming from other sources, may center around child-rearing as one battlefield. (3) One spouse may attempt to enlist a child as an ally against the other spouse. (4) One spouse may react to the other with helplessness and withdrawal, and attempt to get a child to assume adult responsibility.

The possibilities are infinite. There is no reason, however, to suggest that *all* neurotic disorders develop in families with disturbed marital interaction or that disturbed marital interaction *always* results in neurotic disturbances in children. It is quite likely that in some instances rather serious marital discord is kept confined to the husband-wife dyad and not allowed to seriously affect parent-child interactions. Some degree of insight into the nature of displacement mechanisms would probably aid in keeping the marital conflict "encapsulated." It is also likely that there are numerous instances of disturbed parent-child interactions occurring in families where there is little or no marital conflict.

Parent-Child Interaction

No matter what larger systems are operative, they can only impinge on the child in some form of direct interaction. There are many clinical reports about possible neurosis-inducing aspects of family interaction, but unfortunately there are few studies in which a group of families with a young child just beginning to manifest a specific kind of neurotic disorder has been compared with nonneurotic control families on behaviorally oriented measures of relevant family interaction. Most of the research to be reviewed below will fall short of this ideal in several respects, and we shall weight our conclusions on the basis of the quality of research methodology instead of by a simple counting of positive and negative findings. Research will be considered first in which the child grouping seemed to reflect a rather general category of neurotic disturbance, and then we shall discuss research that focused on more specifically delineated categories, such as anxiety reaction and various types of psychosomatic disorders.

General Neurotic Disorders. As was mentioned earlier, research has generally yielded two broad groupings of childhood disorders representing impulsive-aggressive and neurotic-inhibited types of symptoms. Some of the following studies have been referred to in the section on conduct disorders and will be mentioned briefly again here with emphasis on those findings pertinent to neurotic-inhibited behavior. Despite the likelihood that the neurotic-inhibited category includes a diversity of subgroups, there are certain consistencies that emerge from these older studies. In the Hewitt and Jenkins (1946) study a tetrachoric correlation of .52 was found between the presence of family repression (referring generally to high parental control and restriction) and the presence of overinhibited behavior; and a correlation of .46 was found between physical deficiency in the child and overinhibited behavior. A correlation of .73 resulted when these two variables were combined, indicating that parental repression and physical deficiency in the child make independent contributions to the development of overinhibited behavior. More recently, Jenkins (1968) found that mothers of overanxious children were more likely than mothers of other clinic children to be described in the case notes as having an infantilizing, overprotective attitude, as setting an example for the child's pathology, and as sometimes having a marked preference for the child relative to other siblings. The parents of the overanxious child were also less likely to use physical punishment than parents of the average clinic child.

Lewis (1954) found that parents of inhibited-neurotic children showed more "constraint" in their child-rearing practices relative to parents of un-socialized aggressive or socialized delinquent children. Constraint was considered to be present if at least two of the following conditions were met: (1) rigid daily program, (2) excessive discipline, (3) domination and hyper-criticism, (4) lack of warmth in family, (5) enforced isolation, or (6) over-protection. Bennett (1960), in comparing the case histories of 50 delinquent and 50 neurotic children, found that the parents of neurotic children were more likely to have a stable marriage, have neurotic personalities themselves, and to be overly strict in their discipline.

Becker et al. (1959), using ratings based on parent interviews, found no relationship between presence of child personality problem and any mother ratings; but he did find that fathers of children with personality problems were low on readiness to explain things to the child (or thwarted childs' curiosity) and these fathers were themselves rated as maladjusted. Interestingly, in this study measures of parental overprotection were not related to child personality problems. In other studies using clinical populations, Rosenthal et al. (1959) and Rosenthal et al. (1962) also report that parents of neurotic-inhibited children were more restrictive and controlling than parents of aggressive or delinquent children.

Several studies have used "normal" children. Sears (1961) provides some evidence that mothers who were rated from interviews as restrictive and punishing when their sons were age 5, had sons at age 12 who were inclined to self-aggression (self-punishment, suicidal tendencies, and accident prone-ness). Kagan and Moss (1962) found lack of dominance and assertiveness, and more conformity and dependence on adults in children, ages 3–10, whose mothers had been highly protective at ages 1–3. As was previously discussed, McCord, McCord, and Howard (1961) found nonassertive boys to have mothers that were overcontrolling, that insisted that they be close at all times, and that required submission to their direction.

Given the crude methodology employed in the above studies (indirect measures based on interviews or case notes, the lack of nondeviant compari-son groups, the rough grouping of children based frequently on indirect measures, etc.), the general implication of a relation between parent restric-tiveness and neurotic-inhibited symptoms in the child must be viewed as a viable hypothesis, but one that requires a more fine-grained examination. It is, for example, possible that preconceptions on the part of raters and inter-viewers could have slanted the data in this direction in many studies.

Baumrind's (1967) study is relevant to the development of both person-ality disorder and conduct disorders. It will be described in more detail be-cause it incorporates many desirable methodological features such as direct measures of parent-child interaction obtained in both structured and unstructured situations. Three groups of children were selected from a larger group of 110 3- to 4-year-old nursery school children (male and female) on the basis of 14 weeks of behavioral observation. Group I (energetic-friendly, $N = 13$) children were rated higher on each of the following than either of the other two groups: self-reliance, approach to novel or stressful situations with interest and curiosity, self-control, energy level, cheerful mood, and friendly peer relations. The differences between Group II (conflicted-irritable, $N = 11$) and Group III (impulsive-aggressive, $N = 8$) children might be summarized as follows: Group II children showed more self-control and self-reliance than Group III but less than Group I. Group II children were inclined to be less cheerful and recover from expressions of annoyance more slowly than Group III. In general, Group II seemed to involve a more conflicted group of children in which aggressions and unfriendly reactions alternate with more socially withdrawn behavior; and unhappy, irritable, and apprehensive mood states prevail. Group III children seemed to be more purely impulsive and lacking in self-discipline of any kind.

Parent behavior was assessed in three ways: (1) in the homes, (2) in a Structured Observation procedure (mother only), and (3) by interview. The observational procedures permitted the functional analysis of certain interactional patterns. Interaction sequences were identified which were initiated by either the parent or child and involved some demand upon the other person. The various responses were then coded in terms of the way in which the person attempted to gain compliance (for example, a parent might offer positive incentives or use arbitrary power) and whether the other person complied. It was determined whether the parent did or did not persist in his demand after an initial noncompliance from the child, or the extent to which the parent succumbed to the child's "nuisance value," that is, was coerced into complying by the child's whining, pleading, or crying.

The Structured Observation procedure involved two parts: (1) the mother teaching the child some simple mathematical concepts and (2) a free play period. This interaction was coded in a number of ways including compliance or noncompliance to demands as described above.

Results indicated a strong tendency for parents of Group I children (energetic-friendly) relative to both other groups to exert more control over their children and to be less affected by coercive demands based on whining and crying. This kind of control is not necessarily punitive, unduly restrictive, or intrusive. It seems to reflect the parent's ability to resist pressure from the child and a willingness to exert influence on the child.

Parents of Group I children also made more maturity demands in which information and reasons were given for the demands. They also more often explicitly retracted a demand on the basis of the child's arguments. Retracting a demand is different from succumbing to a child's nuisance value in that the parent explicitly indicates that the demand is being modified on the basis of a specific argument advanced by the child. In other words, parents of Group I children permitted and, to some extent, encouraged independent thought and action, but did not allow themselves to be coerced by noxious child behavior. Parents of Group I children were also more nurturant as indicated by a greater percentage of child-initiated sequences that resulted in satisfaction for the child, including those involving the child's request for support and attention. Greater nurturance was also indicated by the tendency for Group I parents to use more positive reinforcement and less punishment than other parents.

In summary, Group I parents, relative to Group II and III parents, provided high nurturance with high control, high demands with clear communication about what was required, and a willingness to listen and occasionally be influenced by the child's point of view.

Groups II (conflicted-irritable) and III (impulsive-aggressive) differed from each other in that parents of Group III were less persistent in the face of child opposition to enforce demands, and succumbed more to child nuisance value. Group III parents also provided fewer maturity demands, and tended to be more nurturant (difference not statistically significant) than Group II parents. A father interview measure indicated greater use of corporal punishment by Group II than Group III fathers, further suggesting lower nurturance as well as greater punitiveness in Group II. The children in Group II would seem to show neuroticlike conflict over the expression of aggression, which would be consistent with the combination of aggression-producing and aggression-inhibiting factors present in the parent behavior.

The children in this study were not selected from clinical populations, but it would seem reasonable to hypothesize that the Group II (conflicted-irritable) children represent a high risk group for more severe personality disturbance at a later time. The operationalized measures of parent-child interaction make it possible to know with some certainty what is involved in the measures labeled control and maturity demands, and it turns out that the parents of children with the most neuroticlike behavior (Group II) exert *less* control and make *fewer* maturity demands than parents of the less maladjusted children (Group I). This finding is opposite to what might have been predicted from the previously reviewed research. On the other hand, the parents of the Group II (conflicted-irritable) children did exert more control and make more maturity demands than did parents of Group III (impulsive-aggressive) children—a finding quite consistent with the earlier studies. If Baumrind had not included the energetic-friendly children, we might have taken this study as another demonstration that parents of neurotic-inhibited children are overcontrolling. As it is, we must conclude that the parents of these possibly preneurotic children show a combination of lower than normal control with very low nurturance. They are also unable to listen to the child and occasionally be influenced by his arguments.

There have been other studies in recent years that compared direct measures of family interaction of normal families with families in which a child was showing some kind of psychological disturbance. Ferreira and Winter (1968) (mentioned briefly before with respect to interparent conflict) asked family triads (mother, father, and child) to reach agreement on a series of seven hypothetical questions such as a country to visit for a year, the meal to choose at a restaurant, etc. These same items had been answered previously by the individual family members, but they were not told what the other persons' preferences had been at the time of the three-way interaction. This procedure might be referred to as the Unrevealed Differences Test in contrast to the Revealed Differences Test described in the methodological section at the beginning of this chapter.

The authors found that the normal families had significantly higher rates of "spontaneous agreement" (agreement on preferences made independently prior to meeting as a group) than did all other groups. Normal families also exchanged more information, took less overall time to reach decisions, and spent proportionately less time in silence than did all other groups. These characteristics held for each family member as well as for the family as a whole. The longer decision times for the deviant families also held up when levels of initial "spontaneous agreement" were partialled out by analysis of covariance. The authors suggest that the inability to exchange appropriate information and resolve differences in a reasonable period of time results from and further contributes to family pathology. The initially low scores on "spontaneous agreement" may reflect, in part, an end result of having insufficient information about the preferences of other members.

Other investigators have also found that families with a deviant child perform problem-solving tasks less efficiently. Murrell and Stachowiak (1967) found that families seeking help at a clinic (child symptoms included poor school achievement, hyperactivity, nervousness, enuresis, etc.) were less productive on tasks such as writing as many adjectives as they could that would describe their family as a group, or in making up joint stories to TAT pictures. In this study, direct measures were obtained on family tetrads (father, mother, and two children). Similar inefficiency in resolving disagreements on a Revealed Differences Test was also obtained for families with a child who was considered to be in the beginning stages of a psychotic process (Schuham, 1970).

In both the Murrell and Stachowiak, and Schuham studies, it was also found that power or influence attempts were more evenly distributed among family members for the disturbed families than for the normal families—a finding that neither of the investigators had anticipated. They had expected a more "democratic" leveling of power in the normal families. As it turned out, the parents exerted more influence over the children in the normal families than in the disturbed families. The authors suggested, post hoc, that some degree of accepted parental leadership facilitated more efficient problem solving. As was pointed out previously, findings have been inconsistent with respect to parent dominance in normal families, and one should accept the above findings with caution. Relevant to this point is the fact that although Murrell and Stachowiak (1967) and Schuham (1970) both report greater *parental* dominance over the children in normal families, mothers were more dominant in the former study and fathers in the latter study.

There is a question as to the ultimate value of the highly structured procedures of the type used in the above studies for the understanding of the family contribution to psychopathology. These particular studies do suggest that there is some breakdown or inefficiency in family communication and decision-making processes. On the other hand, they do not tell us much about how the current family interaction is maintaining a particular kind of child disorder or how it contributed to the past development of the disorder. It may be necessary to move away from these structured "reach-an-agreement" type of tasks to some combination of naturalistic home observations or semi-structured tasks that elicit behavior more directly relevant to the child's symptom, and to analyses of discrete interaction sequences as attempted by Baumrind (1967).

Anxiety Reactions. Anxiety, although present to some extent, was not the primary criterion used to designate children as neurotic in most of the studies reviewed above. In an early study, Langford (1937) found that definite traumatic experiences had preceded the first attack in 16 out of 20 children suffering from acute anxiety symptoms. Such a finding would seem to deemphasize the role of family interaction dynamics. Thus, in 6 of the children, the first anxiety attack followed within a month or two after tonsillectomies given under ether anesthetic; in another 6 children there had been either a death in the family or, in 2 cases, the witnessing of rather violent deaths in the neighborhood. On the other hand, Langford also reported that "they were, with one exception, all timid children who did not mix well with their playmates." If that were so, then the possibility remains that prior social learning experiences in the family, or hereditary characteristics made these children more vulnerable to the traumatic experiences. Without knowledge of base rates of traumatic experiences of this kind one does not know what proportion of children experience these trauma without developing anxiety reactions.

"School phobias" have been studied more intensively than perhaps any other specific type of neurotic disorder in children. Here again, we find many reports suggesting that an overprotective parent has contributed to the development of the phobic anxiety (Eisenberg, 1958; Waldfogel, 1957).

These authors conclude, rather convincingly, that in a high proportion of cases the children and their mothers (in a few cases, fathers) have developed a mutually dependent relationship, where separation is very disturbing to both. Starting to school simply represents the first time that sustained separation is demanded, although there are usually isolated incidents of previous intense anxiety or disturbance on the part of the child when mother has been away temporarily. School phobia is a misnomer in this case. The "phobic situation" might be better described as separation from mother.

Eisenberg (1958) studied 11 preschool children (6 boys and 5 girls) with such separation problems in a special nursery school for emotionally disturbed children. Direct observations were made of the mother and child behavior during the early phases of nursery school attendance. During the first days, a typical child would remain close to mother and then begin to oscillate toward and away from the attractions of the play area. As the child began to look less at mother and move away from her, she would take a seat closer to the child and occasionally use a pretext of wiping his nose or checking his toilet needs for intruding into the child's activity. Separation was as difficult for mother as for the child. Similar resistance to separation was shown by the mother when she was required to move to an adjacent room as part of the program for reducing the mutual separation anxiety.

Interviews with the mothers indicated that in most cases, the child as an infant had been treated with apprehensive oversolicitude. They were not trusted to babysitters outside the immediate family and later were constantly warned of hazards if they ventured away from home. The circumstances in the mother's life that led to this behavior with her child were varied. For example, the child may have been a late arrival after many sterile years, the child may have been seen in terms of the mother's own unhappy childhood with the result that she wished to protect the child from similar experiences, or a frustrated marriage relationship may have caused the mother to turn to her child for a "secure" relationship. In some cases, mothers were also seen as experiencing angry feelings toward the child, displaced, perhaps, from an unhappy marriage or paradoxically from being tied down so much by the child. The occasional awareness of this anger, or its impulsive expression toward the child, would lead to compensatory protectiveness and greater tightening of the symbiotic bond.

Some questions remain about how these separation fears developed; for example, how did the fear response become associated with separation? It is possible that some fear-arousing incident occurred in association with mother's leaving that would account for the initial fear-separation association.

It would seem more likely in the case of Eisenberg's children that the early development of the mother-child symbiotic relationship preceded the fear development.

We might speculate that shortly after birth the mother began the over-protective regime that fostered an unusually close attachment and dependency on her. This overprotective behavior on mother's part might have any of several sources: irrational fear for the child's safety, substitution of the child relationship for an unsatisfactory marriage, etc. For purposes of this analysis, it does not matter what motivates the mother We only assume that the in-dependent or separative tendencies on the part of the child are aversive to the mother and, consequently, any reduction of such tendencies is reinforc-ing to her. Under such a regime the child is increasingly likely to turn to mother for help and as a source of "positive affect" to reduce all sources of "negative affect" such as bodily hurts, illnesses, teasing by other children, etc. The child eventually learns to coerce mother into providing "mothering" at the onset of any disturbing situation by emitting the first signs of distress —a whimper, a few tears, a yell.

An important result of such a system is that the child may not learn to master new fear experiences successfully. Both humans and animals can be observed to master mild to moderate fear in new situations by approaching and withdrawing repeatedly from the feared situation. The repeated arousal of the fear response in small, controlled doses in this way leads eventually to extinction of the fear response. The overprotected child is not allowed to learn the skills involved in mastering new fears in this way, and is in danger of being overwhelmed at some future time by an unavoidable fear-arousing situation. The high prevalence of transitory fears in normal children (Jersild & Holmes, 1935) suggests that no special circumstances have to be hypothe-sized to account for some degree of initial fearfulness. The important factor is whether the child is able to master the fears that would seem to be in-evitably present. Jersild and Holmes, for example, obtained information from parents about how they handled their children's fears. According to these parent reports, reassurance, ridicule, forcing the child to confront the fearful situation, and ignoring the child's fears were all relatively ineffective in removing the fear. Those parents, however, who had with some patience introduced the child to the feared object in small steps reported considerable success.

Thus, an abrupt separation of mother from an overprotected child, especially in a new situation, might well lead to an emotional reaction in the child with a strong fear component. No additional fear-evoking circumstances would have to be present. Once a fear reaction of high intensity had occurred, it could, by classical conditioning, become more strongly associated with the circumstances of separation. If the fear were also reduced by mother's return, then clinging to mother as a response to fear would also be reinforced. Overt manifestations of fear on the child's part would likely become discriminative stimuli for mother's protective behavior. In addition to the factors involved in the above formulation, mother may also further strengthen the separation-fear association by verbal means; for example, by frequent warnings about the various dangers that lie in wait away from mother.

Although the above formulation may seem reasonable, it should be emphasized that it is based on rather indirect sources of data. Formulations of this kind can be made to appear simple and elegant as long as one does not ask for their confirmation by direct measures of the relevant behavior. Then frequently the whole business turns out to be more complicated than the theory implies. For example, careful description of the child's response to separation might reveal that, in some cases, the child is not responding with fear at all but with temper-tantrumlike behavior including crying and other signs of distress. The absence of strong fear would suggest some differences in the past reinforcement contingencies leading to the disorder and also some differences in treatment strategies. It is more likely, for example, that tantrum-like behavior would be learned primarily as an instrumental response aimed at coercing certain kinds of parent behavior, rather than as a classically conditioned emotional response.

Depression-withdrawal.   Depressive reactions are relatively rare in childhood, or at least depressed children do not come to the attention of clinics as frequently as other types of child disorders. A common view is that a major precipitant of depressive reactions is a loss of some kind, usually involving the physical or psychological withdrawal of another person. This loss may be conceptualized in terms of object relations and "narcissistic supplies," as within psychoanalytic theory, or as a relative reduction in available reinforcements from a learning theory viewpoint.

One obvious form that such a loss can take is prolonged physical separation of the child from his parents. Yarrow (1964) provides a good summary of the substantial literature on the effects of such separation during early childhood. For example, Bowlby (1960), Freud and Burlingham (1942), and Heinicke (1956) describe grief reactions as they occurred in normal children age 1–3 years, when separated from their parents because of wartime evacuation of London or extended periods of hospitalization. First there is a period of "protest" during which the child cries a great deal, asks for parents if he can talk, shows a restless hyperactivity, and is easily angered. After about a week some children decrease their overt protests and manifest what has variously been called despair, depression, or withdrawal. They become unresponsive and lose interest in the environment. The facial muscles sag and the face presents the generally accepted features of sadness and dejection. Loud wailing and crying may be replaced with low-intensity whimpering or sobbing. Most children of this age are likely to recover after several weeks from this depression-withdrawal phase and return to a normal interest and responsiveness in their environment.

In studies such as these, the effects of separation from parents are confounded with the effects of living in an institutional setting. Spitz (1946) reported a study in which a constant environment was maintained for the infants except for the temporary withdrawal of the mother. Infants of unwed mothers were kept in a nursery and their mothers were encouraged to spend considerable time with them. From a sample of 123 infants observed during the first year of life, 19 were reported to have developed a clear-cut syndrome of depression-withdrawal. This reaction occurred only in infants whose mothers had to be away from them for about three months when the infants were about 6–10 months of age, but apparently did not occur in all such infants. The reaction began about 4–6 weeks after the mother left, and the availability of a substitute mother did not help much in most cases. The infants were reported to have returned to normalcy when their mothers returned. There are major methodological shortcomings in Spitz's study in terms of research design and reporting of procedures, but viewed as a report on clinical observations, it continues to be quite suggestive.

In a more carefully conducted study, Engel, Reichsman, and Segal (1956) report systematic observations of behavioral and physiological reactions in an infant girl who showed depressive reactions similar to the depression described by Spitz. The infant, Monica, was born with a congenital atresia of the esophagus which necessitated an operation a few days after birth to establish a gastric fistula, an opening into the stomach by which the infant could receive food. Subsequently, she developed a depressive reaction that may have been related to her mother's avoidance of a normal affectional relationship with her. During hospitalization this depressive reaction could be "experimentally" produced by having a stranger enter the room and approach her.

There have been many anecdotal reports of grief reactions in animals following separation from a mate, child, parent, or human master. Nonhuman primates, especially, show a sequence of grief reactions remarkably similar to those seen in humans. Fortunately, in recent years, there have been experimental studies with monkeys to supplement the anecdotal reports (Hinde, Spencer-Booth, & Bruce, 1966; Kaufman & Rosenblum, 1967; Seay & Harlow, 1965). Kaufman and Rosenblum, for example, separated four pigtail monkeys at an average age of 5.6 lunar months from their mothers. Prior to separation, the infant monkeys were reared in a group composed of the feral mother, the sire, and an infantless adult female. During separation, which lasted for four weeks, the infants remained with their sire and the infantless adult female (avoiding the confounding of separation with being put in a strange environment).

The immediate response to separation was vigorous protest involving loud screams, agitated pacing and "searching," and a plaintive distress call referred to as cooing. This lasted for 24–36 hours during which the infant did not sleep.

After 24–36 hours, there was a marked change in three of the four monkeys. These monkeys became inactive, stopped responding to or making social gestures, and ceased play behavior. They frequently sat hunched over, almost in a ball with head between their legs. The facial muscles sagged and they presented the classical facial configuration of human dejection. They occasionally emitted the plaintive cooing sound. Two of the monkeys developed autoerotic activity in the form of penis sucking—a reaction not seen in this monkey colony before except in one case of unplanned separation from the mother.

This depression-withdrawal phase lasted about five to six days after which they gradually began to recover. The posture became more upright, exploration of the inanimate environment began and a gradual increase in contacts with other monkeys occurred. For a while, there were periods of depression that alternated with periods of exploration and play. By the end of the month of separation, the infants had almost returned to normal.

Separation resulting from parent death or divorce might also be expected to produce child disturbances with depression-withdrawal features. Retrospective research does suggest that adult depression is more frequently associated with loss of a parent during childhood than are other psychiatric symptoms. Beck (1967), Brown (1966), Denneby (1966), Earle and Earle (1961), Gay and Tonge (1967), Hill and Price (1967), and Munro (1966) found such a relationship. On the other hand, Pitts, Meyer, Brooks, & Winokur (1965) and Gregory (1966) did not find such an association. The death of a parent per se is probably less important than the general character of the family interaction prior to and subsequent to the death. For example, Hilgard, Newman, and Fisk (1960), in a retrospective study of adults whose fathers had died when they were children, found that the currently well-adjusted adults came from homes that had provided close affectional relationships prior to the father's death.

In summary, prolonged physical separation of a young child from his parent or parents is likely to produce protest followed by a depression-withdrawal reaction. The degree of recovery from this reaction may well depend on the availability of alternative sources of "mothering" or reinforcement (attention, stimulation, affection, etc.). These researches, as well as clinical experience, suggest the possibility that less obvious ways in which parents might withhold expected sources of reinforcement would also instigate depressive-withdrawal reactions in children or predispose them to symptoms of this kind as adults. Coleman and Provence (1957), for example, report features of depression-withdrawal in children living in intact families which provide very little attention, stimulation, and affection.

Low self-esteem, characterized by attitudes of self-worthlessness and self-criticism, is commonly associated with depressive reactions and more generally with neurotic reactions of all kinds Self-criticism responses might be learned in the family context by direct reinforcement, by the association of such responses with punishment termination (Aronfreed, 1964), or by modeling from a parent with low self-esteem. The major empirical research that focuses on family interaction correlates of self-esteem is that of Coopersmith (1967). Boys, ages 10–12, were selected to represent high and low self-esteem groups on the basis of self-report and teacher ratings. Parent variables were largely limited to mother self-reports derived from an interview and a questionnaire. High self-esteem children were found to have higher IQ's, to be more well formed and physically coordinated, to come less often from broken homes, and to have a strong but nonsignificant tendency to come from higher socioeconomic backgrounds. These "reality" characteristics could easily increase expectations of success and probably influenced the author's measure of self-esteem. It is unfortunate that high and low self-esteem groups were not matched on these variables (or subsequent statistical control attempted by partialling out the effect of these variables) in order to study the unconfounded effects of child-rearing variables.

The child-rearing results are, nevertheless, of some interest because they parallel the results obtained by Baumrind (1967) on 3- to 4-year-old children described earlier. On the basis of mother interview ratings, Coopersmith found mothers of high self-esteem boys to have high self-esteem themselves, to be more satisfied with the father's child-rearing practices, to have less conflict with the father, to have higher rapport (a friendly, mutually satisfying relationship) with her son, to demand higher standards of performance, to enforce rules and demands with consistency and firmness, to use reasoning and discussion instead of arbitrary, punitive discipline, and to use more rewards and less punishment in training the child. Baumrind found most of these characteristics to be associated with parents of her energetic-friendly group and the opposite to be true for parents of the conflicted-irritable group.

Hysterical reactions.   Cases of childhood hysteria (both conversion and dissociative reactions) do occur, but not with particularly high frequency. There are no studies that come close to representing a research comparison of family interaction measures in families with a hysterical child disorder and similar measures in other types of families. Clinical reports and individual case studies (for example, Carter, 1937; Proctor, 1958; Schuler & Parenton,

1943) suggest the importance of emotionally stressing circumstances, modeling of certain features of the hysterical symptom by other people, and a generally naive denial by the family or community of the sexual or aggressive meanings inherent in certain situations.

Proctor's study is especially interesting in pointing to cultural influences that include, but go beyond, the immediate family. He found that 13% of 191 children seen consecutively at the University of North Carolina Medical School Psychiatric Unit were diagnosed hysterical. This was a much higher incidence rate than seemed to exist in other parts of the country at that time. Proctor indicated that the largely rural areas from which these children came were characterized by low economic and educational levels with a strong element of dour, pleasure-inhibiting fundamentalist religion that emphasized the sinful nature of smoking, drinking, and sex. But at the same time, children were likely to experience inconsistency with these verbal preachments through the behavior of parents and other adults. For example, they might witness parent sexual intercourse or sleep with the opposite sex parent to an advanced age. The combination of overstimulation with strong verbally induced inhibitions and the lack of psychological sophistication probably contributed to the higher incidence of hysteria.

Psychosomatic Disorders

Although children show most of the psychosomatic disorders that occur in adults, research relevant to family interaction factors exists primarily for asthma and to only a limited extent for other disorders. Accordingly, this section will be devoted largely to the asthma research.

First, however, we shall consider a study by Garner and Wenar (1959), which assessed mother-child interaction for a group of children suffering from a variety of psychosomatic disorders—bronchial asthma, rheumatoid arthritis, ulcerative colitis, peptic ulcer, and atopic eczema. In the psychosomatic group 21 mother-child pairs were compared with matched groups of 21 mother-child pairs in a neurotic group (for example, phobias, learning blocks, minor delinquencies, night terrors, hyperactivity) and 20 mother-child pairs in a nonpsychosomatic illness group (for example, chronic illnesses, such as polio, congenital cardiac disease, nephrosis, hemophilia). Ratings of mother-child interaction were obtained from four procedures: (1) a semistructured interview with mother, (2) stories told by mother to pictures portraying children and adults, (3) direct observation of a 10-minute sample of mother-child interaction in a free-play situation, and (4) stories told by children to pictures of mothers and children.

Results from all four data sources yielded a fairly consistent picture. Following our own methodological preference, the findings from the direct observation procedure can be summarized as follows: Mother-child interaction for the psychosomatic group was rated basically negative in character. There was little positive closeness, mothers obtained high ratings on irritability and anger, and the child was also rated high on anger. The mothers tended to compete with the child and dominate the child. The child in turn was seen as victimized by the mother. The flavor of mutual entanglement is described in the following quotation, "The mother cannot relinquish the techniques of competition and domination which keep her continually reacting to the child, nor can the child find relief in independent or encapsulated task-oriented activity" (p. 72).

In the neurotic group, the general atmosphere was also negative and uncomfortable. Mothers and, to a lesser degree, the children were irritable and angry. The mothers of neurotic children differed from mothers of psychosomatic children in showing much less competition and victimization. Instead, mother and child avoided intense or intimate interaction, maintaining a certain distance and independence from each other: "She [the mother] seems to welcome and even foster a certain degree of remoteness in the situation; from many of the mothers of neurotic children, the magazines on the chair in the far corner were an obvious refuge from an otherwise unpleasantly close association with their offspring" (p. 74).

The mother-child interaction for the nonpsychosomatic illness group was rated as generally more positive than for either of the other groups. There was a relative absence of anger and irritability. Although there was almost as much independence and lack of intense interpersonal interactions in the nonpsychosomatic group as for the neurotic group, in the nonpsychosomatic group this relatively independent behavior occurred in a friendly, relaxed atmosphere instead of in the negative-irritable atmosphere of the neurotic group.

In a subsequent study, Wenar, Handlon, and Garner (1960) used the same procedures to compare a group of psychosomatic children (apparently the same group used in the previous study) with a group of severely disturbed children. The psychopathology in the disturbed group was considerably more severe than was the case for the neurotic group in the previous study, although few of the children would be considered classically autistic or schizophrenic. In the direct observation procedure, the severely disturbed group showed the same highly negative features and lack of positive closeness as the psychosomatic and neurotic groups. The child showed a marked degree of encapsulation and few signs of irritability with mother. The mother was rated very high on obliviousness, in being impervious to the effects of her behavior on the child, or to the ideas and feelings the child was trying to communicate. This quality of insensitivity to the child was much higher in this group than in the psychosomatic group.

These studies, then, certainly suggest that something is going on in the mother-child interaction that plays a role in the development of the psychosomatic disorder in the child. The mutual entanglement, domination, and victimization would seem to be the features especially related to the psychosomatic mothers. The use of heterogeneous groupings of children and global ratings makes it difficult to draw more than this rather general conclusion. It is relevant to note that a higher proportion of both psychosomatic and neurotic mothers report some special stresses during the first year of their child's life (for example, having to work full time to make ends meet, husband away during war, severe marital problems). Perhaps some combination of specific stress for mothers, a biological predisposition in the child, and the development of some variation on the mutual entanglement theme are the distinctive causative factors. The inclusion of a chronic illness group was a major achievement in this research, and it increases the confidence with which one can conclude that the mothers' reactions in the psychosomatic and neurotic groups are not just secondary responses to a chronically incapacitated child.

The relatively independent behavior of the neurotic children appears inconsistent with previous research suggesting an overly close relationship for children with certain phobic reactions, but this behavior is not necessarily inconsistent with Baumrind's (1967) findings for the conflicted-irritable group. The grouping of neurotic children, however, in the Wenar and Garner study included hyperactive, disobedient, aggressive, and delinquent (minor) children as well as phobic and anxious children. The grouping is probably too heterogeneous to permit any conclusions about family interaction characteristics associated with specific neurotic symptoms—especially since other research has indicated definite differences between the inhibited-fearful and the aggressive child.

Asthma

As noted in Chapter Four, an asthmatic attack is characterized by constriction of the bronchial ducts supplying air to the lungs. The individual experiences difficulty in breathing, particularly in exhaling, and manifests a wheezing sound. It is generally agreed that a number of factors can contribute to the development of the disorder. Rees (1964), for example, studied a sample of 388 asthmatic children, and concluded that the dominant cause was infectious (whooping cough, bronchitis, pneumonia, etc.) in 41.5% of the cases, allergic in 17% of the cases, and psychological (precipitated by emotional reactions) in 41.5% of the cases. Mixed causation was common and the above proportions reflect only the most prominent factor.

The common observation that emotionally arousing experiences can precipitate asthma attacks in many individuals undoubtedly gave impetus to the idea that asthma is a psychosomatic disorder. French and Alexander (1941), within the context of psychoanalytic theory, proposed that the asthmatic attack had its childhood origins in a suppressed cry for help associated with real or imagined estrangement from mother. In later life the attack would be precipitated by similar occasions or fantasies of estrangement. Gerard (1946) reported that some asthma patients experience relief from their asthmatic symptoms after being able to express their grief in uninhibited crying.

Many clinical reports have emphasized an overly close relationship between mother and child—the overprotective mother and excessively dependent child syndrome (Gerard, 1946; Long, Lamont, Whipple, Bandler, Blom, Burgin, & Jessner, 1958; Mohr, Tausend, Selesnick, & Augenbraun, 1963). Rees (1964) used global ratings based on interviews to compare attitudes of mothers of 170 asthmatic children with mothers of 160 control children. Of the mothers of the asthmatic children, 44.5% were rated as overprotective compared with 14% of the control mothers. Rees also attempted to determine whether the overprotective tendencies (for this subsample of 44.5% of the mothers) were present in the mother *prior* to the onset of asthma. This determination was made, however, on the basis of retrospective information given by the mother after the asthma had begun. Rees concluded that in 75% of these cases the mother had been overprotective before onset of the asthma. This conclusion was based on evidence suggesting that 22% of these mothers were chronically neurotic before the asthma began, 12% had been experiencing marital difficulties, and 41% had experiences such as pregnancy or birth difficulties, loss of previous children, or feeding difficulties that would instigate overconcern for the child. Rees also reported that when allergic factors were considered to be the dominant causative factor, 41% of the mothers were rated as having an unsatisfactory (primarily overprotective in nature) relation with their child; when infectious factors were dominant, 73% had an unsatisfactory relationship, and when psychological factors (asthma precipitated by emotional reactions) were dominant, 80% had an unsatisfactory relationship. There was no indication that raters were not aware of the asthma or control-group status of the mothers, or the dominant causative factors assessed for the children in this study. Nevertheless, the study strongly suggests that a disturbed mother-child interaction plays a significant role in the causation of *some* cases of asthma.

Another line of research that implicates family interaction as a contributing factor in asthma is the repeated finding that removal of the child from the home and placement in a hospital often results in immediate and dramatic improvement for *some* children (Long et al., 1958; Purcell, 1963; Purcell, Bernstein, & Bukantz, 1961; Purcell, Turnbull, & Bernstein, 1962; Peshkin, 1963). It is, of course, possible that removal of the child from the home involves removal from allergens such as house dust, animals, feathers, etc. as well as from the family. In the Long et al. study, a number of children placed in a hospital experienced almost immediate relief from asthma symptoms. The hospital rooms of these children were then sprayed with house dust taken from their respective homes, and none of the children developed asthmatic symptoms. Fourteen of the 18 children had previously shown skin sensitivity to house dust. Of course, other allergens may have been responsible for the asthma at home, but again the results are strongly suggestive of familial causes.

Relevant to the question of family etiology are studies which indicate that psychological and familial factors are more highly associated with children who show rapid remission of symptom when hospitalized. Rapid remission includes the capacity to remain symptom-free after drugs (usually steroids) are withdrawn. The nonrapidly remitting children are frequently referred to as steroid dependent. Purcell (1963) reported that 15 of 20 rapidly remitting children considered such emotions as anger and worry to be factors in precipitating asthma attacks, whereas only 6 of 18 steroid-dependent children reported similar emotional precipitants. Purcell et al. (1961) compared 54 rapidly remitting children with 59 steroid-dependent children. They found more neurotic type symptomatology in the rapid-remitters, and also found that mothers of rapid-remitters scored higher on scales of authoritarian-controlling and hostile-rejecting on the Parent Attitude Research Instrument than mothers of steroid dependents.

Block, Jennings, Harvey, & Simpson, (1964) in a methodologically improved study, followed up Rees' (1964) finding that psychological factors seemed to play a less important role when allergic predisposition was high. Children were divided into those for whom allergic predisposition seemed to play an important part and those for whom such predisposition seemed minimal. The Allergic Potential Scale, on which this discrimination was made, consists of five subscales: (1) family history of allergic reactions, (2) blood eosinophile counts, (3) skin test reactivity, (4) total number of allergies, and (5) ease of diagnosis of specific allergens. The 35 children who scored above the mean on this scale were similar in age, race, intelligence, socioeconomic level, severity of asthma, and age of onset of asthma to the 27 children scoring below the mean.

More severe indications of neuroticlike symptomatology were reported for the low (on the Allergic Potential Scale) children by both parents on Q-sort descriptions than for high children. Thus, mothers described children with low allergic predisposition as significantly more rebellious, clinging, intelligent, jealous, nervous and whiny. Mothers described children with high allergic predisposition as significantly more self-confident, reasonable, and masculine (or feminine as the case may be). Father ratings and child productions on a TAT and in a doll-play situation yielded similar results. Raters did Q-sorts of mother characteristics based on an interview and psychological tests (Rorschach, TAT, and MMPI). A sampling of items that significantly discriminated mothers of high and low children is as follows: High mothers were rated more frequently as being socially poised, assertive, candid, cheerful, and directly expressive of hostility. Low mothers were rated more frequently as having a lack of personal meaning in life, being vulnerable to real or fancied threats, generally fearful, self-defeating, giving up and withdrawing in the face of frustration, brittle ego-defenses, and feeling victimized by life.

Raters directly observed a sample of mother-child interaction and did Q-sort descriptions of the interaction. Mothers of highs were rated more frequently as responsive to child, cautioning child, defending child, wanting child to make decisions, and more comfortable and at ease. Mothers of lows were described more frequently as competitive and condescending, disappointed in the child's performance, angry with child, rejecting, and expecting obedience.

Marital interaction assessed by interviews of mothers indicated that low mothers experienced more friction with husband, excluded husband from the mother-child relation, and were domineering and depreciating toward the husband. Q-sort ratings based on direct observation of husband-wife interaction indicated that low wives were more demanding and belittling of self, and high wives showed more pride in their husbands. Low husbands tried to embarrass and belittle wife, and high husbands showed more pride in their wives, and were more cooperative and considerate.

The general findings of the Block et al. study are strongly reminiscent of the findings in the Wenar, Handlon, and Garner (1960) study in which children with a variety of psychosomatic complaints were grouped together. Dubo, McLean, Ching, Wright, Kaufman, & Sheldon (1961) did not find a relationship between family variables assessed by interview and severity or age of onset of the child's asthma. This finding is not necessarily inconsistent with those of Rees (1964), Purcell (1963), and Block et al. (1964) in that these latter authors generally found that severity and age of onset of asthma were not related to the remitter-nonremitter on allergic predisposition variables.

Purcell, Brady, Chai, Muser, Molk, Gordon, & Means (1969) have recently reported an excellent study showing that family interaction variables strongly contribute to asthma in children whose attacks are frequently precipitated by emotional reactions. Parents of 60 asthmatic children were interviewed with respect to the frequency of asthmatic attacks and whether emotional reactions were important in instigating attacks. The selection procedure resulted in 13 families in which emotional factors were important and 12 families in which they were not important. These families then participated in an experiment involving five two-week periods: (1) qualification (no mention made of separation), (2) preseparation, (3) separation, (4) reunion, and (5) a postreunion follow-up for most subjects. During separation, the entire family, except for the asthmatic child, moved out of the home, and lived in a motel. A substitute mother was provided to live with the child. No contacts were permitted between the parents and child during this period. Various measures of asthma were obtained during all these periods: (1) expiratory peak flow rate, measuring how rapidly the child could expel air, was obtained 4 times a day, (2) ratings of degree of wheezing was made once a day at the institute, (3) amount of daily medication as reported by the adult (mother or mother substitute), and (4) daily record of frequency and intensity of asthma attacks as reported by the adult.

Results showed a dramatic drop on *all* of these measures of asthma during the separation period for the group of children for whom the emotional factors played an important role. There were no differences between the qualification and preseparation periods—a difference that might have been expected if the child's *anticipation* of separation from parents was a contributing factor. For the group of children in which emotional factors were considered unimportant, only one variable, adult reported frequency of attacks, was significantly affected by separation. Unfortunately, the authors did not report direct statistical comparisons between the two groups. However, the most objective measure used, expiratory peak flow rate, showed an increase significant at $p < .001$ for the emotional factor group and a nonsignificant *decrease* for the other group.

The authors plan to describe additional findings related to parent and child reactions to anticipated and actual separation in a later publication, and reported only anecdotal findings at this time. However, one of these qualitative reports is of considerable interest. Strong emotional reactions were precipitated in many mothers by the separation. Several had frank anxiety reactions. One mother crawled onto the roof of her house to peek through a window to see her boy without his knowledge. Another mother alternated between critical attack on the mother substitute and self-condemnation with suicidal ideation. The authors further suggest that it is the presence of specific emotional reactions in the child that are important, not general personality traits or styles of interpersonal interaction.

A theme that occurs many times in speculations about the childhood origins of psychopathology is the symbiotic mother-child relationship—the overprotective mother and excessively dependent child. Not only has this type of relationship been given etiological significance for asthma and other psychosomatic disorders, but also for a number of other disorders such as school phobia (separation anxiety), childhood psychosis (Mahler, 1955), and homosexuality (Bieber, Dain, Dince, Drellich, Grand, Gundlach, Kremer, Rifkin, Wilbur, & Bieber, 1962; Evans, 1969). Obviously, a theory about etiology is of little use if it is used to explain the development of so diverse a group of disorders. We believe that future studies that use direct observation of relevant family interaction with appropriate manipulations of the situational context can provide the kind of data that will permit a more fine-grained analysis. The rather vague concept of a symbiotic mother-child relationship may then be resolved into qualitatively distinct patterns as well as quantitative degrees of intensity.

Summary

This chapter has focused on familial correlates of psychopathology in children. The artificiality of separating social learning experiences in the family from extrafamilial social factors, specific traumatic experiences, and hereditary or constitutional factors must be emphasized. Although any one of these factors may initiate a developmental process, unidirectional causality quickly gives way to an interactive process between the child and other family members.

Deficiencies and variations in methodology do not permit broad generalizations across the many studies dealing with these problems. Recent methodological refinements such as greater use of multiple procedures to assess family interaction, concern with convergent validity of measures, greater use of observational and fewer self-report procedures, and assessment of actual sequences of behavior and response contingencies within family interaction sessions offer hope of clarifying the many problems that still remain in this area.

References

Ackerson, L. *Children's behavior problems.* Chicago: The University of Chicago Press, 1942.

Alkire, A. Social power and communication within families of disturbed and non-disturbed preadolescents. *Journal of Personality and Social Psychology,* 1969, **13**, 335–349.

Andry, R. G. *Delinquency and parental pathology.* London: Methuen, 1960.

Aronfreed, J. The origin of self-criticism. *Psychological Review,* 1964, **71**, 193–218.

Aronfreed, J. The concept of internalization. In D. Goslin (Ed.), *Socialization theory and research.* New York: Rand McNally, 1969, 263–324.

Bacon, H. K., Child, I. L., & Barry, H. A. A cross-cultural study of correlates of crime. *Journal of Abnormal and Social Psychology,* 1963, **66**, 291–300.

Bandura, A., & Walters, R. H. *Adolescent aggression.* New York: Ronald, 1959.

Bandura, A., & Walters, R. H. *Social learning and personality development.* New York: Holt, Rinehart and Winston, Inc., 1963.

Baruch, D. W., & Wilcox, J. A. A study of sex differences in pre-school children's adjustment coexistent with interparental tensions. *Journal of Genetic Psychology,* 1944, **64**, 281–303.

Baumrind, D. Child care practices anteceding three patterns of pre-school behavior. *Genetic Psychology Monographs,* 1967, **75**, 43–88.

Beck, A. T. *Depression.* New York: Harper and Row, 1967.

Becker, J., & Iwakami, E. Conflict and dominance within families of disturbed children. *Journal of Abnormal Psychology,* 1969, **74**, 330–335.

Becker, W. C. The relationship of factors in parental ratings of self and each other to the behavior of kindergarten children as rated by mothers, fathers, and teachers. *Journal of Consulting Psychology,* 1960, **24**, 507–527.

Becker, W. C. Consequences of different kinds of parental discipline. In M. L. Hoffman and L. W. Hoffman (Eds.), *Review of child development research.* New York: Russell Sage Foundation, 1964, **I**, 169–208.

Becker, W. C., & Krug, R. S. The parent attitude research instrument—a research review. *Child Development,* 1965, **36**, 329–365.

Becker, W. C., Peterson, D. R., Hellmer, L. A., Shoemaker, D. J., & Quay, H. C.

Factors in parental behavior and personality as related to problem behavior in children. *Journal of Consulting Psychology,* 1959, **23,** 107–118.

Becker W. C., Peterson, D. R., Luria, Z., Shoemaker, D. J., & Hellmer, L. A. Relations of factors derived from parent-interview ratings to behavior problems of five-year-olds. *Child Development,* 1962, **33,** 509–535.

Bell, R. Q. Structuring parent-child interaction situations for direct observation. *Child Development,* 1964, **35,** 1009–1020.

Bell, R. Q. A reinterpretation of the direction of effects in studies of socialization. *Psychological Review,* 1968, **75,** 81–95.

Bene, E. On the genesis of female homosexuality. *British Journal of Psychiatry,* 1965, **3,** 815–821.

Bennett, I. *Delinquent and neurotic children: A comparative study.* New York: Basic Books, Inc., 1960.

Berkowitz, L. *Aggression: A social psychological analysis.* New York: McGraw-Hill, 1962.

Bieber, I., Dain, H. J., Dince, P..R., Drellich, M. G., Grand, H. G., Gundlach, R. H., Kremer, M. W., Rifkin, A. H., Wilbur, C. B., & Bieber, T. B. *Homosexuality.* New York: Basic Books, Inc., 1962.

Biller, H. B. Father absence and the personality development of the male child. *Developmental Psychology,* 1970, **2,** 181–201.

Block, J., Jennings, P. H., Harvey, E., & Simpson, E. Interaction between allergic potential and psychopathology in childhood asthma. *Psychosomatic Medicine,* 1964, **26,** 307–320.

Bostow, D. E., & Bailey, J. B. Modification of severe disruptive and aggressive behavior using brief timeout and reinforcement procedures. *Journal of Applied Behavior Analysis,* 1969, **2,** 31–37.

Bowlby, J. Grief and mourning in infancy and early childhood. *Psychoanalytic Study of the Child,* 1960, **15,** 9–52.

Bowlby, J., Ainsworth, M., Boston, M., & Rosenbluth, D. The effects of mother-child separation: A follow-up study. *British Journal of Medical Psychology,* 1956, Vol. 29.

Boyle, R. H., Dykman, R. A., & Ackerman, P. T. Relationship of resting autonomic activity, motor impulsivity, and EEG tracings in children. *Archives of General Psychiatry,* 1965, **12,** 314–323.

Bronfenbrenner, U. Some familial antecedents of responsibility and leadership in adolescents. In L. Petrullo and B. M. Bass (Eds.), *Leadership and interpersonal behavior.* New York: Holt, 1961a.

Bronfenbrenner, U. Toward a theoretical model for the analysis of parent-child relationships in a social context. In J. C. Glidewell (Ed.), *Parental attitudes and child behavior.* Springfield, Ill.: Charles C Thomas, 1961b.

Bronson, Wanda. Stable patterns of behavior: The significance of enduring orientations for personality development. In John P. Hill (Ed.), *Minnesota Symposia on child psychology,* Vol. 2. University of Minnesota Press, Minneapolis, Minnesota, 1969, 3–27.

Brown, F. Childhood bereavement and subsequent psychiatric disorder. *British Journal of Psychiatry,* 1966, **112,** 1035–1041.

Buck, C. W., & Ladd, K. L. Psychoneurosis in marital partners. *British Journal of Psychiatry*, 1965, 111, 587–590.

Burt, C. *The young delinquent*. New York: Appleton, 1929.

Caldwell, B. The effects of infant care. In M. L. Hoffman and L. W. Hoffman (Eds.), *Review of child development research*, Vol. I, 1964, 9–87.

Carter, J. W. A case of reactional dissociation. *American Journal of Orthopsychiatry*, 1937, 7, 219–224.

Chess, S., Thomas, A., & Birch, H. G. Behavior problems revisited. In S. Chess and T. Birch (Eds.), *Annual progress in child psychiatry and child development*. New York: Brunner and Mazel, 1968, 335–344.

Chess, S., Thomas, A., Birch, H. G., & Hertzig, M. Implications of a longitudinal study of child development for child psychiatry. *American Journal of Psychiatry*, 1960, 117, 434–441.

Coleman, R. W., & Province, S. Environmental retardation (hospitalism) in infants living in families. *Pediatrics*, 1957, 19, 285–292.

Coopersmith, S. *The antecedents of self-esteem*. San Francisco: W. H. Freeman, 1967.

Cummings, S. T., Bayley, H. C., & Rie, H. E. The effects of the child's deficiency on the mother: A study of mothers of mentally retarded, chronically ill and neurotic children. *American Journal of Orthopsychiatry*, 1966, 36, 595–608.

Darling, R. P. Autonomic action in relation to personality traits in children. *Journal of Abnormal and Social Psychology*, 1940, 35, 246–260.

Denneby, C. M. Childhood bereavement and psychiatric illness. *British Journal of Psychiatry*, 1966, 112, 1049–1069.

Dennis, W. Infant development under conditions of restricted practice and of minimal social stimulation. *Genetic Psychology Monographs*, 1941, 23, 143–191.

Docter, R. F., Kaswan, J. W., & Nakamura, C. Y. Spontaneous heart rate and GSR changes as related to motor performance. *Psychophysiology*, 1964, 1, 73–78.

Dubo, S., McLean, J. A., Ching, A. Y. T., Wright, H. L., Kaufman, P. E., & Sheldon, J. M. A study of relationships between family situation, bronchial asthma, and personal adjustment in children. *Journal of Pediatrics*, 1961, 59, 402–414.

Earle, A. M., & Earle, B. V. Early maternal deprivation and later psychiatric illness. *American Journal of Orthopsychiatry*, 1961, 31, 181–186.

Eisenberg, L. School phobia: A study in the communication of anxiety. *American Journal of Psychiatry*, 1958, 114, 712–718.

Engel, G. L., Reichsman, F., & Segal, H. L. A study of an infant with a gastric fistula. *Psychosomatic Medicine*, 1956, 5, 374–398.

Eron, L. D. Psychosocial development of aggressive behavior. *USPHS Progress Report*, M-1726, Hudson, New York: Rip Van Winkle Foundation, May 15, 1961.

Eron, L. D., Banta, T. J., Waller, L. O., & Laulicht, J. H. Comparison of data obtained from mothers and fathers on childbearing practices and their relation to child aggression. *Child Development*, 1961, 32, 457–472.

Escalona, S., & Heider, G. M. *Prediction and outcome*. New York: Basic Books, 1959.

Evans, R. B. Childhood parental relationships of homosexual men. *Journal of Consulting and Clinical Psychology*, 1969, 33, 129–135.

Eysenck, S. B. G. An experimental study of psychogalvanic reflex responses of normal neurotic and psychotic subjects. *Journal of Psychosomatic Research*, 1956, **1**, 258–272.

Farina, A. Patterns of role dominance and conflict in parents of schizophrenic patients. *Journal of Abnormal and Social Psychology*, 1960, **61**, 31–38.

Ferreira, A. J., & Winter, W. D. Stability of interactional variables in family decision making. *Archives of General Psychiatry*, 1966, 352–355.

Ferreira, A. J., & Winter, W. D. Information exchange and silence in normal and abnormal families. *Family Process*, 1968, **7**, 251–276.

Fontana, S. F. Familial etiology of schizophrenia. *Psychological Bulletin*, 1966, **66**, 214–227.

Frank, G. H. The role of the family in the development of psychopathology. *Psychological Bulletin*, 1965, **64**, 191–205.

Freedman, D. G., & Keller, A. Inheritance of behavior in infants. *Science*, 1963, **140**, 196–198.

French, T., & Alexander, F. Psychogenic factors in bronchial asthma. *Psychosomatic Medicine Monograph*, 1941, No. 4.

Freud, A., & Burlingham, D. T. *War and children*. New York: Willard, 1943.

Garner, A. M., & Wenar, G. *The mother-child interaction in psychosomatic disorders*. Urbana: University of Illinois Press, 1959.

Gassner, S., & Murray, E. J. Dominance and conflict in the interactions between parents of normal and neurotic children. *Journal of Abnormal and Social Psychology*, 1969, **74**, 33–41.

Gay, M. J., & Tonge, W. L. The late effects of loss of parents in childhood. *British Journal of Psychiatry*, 1967, **113**, 753–759.

Gerard, M. W. Bronchial asthma in children. *Nervous Child*, 1946, **5**, 327–331.

Glueck, S., & Glueck, E. T. *Unraveling juvenile delinquency*. New York: Commonwealth Fund, 1950.

Glueck, S., & Glueck, E. T. Working mothers and delinquency. *Mental Hygiene*, 1957, **41**, 327–352.

Goddard, K. E., Broder, G., & Wenar, C. Special article—reliability of pediatric histories, a preliminary study. *Pediatrics*, 1961, **28**, No. 6.

Goldfarb, W. Psychological privation in infancy and subsequent adjustment. *American Journal of Orthopsychiatry*, 1945, **15**, 247–255.

Gottesman, I. Differential inheritance of the psychoneuroses. *Eugenics Quarterly*, 1962, **9**, 223–227.

Gottesman, I. Genetic variance in adaptive personality traits. *Journal of Child Psychology and Psychiatry*, 1966, **7**, 199–208.

Gregory, I. W. Retrospective data concerning childhood loss of a parent: II. Category of parental loss by decade of birth, diagnosis and MMPI. *Archives of General Psychiatry*, 1966, **15**, 362–367.

Grim, P. F., Kohlberg, L., & White, S. Some relationships between conscience and attentional processes. *Journal of Personality and Social Psychology*, 1968, 239–249.

Grinder, R. E. Parental child rearing practices, conscience and resistance to temptation of sixth-grade children. *Child Development*, 1962, **33**, 803–820.

Haggard, E. A., Brekstad, A., & Skard, A. G. On the reliability of the anamnestic interview. *Journal of Abnormal and Social Psychology*, 1960, **61**, 311–318.

Haley, J. Research on family patterns: An instrument measurement. *Family Process*, **3**, 1964, 141–165.

Hamburg, D. A., & Lunde, D. T. Sex hormones in the development of sex differences in human behavior. In E. Maccoby (Ed.), *The development of sex differences*. Stanford: Stanford University Press, 1966, 1–24.

Hatfield, J. S., Ferguson, L. R., & Alpert, R. Mother-child interaction and the socialization process. *Child Development*, 1967, **38**, 365–414.

Heinecke, C. M. Some antecedents and correlates of guilt and fear in young boys. Unpublished doctoral dissertation, Harvard University, 1953.

Heinecke, C. M. Some effects of separating two-year-old children from their parents: A comparative study. *Human Relations*, 1956, **9**, 105–176.

Helper, M. M. Parental evaluations of children and children's self-evaluations. *Journal of Abnormal and Social Psychology*, 1958, **56**, 190–194.

Hetherington, E. M., & Deur, J. Effects of father absence on the personality development of daughters. Unpublished manuscript, University of Wisconsin, 1970.

Hetherington, E. M., & Frankie, G. Effects of parental dominance, warmth and conflict on imitation in children. *Journal of Personality and Social Psychology*, 1965, **2**, 188–194.

Hetherington, E. M., Stouwie, R., & Ridberg, E. H. Patterns of family interaction and child rearing attitudes related to three dimensions of juvenile delinquency. Unpublished manuscript, University of Wisconsin, 1970.

Hewitt, L. E., & Jenkins, R. L. *Fundamental patterns of maladjustment: The dynamics of their origin*. Springfield, Ill.: Green, 1946.

Hilgard, J. R., Newman, M. F., & Fisk, F. Strength of adult ego following childhood bereavement. *American Journal of Orthopsychiatry*, 1960, **30**, 788–798.

Hill, O. W., & Price, J. S. Childhood bereavement and adult depression. *British Journal of Psychiatry*, 1967, **113**, 743–751.

Hinde, R. A., Spencer-Booth, Y., & Bruce, M. Effects of 6-day maternal deprivation on rhesus monkey infants. *Nature*. 1966, **210**, 1021–1023.

Hoffman, L. W. Effects on children: Summary and discussion. In F. I. Nye and Lois W. Hoffman (Eds.), *The employed mother in America*. Chicago: Rand McNally, 1963, 190–212.

Holz, W. C., Azrin, N. H., & Ayllon, T. Elimination of behavior of mental patients by response-produced extinction. *Journal of Experimental Analysis of Behavior*, 1963, **6**, 407–412.

Jenkins, R. L. Psychiatric syndromes in children and their relation to family background. *American Journal of Orthopsychiatry*, 1966, **36**, 450–457.

Jenkins, R. L. The varieties of children's behavioral problems and family dynamics. *American Journal of Psychiatry*, 1968, **124**, 1440–1445.

Jersild, A. T., & Holmes, F. B. Children's fears. *Child Development Monograph*, 1935, No. 20.

Jost, H., & Sontag, L. W. The genetic factor in autonomic nervous system function. *Psychosomatic Medicine*, 1944, **6**, 308–310.

Kagan, J. Socialization of aggression and the perception of parents in fantasy. *Child Development*, 1958, **29**, 311–320.

Kagan, J., & Moss, H. A. *Birth to maturity: A study in psychological development.* New York: Wiley, 1962.

Kagan, J., & Rosman, B. L. Cardiac and respiratory correlates of attention and an analytic attitude. *Journal of Experimental Child Psychology*, 1964, **1**, 50–63.

Kaufman, I. C., & Rosenblum, L. A. The reaction to separation in infant monkeys: Anaclitic depression and conservation-withdrawal. *Psychosomatic Medicine*, 1967, **29**, 648–675.

Kohn, M. L., & Carroll, E. E. Social class and the allocation of parental responsibilities. *Sociometry*, 1960, **23**, 372–392.

Kris, M. The use of prediction in a longitudinal study. *The Psychoanalytic Study of the Child*, 1957, **12**, 175–189. New York: International Universities Press.

Lacey, J. I. Individual differences in somatic response patterns. *Journal of Comparative and Physiological Psychology*, 1950, **43**, 338–350.

Lacey, J. I., & Lacey, B. The relationship of resting autonomic activity to motor impulsivity. In H. Solomon, S. Cobb, and W. Penfield (Eds.), *The brain and human behavior*. Baltimore: Williams and Wilkens, 1958, 144–209.

Lader, M. H., & Wing, L. Physiological measures, sedative drugs, and morbid anxiety. *Maudsley Monographs No. 14*, London: Oxford University Press, 1966.

Langford, W. Anxiety attacks in children. *American Journal of Orthopsychiatry*, 1937, **7**, 210–219.

Lapouse, R., & Monk, M. A. An epidemiologic study of behavior characteristics in children. *American Journal of Public Health*, 1958, **48**, 1134–1144.

Leonard, M. R. Fathers and daughters. *International Journal of Psychoanalysis*, 1966, **47**, 325–333.

Levitt, E. E. A comparison of parental and self-evaluations of psychopathology in children. *Journal of Clinical Psychology*, 1959, **15**, 402–404.

Levy, D. M. *Maternal overprotection.* New York: Columbia University Press, 1943.

Levy, P., & Lang, P. Activation, control, and the spiral after-movement. *Journal of Personality and Social Psychology*, 1966, **3**, 105–112.

Lewis, H. *Deprived children.* London: Oxford University Press, 1954.

Liverant, S. MMPI differences between parents of disturbed and nondisturbed children. *Journal of Consulting Psychology*, 1959, **23**, 256–260.

Long, R. T., Lamont, J. H., Whipple, B., Bandler, L., Blom, G. E., Burgin, L., & Jessner, L. A psychosomatic study of allergic and emotional factors in children with asthma. *American Journal of Psychiatry*, 1958, **114**, 890–899.

Lowry, L. G. Personality distortion and early institutional care. *American Journal of Orthopsychiatry*, 1940, **10**, 576–586.

MacFarlane, J. W. Studies in child guidance. I. Methodology of data collection and organization. *Monograph of the Society for Research in Child Development*, 1938, 3, No. 6.

MacFarlane, J. W., Allen, L., & Honzik, M. P. *A developmental study of the behavior problems of normal children between twenty-one months and fourteen years.* (University of California Publications in Child Development, Vol. II.) Berkeley: University of California Press, 1954.

Mahler, M. S. On childhood psychosis and schizophrenia: Autistic and symbiotic infantile psychosis. *Psychoanalytic study of the child,* Vol. X. New York: International University Press, 1955.

Martin, B., & Hetherington, E. M. Family interaction in withdrawn, aggressive and normal children. Unpublished manuscript, 1970.

McCord, J., & McCord, W. The effects of parental role model on criminality. *Journal of Social Issues,* 1958, **14,** 66–75.

McCord, J., & McCord, W. Cultural stereotypes and the validity of interviews for research in child development. *Child Development,* 1961, **32,** 171–185.

McCord, W., McCord, J., & Gudeman, J. *Origins of alcoholism.* Palo Alto: Stanford University Press, 1960.

McCord, W., McCord, J., & Howard, A. Familial correlates of aggression in non-delinquent male children. *Journal of Abnormal and Social Psychology,* 1961, **62,** 79–93.

McCord, W., McCord, J., & Thurber, E. Some effects of paternal absence on male children. *Journal of Abnormal and Social Psychology,* 1962, **64,** 361–369.

McCord, W., McCord, J., & Zola, I. K. *Origins of crime.* New York: Columbia University Press, 1959.

Merrill, M. A. *Problems of child delinquency.* Boston: Houghton Mifflin, 1947.

Mishler, E. G., & Waxler, N. E. *Interaction in families: An experimental study of family processes and schizophrenia.* New York: Wiley, 1968.

Mohr, G. J., Tausend, H., Selesnick, S., & Augenbraun, B. Studies of eczema and asthma in the preschool child. *Journal of American Academic Child Psychiatry,* 1963, **2,** 271–291.

Monahan, T. P. Family status and the delinquent child: A reappraisal and some new findings. *Social Forces,* 1957, **35,** 250–258.

Monahan, T. P. Broken homes by age of delinquent children. *Journal of Social Psychology,* 1960, **51,** 387–397.

Moss, H. A. Sex, age, and state as determinants of mother-infant interaction. *Merrill-Palmer Quarterly,* 1967, **13,** 19–36.

Moustakas, C. E., Sigel, I. E., & Schalock, H. D. An objective method for the measurement and analysis of child-adult interaction. *Child Development,* 1956, **27,** 109–134.

Munro, A. Parental deprivation in depressive patients. *British Journal of Psychiatry,* 1966, **112,** 443–457.

Murphy, L. B. *The widening world of childhood.* New York: Basic Books, 1962.

Murrell, S. A., & Stachowiak, J. G. Consistency, rigidity, and power in the interaction patterns of clinic and nonclinic families. *Journal of Abnormal and Social Psychology,* 1967, **72,** 265–272.

Neubauer, P. B. The one-parent child and his oedepal development. *Psychoanalytic Study of the Child,* 1960, **15,** 286–309.

Nye, F. I. The rejected parent and delinquency. *Marriage and Family Living,* 1956, **18,** 291–296.

Nye, F. I. *Family relationships and delinquent behavior.* New York: Wiley, 1958.

O'Connor, F. J. Aetiological factors in homosexuality as seen in RAF psychiatric practice. *British Journal of Psychiatry,* 1964, **110,** 381–391.

O'Rourke, J. F. Field and laboratory: The decision making behavior of family groups in two experimental conditions. *Sociometry*, 1963, 4.

Perry, D. G. Verbal interaction processes in families containing an aggressive withdrawn or normal boy. Unpublished Master's thesis. University of Wisconsin, 1970.

Peshkin, M. M. Diagnosis of asthma in children: past and present. In H. I. Schneer (Ed.), *The asthmatic child*. New York: Harper and Row, 1963.

Peterson, D. R., & Becker, W. C. Family interaction and delinquency. In H. C. Quay (Ed.), *Juvenile delinquency*. New York: Van Nostrand Co., 1965.

Pitts, Jr., F. N., Meyer, J., Brooks, M., & Winokur, G. Adult psychiatric illness assessed for childhood parental loss, and psychiatric illness in family members. A study of 748 patients and 250 controls. *American Journal of Psychiatry*, 1965, Supplement 121: i-x.

Pond, D., Ryle, A., & Hamilton, M. Marriage and neurosis in a working-class population. *British Journal of Psychiatry*, 1963, **109**, 592–598.

Proctor, J. T. Hysteria in childhood. *American Journal of Orthopsychiatry*, 1958, **28**, 394–406.

Purcell, K. Distinctions between subgroups of asthmatic children: Children's perceptions of events associated with asthma. *Pediatrics*, 1963, **31**, 486–494.

Purcell, K., Bernstein, L., & Bukantz, S. C. A preliminary comparison of rapidly remitting and persistently "steroid dependent" asthmatic children. *Psychosomatic Medicine*, 1961, **23**, 305–310.

Purcell, K., Turnbull, J. W., & Bernstein, L. Distinctions between subgroups of asthmatic children: Psychological test and behavior rating comparisons. *Journal of Psychosomatic Research*, 1962, **6**, 283–291.

Purcell, K., Brady, K., Chai, H., Muser, J., Molk, L., Gordon, N., & Means, J. The effect on asthma in children of experimental separation from the family. *Psychosomatic Medicine*, 1969, **31**, 144–164.

Quay, H. C., & Peterson, D. R. The questionnaire measurement of personality dimensions associated with juvenile delinquency. Unpublished manuscript, 1964.

Raush, H. Interaction sequences. *Journal of Personality and Social Psychology*, 1965, **2**, 487–499.

Read, K. H. Parents' expressed attitudes and children's behavior. *Journal of Consulting Psychology*, 1945, **9**, 95–100.

Rees, L. The importance of psychological, allergic and infective factors in childhood asthma. *Journal of Psychosomatic Research*, 1964, **7**, 253–262.

Reid, J. B. Reliability assessment of observation data: A possible methodological problem. *Child Development*, 1970, **41**, 1143–1150.

Richmond, J. B., & Lustman, S. L. Autonomic function in the neonate: Implications for psychosomatic theory. *Psychosomatic Medicine*, 1955, **17**, 269–275.

Robins, L. N. *Deviant children grown-up*. Baltimore: Williams and Wilkins Co., 1966.

Rohrbaugh, P. J. Family interaction patterns in families containing an aggressive withdrawn or sociable boy. Unpublished doctoral dissertation, University of Wisconsin, 1966.

Rosenthal, M. J., Finkelstein, M., Ni, E., & Robertson, R. E. A study of mother-child relationships in the emotional disorders of children. *Genetic Psychology Monographs*, 1959, **60**, 65–116.

Rosenthal, M. J., Ni, E., Finkelstein, M., & Berkwits, G. K. Father-child relationships and children's problems. *AMA Archives of General Psychiatry*, 1962, **7**, No. 5.

Satir, V. *Conjoint family therapy*. Palo Alto: Science and Behavior Books, 1964.

Scarr, S. The inheritance of sociability. Paper presented at American Psychological Association meeting in Chicago, September 5, 1965.

Schaefer, E. S. Converging conceptual models for maternal behavior and for child behavior. In J. C. Glidewell (Ed.), *Parental attitudes and child behavior*. Springfield, Ill.: Charles C Thomas, 1961.

Schaffer, H. R., & Emerson, P. E. The development of social attachments in infancy. *Monographs of the Society for Research in Child Development*, 1964, **29**, No. 3, (Serial 94) (a).

Schuham, A. I. Power relations in emotionally disturbed and normal family triads. *Journal of Abnormal and Social Psychology*, 1970, **75**, 30–37.

Schuler, E. A., & Parenton, V. J. A recent epidemic of hysteria in a Louisiana High School. *Journal of Social Psychology*, 1943, **17**, 221–235.

Sears, R. R. Relation of early socialization to aggression in middle childhood. *Journal of Abnormal and Social Psychology*, 1961, **63**, 466–492.

Sears, R. R., Maccoby, E. E., & Levin, H. *Patterns of child rearing*. Evanston, Ill.: Row and Peterson, 1957.

Sears, R. R., Rau, L., & Alpert, R. *Identification and child training*. Stanford, Cal.: Stanford University Press, 1965.

Sears, R. R., Whiting, J. W. M., Nowlis, V., & Sears, P. S. Some child-rearing antecedents of aggression and dependency in young children. *Genetic Psychology Monographs*, 1953, **47**, 135–234.

Seay, B., & Harlow, H. F. Maternal separation in the rhesus monkey. *Journal of Nervous and Mental Diseases*, 1965, **140**, 434–441.

Shaw, C. R., & McKay, H. D. *Juvenile delinquency and urban areas*. Chicago: University of Chicago Press, 1942.

Shields, J. Personality differences and neurotic traits in normal twin school children. *Eugenics Review*, 1954, **45**, 213–245.

Shields, J. Monozygotic twins, *Brought up apart and brought up together*. London: Oxford University Press, 1962.

Shields, J., & Slater, E. Heredity and psychological abnormality. In H. J. Eysenck (Ed.), *Handbook of abnormal psychology*. New York: Basic Books, 1961.

Siegman, A. Father absence during early childhood and anti-social behavior. *Journal of Abnormal Psychology*, 1966, **71**, 71–74.

Slater, E., & Shields, J. Genetical aspects of anxiety. In M. H. Lader (Ed.), *Studies of anxiety*, Ashford, Kent, England: Headley Brothers, 1969.

Spitz, R. A. Anaclitic depression. *The Psychoanalytic Study of the Child*, 1946, **2**, 313–342.

Stolz, L. M. Effects of maternal employment on children: evidence from research. *Child Development*, 1960, **31**, 749–782.

Theron, P. A. Peripheral vasomotor reactions as indices of basic emotional tension and lability. *Psychosomatic Medicine*, 1948, **10**, 335–346.

Thomas, A., Chess, S., Birch, H. G., Hertzig, M., & Korn, S. *Behavioral individuality in early childhood.* New York: New York University Press, 1963.

Toby, J. The differential impact of family disorganization. *American Sociological Review,* 1957, **22,** 505–512.

Vandenberg, S. G., Clark, P. J., & Samuels, I. Psychophysiological reactions of twins: Heritability factors in galvanic skin resistance, heartbeat, and breathing rates. *Eugenics Quarterly,* 1965, **12,** 7–10.

Wahler, R. G. Oppositional children: A quest for parental reinforcement control. *Journal of Applied Behavior Analysis,* 1968, **3,** 159–170.

Waldfogel, S. The development, meaning, and management of school phobia. *American Journal of Orthopsychiatry,* 1957, **27,** 754–780.

Waxler, N. E., & Mishler, E. Experimental studies of families. In L. Berkowitz (Ed.), *Advances in experimental social psychology,* Vol. 5. New York: Academic Press, 1970.

Wenar, C. The reliability of mother's histories. *Child Development,* 1961, **32,** 491–500.

Wenar, C., Handlon, M. W., & Garner, A. M. Patterns of mothering in psychosomatic disorders and severe emotional disturbances. *Merrill-Palmer Quarterly,* 1960, **6,** No. 3.

Wenger, M. A., Clemens, T. L., Coleman, D. R., Cullen, T. L., & Engel, B. T. Autonomic response specificity. *Psychosomatic Medicine,* 1961, **23,** 185–193.

West, D. J. *Homosexuality.* Chicago: Aldine, 1967.

Williams, T. A., Schachter, J., & Rowe, R. Spontaneous autonomic activity, anxiety, and "hyperkinetic" impulsivity. *Psychosomatic Medicine,* 1965, **27,** 9–18.

Winder, C. L., & Rau, L. Parental attitudes associated with social deviance in preadolescent boys. *Journal of Abnormal and Social Psychology,* 1962, **64,** 418–424.

Yarrow, L. J. Maternal deprivation. *Psychological Bulletin,* 1961, **58,** 459–490.

Yarrow, L. J. Separation from parents during early childhood. In M. L. Hoffman and L. W. Hoffman (Eds.), *Review of child development research.* New York: Russell Sage Foundation, 1964.

Yarrow, M. R. Problems of methods in parent-child research. *Child Development,* 1963, **34,** 215–226.

Yarrow, M. R., Campbell, J. D., & Burton, R. V. *Child rearing:* An inquiry into research and methods. California: Jossey-Bass, Inc., 1968.

Chapter Three

Organic Factors in Childhood Psychopathology
John S. Werry

Historical

The effect of brain damage on animal behavior, notably changes in activity and emotional reactivity (Schulman, Kaspar, & Throne, 1965, pp. 21–39), has been well demonstrated.

The idea that organic factors are equally important determinants of human behavior is of great antiquity. Greek physicians saw the human personality as the result of the interactions of four bodily fluids or humors. The case of the New England railroad workman, Phineas Gage, who in 1848 suffered an injury to the frontal lobes and reputedly became a moral degenerate thereafter, is well-known. During the second half of the nineteenth century, the idea of hereditary progressive degeneration of the central nervous system (CNS) was prevalent. Behavioral disorder in one generation was seen as the harbinger of insanity and idiocy in succeeding generations.

With the popularization of psychoanalytic theory and the birth of the mental hygiene movement in the United States shortly after World War I, interest in the role of organic factors in psychopathology appears to have waned, even though lethargic encephalitis, which was pandemic in 1917–1918, was generally considered to have produced a particularly severe kind of antisocial disorder in many afflicted children. Shortly after World War II,

Strauss (Strauss & Lehtinen, 1947) published his now classical treatise on the "brain-injured child" in which he advanced the hypothesis that brain damage in children resulted in a specific cognitive and behavioral syndrome, the hyperactivity perceptual-confusion syndrome. Since that time the role of organic brain factors in the etiology of certain children's behavior disorders has become increasingly accepted so that the literature in this area is now vast. Unfortunately, the quality of studies is not matched by their quantity. Many are difficult to read and to evaluate and, perhaps not surprisingly, results are often contradictory, making definite statements difficult.

Concepts of Brain-Behavior Relationships

Teuber (1960), in discussing the relationship between cerebral damage or dysfunction and personality, has described two points of view—the "hard" and the "soft." In the hard, the lesion is seen as directly instrumental in producing the behavioral disorder, either a general brain-damage syndrome (Bakwin, 1949; Strauss & Lehtinen, 1947) or a series of specific syndromes depending on the site or type of the lesion. In the "soft" view, cerebral status is a relatively minor variable, the behavioral effect of which is made quite unpredictable by the overriding importance of the individual personality (e.g., Blau, 1954).

Intermediate views (e.g., Bender, 1959; Birch, 1964, pp. 3–11; Eisenberg, 1957) suggest that certain primary deficits, especially of cognitive and motor function, are directly the result of cerebral pathology, but that the specific behavioral syndromes are largely determined by the reaction of the individual child and his environment to these primary deficits. Other factors of demonstrated importance in animals (Schulman et al., 1965, pp. 21–39) suggested as equally important in influencing the effect of brain damage on the psychopathology of childhood are the site and extent of the lesion, and the age at which it is suffered (Benton, 1962; Eisenberg, 1957; Ernhart, Graham, Eichman, Marshall, and Thurston, 1963; Meyer, 1961; Schulman et al., 1965; Teuber, 1960). Nevertheless, most experimental or clinical studies relevant to children have been concerned with answering relatively simplistic questions, principally whether "brain damage" in children, independent of site, size, or age of onset (1) has discernible effects on behavior or personality, and if so (2) whether it tends to produce specific types of psychopathology.

This review will be restricted to a consideration of the relationship between abnormal structure (damage) or abnormal physical functioning (dysfunction) of the brain on the one hand, and behavioral or personality status on the other. Other physical conditions and handicaps which, even though quite severe, do not nevertheless interfere with the physiological functions of the CNS will not be considered here since their impact on behavior can be interpreted in a manner similar to that of any other kind of psychological stress. Nor will we discuss slight individual variations in structure or function that cannot be classified as definite abnormalities.

Methodological Problems

Since this review considers the interaction of two variables, psychopathology and brain damage/dysfunction, methodological problems may be grouped into those associated with each variable plus those that arise out of the interaction of the two. The problems of measurement of behavioral disorders are discussed in Chapters One and Six. Before considering problems associated with the diagnosis and measurement of brain damage, the problem of interaction between brain damage and psychopathology will be noted briefly. Both "brain damage" as customarily defined and psychopathology are relatively common conditions so that their joint occurrence in a significant number of cases must be simply one of coincidence (e.g., EEG abnormalities and behavior disorders). At present, it is seldom possible in an individual case to determine whether the relationship is causal or coincidental (Pond, 1961), despite the facility with which correlation is assumed to be causality. Even where the relationship between the brain damage and the behavior seems to be causal, it has to be remembered that brain damage has a psychological as well as a physical impact, and probably in many cases brain damage is not pathogenic because of its alteration in the physical substrate, but rather because of its psychological stimulus value (Blau, 1954), or because of impaired adaptation, and it thus leads to secondary behavioral disturbance (Wolff and Hurwitz, 1966). The problem is further complicated in children by the reasonable expectation that other variables such as the age at which brain damage occurs may greatly influence its effect (Hebb, 1949).

Diagnosis of Brain Damage

Deciding definitely whether there is a structural abnormality or physiological dysfunction in the brain is much more difficult than it may ordinarily appear. In general, medical diagnostic techniques suffer from inadequate validation and tend to be based more on tradition or authority than on the accurate ascertainment of reliabilities and validities. Because of the delicacy, complexity, and inaccessibility of the brain, most of the diagnostic techniques aimed at evaluating its status are necessarily indirect and inferential. Large sections of the brain are "silent"—i.e., they seem to have no externally measurable functions, either input (sensory-perceptual) or output (motor-vocal-autonomic). Compensation for deficit seems common, probably particularly so in younger age groups. For these reasons, many of the diagnostic techniques may be negative in the presence of substantial brain damage or dysfunction (Pond, 1961). Conversely, particularly with tests of higher or more subtle function, there is reason to suspect that positive results often occur in the absence of brain damage or dysfunction (Herbert, 1964).

The usual methods of diagnosis follow:

1. *Autopsy and Biopsy.* Autopsy, the surest of all techniques, is available only in a small minority of cases and then usually only where the diagnosis is already clear so that its value in settling some of the controversies in this area is negligible. Biopsy, usually done only where there is established major disease, does not eliminate the possibility of damage in areas other than those viewed at the time of surgery.

2. *History.* This is one of the least useful yet most often used of all diagnostic criteria. First, the information is often inaccurate because of the fallibility of human memory. Wenar (1963) has reviewed the literature on the reliability of mothers' developmental histories. He found that with the exception of the length of gestation and some global estimate of the difficulty of delivery and birthweight, most of the important details of pregnancy, delivery and neonatal status cannot be reliably recalled. Minde, Webb, and Sykes (1968) found similar discrepancies between mothers' histories and medical records. Second, even when medical records are used, there usually proves to be a distressing absence of necessary data and that which is recorded is neither objective nor quantifiable. Third, the probabilities of damage consequent on most of the potentially traumatic events such as those during pregnancy or the perinatal period are unknown. The studies by F. Graham (Graham, Ernhart, Thurston, & Craft, 1962) indicate how the value of historical data might be greatly enhanced both by the development of reliable techniques and by the weighting of potentially noxious events.

3. *Neurological Examination.* This can detect major degrees of cerebral damage with a significant degree of accuracy when the lesion impinges on non-silent areas of the brain. Unfortunately, however, in patients where other diagnostic aids have proved most ambiguous, the neurological examination is also often ambiguous. Children with psychiatric problems are prone to exhibit so-called "equivocal" or "soft" neurological signs, the significance of which is obscure (Bender, 1958; Kennard, 1960; Clements & Peters, 1962; Lucas, Rodin, & Simson, 1965; Werry, 1968). What is urgently needed is a wide-range system of pediatric neurological examination which has been properly systematized (such as that by Ozer, 1968), its reliability estimated, and then standardized in the general population as have been intelligence tests. This would guarantee that a full examination of all areas had indeed been carried out by the neurologist, and that techniques of eliciting and

estimating findings were general instead of idiosyncratic to each neurologist. It would also permit proper evaluation of the normative significance of the findings in terms of their frequency in the general population.

4. *The Electroencephalogram* (*EEG*). Ellingson (1954) and Freeman (1967) have reviewed some of the problems of reliability and interpretation of EEG abnormalities in children. These are essentially similar to those already described for the neurological examination, namely, lack of agreement on criteria of abnormality (Freeman cites one of the few studies of the reliability of the EEG as showing an agreement of only 40% in a simple three-point normal-borderline-abnormal classification) and on the significance in terms of damage or dysfunction of many of these abnormalities. As with the neurological examination, the type of EEG abnormalities common among children with behavior problems fall largely in a no-man's-land between normality and undeniable pathology. An example is that of the controversial 14 and 6 positive spike abnormality taken by some to be *prima facie* evidence of an organic etiology (Kellaway, Crawley, & Maulsby, 1965) which has been shown to occur with a frequency of up to 25% in normal children (Demerdash, Eeg-Olofsson, & Petersen, 1968) and which does not differentiate delinquents from normal adolescents (Weiner, Delano, & Klass, 1966). The frequency of these abnormalities tends to decrease with age (Ellingson, 1954; Weiner et al., 1966), which suggests that they might be a result, in part, of the greater difficulty of interpretation of the EEG in children or simply because of immaturity rather than abnormality. Ellingson (1954) states that although there are positive relationships between these EEG abnormalities and a history suggestive of, neurological signs of, or psychometric indications of structural brain defect, these relationships are of moderate size only. Although Aird and Yamamoto (1966) found some relationship between prenatal history, abnormal EEG and abnormal neurological studies, Schulman et al. (1965) found no correlation between the EEG and neurological examination in their careful study. Ellingson hypothesized that the EEG abnormalities could reflect any one or any combination of three etiological factors: (a) a maturational retardation of the CNS (which could, of course, be psychologically or experientially determined [Hebb, 1949]), (b) a psychophysiological reaction to the testing procedure, particularly in children, since the EEG pattern is ordinarily unstable, and (c) actual cerebral defect. Ellingson concludes that of these three variables, structural brain damage is probably more important though to an unknown degree. Freeman (1967) has deplored the uncritical manner in which EEG findings have been interpreted etiologically in behavioral and learning disorders with a complete disregard for the unreliability of the technique and the contradictory interpretation of the significance of abnormal patterns.

5. *Other Special Medical Investigations.* Skull X-rays, pneumoenceph-

alograms (in which the cerebral ventricular system and the subarachnoid system are outlined radiologically by replacing the cerebrospinal fluid with air), cerebral angiograms (where the blood vessels of the brain are outlined by injecting a radio-paque substance intra-arterially), and other such radiological techniques require gross distortions of the structure of the brain in order to show any abnormalities (Pond, 1961). Since many of the behavior disturbances in children are attributed to *minimal brain damage* (Pasamanick, Rogers, & Lilienfeld, 1956) spread diffusely throughout the brain instead of localized, these particular investigations would be predicted to have very limited application to the study of the so-called organic behavior disorders. Biochemical tests are not yet able to detect other than gross kinds of cerebral dysfunction and, to date, most of the studies that purport to have demonstrated subtle differences in the metabolism of patients with psychiatric problems have been shown to be a result of experimental error (Kety, 1965).

6. *Psychodiagnostic Techniques.* Although psychological tests are used extensively in making diagnoses of brain damage and, to a lesser extent, in localizing it (e.g., Reitan, 1968), their validity is largely unestablished. Herbert (1964), in a comprehensive review of this area as it applies to children, points out that most of the studies aimed at ascertaining differences in performance on psychological tests between brain-damaged and normal groups relied on a neurological diagnosis, itself of limited validity, to delineate criterion groups. Other problems raised by Herbert are poor test construction, lack of standardization of tests, lack of cross-validation studies, preoccupation with mentally retarded criterion groups, lack of control for visual field defects or external stimulus variables and, most serious of all, the considerable overlap in scores between brain damaged and normal children. Graham and Berman (1964), in their review of tests for brain damage in infants and preschool children, concluded much as did Herbert that there were no tests which presently discriminate well between brain damaged and normal children. Thus, while these tests may provide some evidence suggestive of brain damage, they can by no means be used as the sole criterion for diagnosing cerebral pathology. The careful attempts of Reitan and his co-workers (Reitan, 1966; Kløve, 1963; Reitan & Heineman, 1968) and Knights (Knights & Watson, 1968) to develop a neuropsychological diagnostic battery for children appear to be one of the more promising developments in this area, although the absence of norms and typically the severely neurologically abnormal validating populations presently limit their usefulness in psychiatric populations.

Thus, the diagnosis of brain damage or dysfunction, unless gross, depends on a group of medical, historical, and psychological measures most of which are of low or untested reliability, which discriminate poorly between normal and brain damaged populations, and which apparently measure a variety of unrelated functions instead of a homogeneous variable "brain damage" (Rodin,

Lucas, & Simson, 1963; Paine, Werry, & Quay, 1968; Schulman et al., 1965; Werry, 1968). Very often, as an illustration of the adage that a prophet is not without honor except in his own country, one profession overvalues the validity of another's diagnostic methods. Thus, psychologists and educators lend ultimate credence to medical tests and physicians to psychological tests.

Under the circumstances the diagnosis of brain damage or dysfunction in the majority of children with behavior disorders is no more than an enlightened guess. Further, as has already been pointed out, even where the diagnosis of brain damage can be firmly established, there is as yet usually no way of proving that it is causally related to the behavior observed (Pond, 1961).

Clinical Studies of Organic Factors and Childhood Psychopathology

For the purposes of orderly discussion, studies will be grouped in the following manner: (1) those in which *brain damage* is the independent variable or means for selecting the abnormal group, (2) those in which unspecified *behavioral* abnormality is the independent variable, (3) those concerned with *specific behavioral* syndromes, (4) those concerned with *specific brain damage variables* such as etiology, site, and age of the lesion.

Brain Damage as an Independent Variable

In this type of study, the starting point has been the selection of a group of children differentiated from normal children by the presence of proven or suspected brain damage. Studies of this type are fewer than those which take psychopathology as the independent variable, and the results in general differ. Most of these studies are retrospective concerning establishment of the diagnosis of brain injury which antedated the investigations of behavioral status or other dependent variables by some years, but a few are prospective. Since the prospective studies are potentially more reliable, they will be discussed first.

1. *Parental Damage, Anoxia or Unspecified Damage.* In a prospective study remarkable for the care with which the investigators attempted to develop accurate methods of establishing and measuring their variables, Graham et al. (1962) investigated the effect of clearly established anoxia or other severe pre- or perinatal complications on later personality and cognitive development in 350 preschool-age children. They then compared their findings with three other similar studies. In two of the three, those by Schacter and Apgar (1959) and Fraser and Wilks (1959) involving a total of 250 children reexamined at about 8 years of age, the findings were similar to their own. The criterion groups showed evidence of slight but significant impairment of

cognitive function, but no or very questionable differences in the frequency of psychopathology as judged by mothers' reports and examiners' ratings (of satisfactory reliability).

A fourth study, that by Prechtl and his group (Prechtl & Dijkstra, 1960; Prechtl, 1960) produced entirely different results as far as subsequent behavior difficulties were concerned. Of 400 infants who had suffered pre- or perinatal complication, the frequency of symptoms of the brain damage behavior syndrome (Strauss & Lehtinen, 1947), such as short attention span, lability of mood, hyperactivity, anxiety, negativism, and disturbances in social interaction, were found on reexamination between the ages of two to four years to be most frequent (70%) in the group that had both a history of complications *and* an abnormal neonatal neurological status; least (12%) in the group that was normal in both these respects; while the group with only an abnormal history was intermediate (38%). Behavior abnormalities were judged in a manner similar to the other studies: by mothers' reports and by observers' ratings particularly during the administration of psychological tests. Unlike the study by Graham et al. (1962), no figures for the reliabilities of the tests used is given nor is there any information as to whether the examiner was kept unaware of the criterion group to which an individual child belonged.

Ucko (1965) compared 29 boys with a history of neonatal anoxia as defined anecdotally by nurses on the obstetrical record with 29 controls matched for age, sex, social class, birth order and approximately matched for maternal age. Data came from a more comprehensive prospective longitudinal study covering the period of birth to eight years and comprised detailed specific questioning of mothers at regular intervals about a number of developmentally appropriate behavioral and adjustment areas with the addition of some psychometric and personality tests and behavior ratings by examiners. There was no difference in overall cognitive and behavioral development in the two groups, but the asphyxiated children were significantly more reactive temperamentally, especially to changes in routine, to frustration, and to enjoyment and, hence, were much more difficult to manage without actually being behaviorally abnormal. This reactivity was positively correlated with the severity of the asphyxia. Ucko points out that this temperamental reactivity had strong positive aspects as well as negative ones, as seen in the strong affectional repressions and enjoyment of pleasurable experiences some of the children exhibited. Ucko's results are thus intermediate between those of Prechtl and of the first three studies cited (Graham et al., 1962; Fraser & Wilkes, 1959; Schachter & Apgar, 1959).

Two other prospective studies, although as yet incomplete, deserve mention. These are the Collaborative Study presently being conducted by the National Institutes of Neurological Diseases & Blindness of the U.S. Public Health Service (NINDB 1968) and the English Perinatal Study (Butler &

Bonham, 1963) both of which involve large populations of children. Neither has yet published any of its follow-up findings, though many of the subjects of both studies are already in middle childhood. Hopefully these studies should provide data on the frequency and type of behavioral abnormalities following complications of pregnancy and the perinatal period and also enable weighting of these complications in terms of the probability of their causing significant brain damage.

The other broad group of studies which still takes brain damage rather than behavioral status as the selective criterion are those that are retrospective in terms of establishing brain damage and are hence probably less reliable. In their now classical studies, Strauss and Lehtinen (1947) demonstrated that in a group of institutionalized, mildly retarded children, those designated by neurological examination or history as being "brain injured" or "exogenously" retarded displayed certain behavioral differences when compared with non-brain injured or "endogeneous" retardates on behavior symptom ratings made by teachers and by cottage parents. The behaviors characteristic of the *brain-injured child* were erratic, uncoordinated, uncontrolled, uninhibited, socially unacceptable, hyperactive, stereotyped behaviors; catastrophic emotional reactions to frustrations; lack of fear or prudence; and sometimes, emotional shallowness, and bladder and bowel difficulties (Strauss & Lehtinen, 1947, p. 84). Sarason (1949, p. 52–58) has criticized Strauss and Lehtinen's method of diagnosing brain injury because of excessive reliance on history taken mostly from parents and on psychological tests results neither of which has a sufficient degree of reliability or validity to use in making such a diagnosis (*vide supra*). Sarason concludes that the behavioral abnormalities described by Strauss have not been demonstrated to be either the result of brain damage or conversely characteristic of every brain-damaged child. Gallagher (1957) also points out that Strauss and Lehtinen appear to have developed their behavior rating scale by choosing items that seemed to discriminate between his two original groups and to have then validated the scale by testing it on the same two groups. Evidence that any attempt was made to cross-validate the scale is lacking.

In his own study of 48 mentally retarded children (IQ 35 to 76), Gallagher (1957) found that the brain-injured group, so defined with unusual care, did differ significantly from the familial or endogenous group when their behavior was evaluated on a specially designed teacher-rating scale of 11 behavioral dimensions. The brain-injured group was found to be more demanding, less able to postpone gratification, more anxious, more deficient in socialization, and more hyperactive. Like most other studies, perceptual and cognitive differences of a slight but significant degree were also present. Gallagher considered that the behavioral differences were not due to lack of accurate perception of social situations (Bender, 1959), since they seemed uncorrelated with degree of perceptual deficit. He felt they were more likely the result of a general lack of impulse control thus making the child socially unacceptable to both adult and peer groups. The anxiety and attention-seeking were thus most probably reactive to rejection as a result of the primary symptom of poor impulse control.

In another study by Graham (Ernhart et al., 1963), a group of preschool children with independently established (that is, by valid criteria other than behavioral or psychological) lesions in the cerebral hemispheres was compared on personality and cognitive measures with a non-brain-damaged group. Slight behavioral impairment as judged by reliable parent and examiner ratings was found in the brain-damaged group, though these differences were slight as compared with the differences in perceptual and cognitive functioning and covered a wide range of unfavorable personality characteristics—not just those described by Strauss and others as typical of brain-injured behavior.

In an inadequately described study of 58 children seen at a psychiatric clinic in whom brain damage could be established with some degree of certitude, Pond (1961) found that the organic group resembled the ordinary child psychiatric population at the same clinic both in symptomatology (very few presented with the typical brain-damage syndrome) and in sociofamilial background. The only significant difference between the two groups was that the brain-damaged children were in general of lower intelligence.

Conversely, in a well-designed epidemiological study using specially developed diagnostic instruments of demonstrated reliability and validity, P. Graham and Rutter (1968) found children with major neurological disease (epilepsy, cerebral palsy, etc.) to have a frequency of psychiatric disorder five times as high as in the normal population and three times as high as 117 children with other physical handicaps. No specific brain-damage behavioral syndrome was found.

Hutt, Hutt, and Ounsted (1965) studied two groups of hospitalized children aged 3 to 8 years in a "free field situation" of systematically increasing complexity. One group had clear evidence of upper CNS lesions, mostly seizures, and the other, matched for age and sex but not IQ, was comprised of emotionally disturbed children in the same hospital. Significant differences in behavior were found in the brain-damaged group—principally greater degrees of locomotion, gesturing, and other types of motor behavior, increased manipulation of fixtures instead of task materials, a tendency to return repeatedly to the same stimulus material, and relatively repetitive unvarying types of behavior despite increasing complexity of the environment. Though this is strictly an experimental situation, it is easy to understand how these elements of behavior could, in the larger social environment, lead to such psychopathological symptoms as hyperactivity, short attention span, stereotyped behaviors, and distractibility. However, how typical these findings are of all brain-damaged children (especially the so-called "minimally brain-damaged" child of normal intelligence), is by no means clear since the sample size was small and highly selected—most of the children had major neurological handicaps and were severely retarded. But this method of analyzing behavior seems likely to prove more fruitful in detecting subtle differences of behavior than the questionnaire or other global observational techniques employed in most studies.

Discussion thus far has centered on studies in which the cerebral damage or dysfunction has been due in the main to birth injury, neonatal anoxia, or brain insult of unspecified etiology. However, several studies have concerned themselves with other specific etiological conditions, and they will now be reviewed.

2. *Prematurity.* Prematurity, defined as a birth weight of less than five pounds, though not necessarily followed by brain damage, is generally regarded as one of the more important causes of brain damage in children. Studies of prematurity would therefore be expected to show effects on behavior qualitatively similar to those purportedly resulting from brain damage, particularly hyperactivity, aggressivity, and distractibility, and this seems to be the case in eight studies reviewed by Wiener (1962). He does point out, however, that whether this association is due to brain damage, to sensory and maternal deprivation accompanying the prolonged hospitalization of the early months, or to the social pathology so highly correlated with prematurity is not clear. Robinson and Robinson (1965, pp. 148–150) state that more recent work has shown that much of the supposed cognitive and behavioral differences between prematures and full-term infants is probably attributable to this social pathology. They report one of their studies of 135 prematures and 92 matched controls which showed that when corrections were made for differences in socioeconomic class, the slight excess of behavior problems in the premature group disappeared. In one of the few other studies of prematures that did attempt to control for socioeconomic factors albeit rather crudely (type of hospital accommodation at delivery) Caplan, Bibace, and Rabinovitch (1963) found that the premature group had an excess (75% versus 57%) of problem children. This difference could well have been due to failure of exact control of socioeconomic variables, to the higher number of psychologically less adequate parents in the premature group, or the unstated (but probably high in view of the large number of problem children in the control group) error in the measurement of psychopathology (psychoanalytically oriented interviews by one psychiatrist).

3. *Encephalitis.* The pandemic of lethargic encephalitis at the end of World War I gave rise to a series of reports that permanent behavioral disturbances could result particularly when the encephalitis occurred in child-

hood (Ebaugh, 1923; Kennedy, 1924; Strecker, 1929). Symptoms emphasized were total change in character usually with marked antisocial behavior, hyperkinesis and nocturnal restlessness, affective disorders such as depression and emotional instability, hysterical reactions especially hyperventilation, tics, and mental deficiency. The general feeling appeared to be that these behavior disturbances were intractable and such children required institutionalization. Strecker (1929) offered evidence that the severity of the problem was correlated positively with the number of neurological sequelae, male sex, and age.

These studies have several defects. First, the diagnosis of encephalitis was not adequately established in a significant number of cases. Second, no attempt appears to have been made to separate social immaturity due to commonly coexistent mental deficiency from psychopathology. Third, all these studies suffer from biased sampling, having usually studied only children referred because of sequelae. Finally, there is reason to be suspicious of parents' reports of "total change in character" especially when there has been some dramatic event to which it may be erroneously or gratefully attributed (Blau, 1954). So strongly entrenched is the association of this behavioral syndrome of hyperkinesis and antisocial disorder with encephalitis (see Mayer-Gross, Slater, & Roth, 1960, p. 446) that some apparently even consider it legitimate to make a diagnosis of a history of encephalitis from the behavioral syndrome alone (Levy, 1959). However, as early as 1924, Strecker and Ebaugh had noted the similarity of post-traumatic and post-encephalitic disturbances.

Gibbs, Gibbs, Spies, and Carpenter (1964) followed 250 children who had suffered from encephalitis of various kinds and found a 10% overall frequency of behavior disorders, established by unidentified means, at follow-up. In an all too common logical error, the authors attributed these disorders and the EEG abnormalities to the encephalitis, which seems unwarranted since there were no pre-hoc measurements and a 10–15% prevalence of behavior disorders seems to be the usually accepted level in the general population (Bower, 1960, pp. 21–28). Sabatino and Cramblett (1968) studied the behavioral sequelae by means of a modified Quay and Petersen Problem Checklist (see Chapter Six) in 14 children 7 months to 2 years after what appear to be serologically and clinically well-authenticated attacks of California viral encephalitis (Cramblett, Stegmiller, & Spencer, 1966). Though the authors concluded that a significant proportion of the children exhibited many symptoms of hyperkinetic syndrome, these symptoms are also common in normal children. The norms for the checklist (Quay and Peterson, 1967, see also Chapter Six) suggest that scores for most of the children probably fell well within one standard deviation on conduct disorder, personality disorder, and immaturity and thus that the degree of psychopathology was slight and well below that observed in psychiatric populations. Furthermore, this study also suffers from the defect of being purely post hoc and the scores no doubt were influenced by the dramatic event of a serious illness. It is interesting in this respect to note that personality disorder (neurotic) symptoms were as much increased as conduct or hyperkinetic. There is no doubt, however, that this study and that by Gibbs et al. (1964) will be incorrectly cited as evidence of post-encephalitic behavior disorder.

4. *Epilepsy.* In view of the prevalence of epilepsy and the frequency with which personality disorders are attributed to it, especially to the temporal lobe kind, it is somewhat surprising to find that there are almost no adequate studies that attempt to assess the prevalence of behavior disorders in children with this disease particularly as compared with normal controls (Tizard, 1962). Standard texts on epilepsy (Lennox & Lennox, 1960), while admitting that behavior difficulties may occur, explicitly or implicitly refute the contention that even a majority of epileptic children exhibit symptoms of psychopathology. The epidemiological study by Graham and Rutter (1968) cited earlier did find an increased frequency of disorder (28%), but this is still a minority of epileptic children.

Ounsted, Lindsay, and Norman (1966) studied 100 children ranging in age from 3 to 15 years, who had an unequivocal diagnosis of temporal lobe epilepsy. They found that 26% exhibited the hyperkinetic (or brain-damaged behavior) syndrome although no information is given on how this diagnosis was established other than that the authors consider it fairly easily made. The hyperkinetic group had a significant excess of gross damage to the brain with early onset of seizures. However, since activity level and mental age are probably negatively correlated (though Ounsted et al. consider the low intelligence to be a result of the overactivity rather than vice versa), the significance of these findings is diluted by the fact that the hyperkinetic group proved to have a mean IQ of 66 as against 94.4 in the non-hyperkinetic group. Ounsted et al. also concluded that although the majority of temporal lobe epileptics were *not* hyperkinetic, there was some correlation and this correlation was higher than in other forms of epilepsy. Catastrophic rage reactions were found in one third of the group and were common in the clearly brain-injured group and the hyperkinetic group.

Epileptics seen in hospitals constitute a sample biased toward overinclusion of the behaviorally disturbed (Tizard, 1962). A study by Pond (1961) of 100 epileptic children seen by family doctors revealed that approximately one-quarter had psychological difficulties, which is somewhat higher than the probable distribution of behavioral disorders in the total population (Bower, 1960, pp. 21–28), but still suggests that the majority are behaviorally normal. Pond, in the same paper (1961), cites an earlier study in which epileptic children with behavior disorders were compared with both a group of epileptic children without psychopathology and a group of children with behavior problems. The crucial determinants of the behavior disorder were seen clearly to be related to a disturbed environment and to be unrelated to epilepsy. Unfortunately Pond's studies are difficult to evaluate since he does not give details of the critical methodological problems of establishment of psychopathological status and whether or not raters were blind. Tizard (1962), in her extensive review of the personality of epileptics, felt able only to conclude that (a) there was no evidence that all or most epileptics have a characteristic personality and (b) although the prevalence of psychopathology *might* be higher in epileptics or some types of epileptics (e.g., temporal lobe), the evidence available scarcely permitted definitive statements.

5. *Cerebral Palsy.* Remarks on the infrequency of behavioral studies similar to those made about epilepsy may be made about cerebral palsy (i.e., brain damage with motor involvement). Cruickshank and Bice (1966) cite several twin studies where psychopathology was found to be equally common in the non-cerebral palsy twin, to show that the psychological rather than the neurophysiological impact of, and the parents' reaction to the cerebral palsy is the more probable explanation of most psychopathology which occurs on this condition. This does not agree with Graham and Rutter's (1968) findings.

6. *Head Injury.* Strecker and Ebaugh (1924) studied behaviorally disturbed children with post-traumatic behavior disorders marked especially by aggressive and antisocial behavior. No control groups, especially of emotionally disturbed children without head injuries, were used. Blau subsequently (1954) confessed that he had been misled in an earlier study (1938) in attributing the behavioral disturbance to head injury instead of to reaction by parents or child to head injury. In a study of postnatal head injury in children and young adults, all of whom were twins, in which the co-twin served as uninjured control, Dencker (1958) showed that head injury appeared to be playing no significant part in the development of psychopathology. Similarly, Harrington and Letemendia (1958) showed that children who suffered head injuries during childhood and were subsequently presented at child guidance clinics were distinguishable from children with head injuries who were not so referred, by their pre-traumatic adjustment or family adjustment at the time of presentation at the clinic. The psychopathology thus reflected either something which had antedated the injury or was the result of family or child reaction to the injury as a psychological rather than a physical stress. Interestingly, the head injuries suffered by the group without behavior difficulties were much more severe than those of the group seen at the child psychiatric clinic.

Summary

Although somewhat contradictory, studies on the effect of carefully established brain damage or a history of events which purportedly carry a strong risk of brain damage show that any increased frequency of childhood psychopathological disorder as compared with a properly matched control group is at best small and difficult to detect. In general, the better the study methodologically, the smaller the effect observed. Slight perceptual, cognitive, or other intellectual differences are generally found and raise the possibility that some of the psychopathological symptoms such as distractibility which are frequently attributed directly to brain damage, may in fact be secondary to intellectual impairment or may be normal for the child's level of mental development. However, since techniques for the measurement of behavior in children have not yet achieved the sophistication of those that measure intellectual function, it is possible that subtle behavioral changes such as increased reactivity (Ucko, 1965) may occur as a consequence of brain injury. Longitudinal studies by Chess and Thomas (Chess, Thomas, Rutter, & Birch, 1963) show that subtle temperamental differences may be augmented into behavioral disorder or mitigated by patterns of parenting making any effect from brain damage unpredictable. Also, if direct effects of brain injury on personality are as weak as they appear to be, differences might be revealed only by large sample studies. There is good evidence to show that when psychopathology is associated with brain damage it can take any form, the *least* common of which is the hyperkinetic syndrome.

Psychopathology as an Independent Variable

Here the criterion by which children to be studied have been selected has been *psychopathology* rather than *brain damage* and attempts have been made to determine the frequency or significance of abnormal brain status in the etiology of the observed behavior disorder. Such studies are more numerous than those that take brain damage as the independent variable since the latter are usually undertaken by investigators whose primary interest is in areas other than behavior, notably neurological status.

1. *General Psychiatric Populations.* Pasamanick and his group (Rogers, Lilienfeld, & Pasamanick, 1955; Pasamanick & Knobloch, 1960) studied about 500 children who had been referred because of behavior problems to the special services division of the Baltimore Department of Education. Forty percent exhibited hyperactivity, or confusion-disorganization (the so-called *brain damage behavior syndrome*), while the remainder exhibited a variety of other psychopathological conditions ranging from antisocial behavior to neurotic symptoms. Through inspection of medical rec-

ords, the frequency of pre- and perinatal complications in this group was compared with that in a normal control group of 350 children from the same classrooms matched for race, sex, and birthplace. The behaviorally deviant group as a whole exhibited a statistically significant excess of certain complications, notably prematurity and abnormalities of pregnancy prone to cause chronic fetal anoxia such as toxemia and antepartum bleeding. The behavioral syndrome most significantly associated with complications was hyperactivity-confusion, which was found to be responsible for all of the statistically significant difference observed between the two groups in the case of white children. The findings of this and additional studies of children with other behavioral, neurological, and educational disorders such as epilepsy, cerebral palsy, mental deficiency, tics, reading and speech disorders led Pasamanick and Knobloch (1960) to postulate a *continuum of reproductive casualty* in which the effect of damage to the brain is seen as varying according to its extent: when severe, death, mental retardation or cerebral palsy result. When minimal, mild cognitive perceptual and other CNS integrative difficulties obtain, leaving a group of children—the "minimally brain injured"—predisposed to develop behavioral difficulties depending on individual socio-familial or educative experience.

This widely cited group of studies is generally accepted as evidence of the importance of brain injury in the genesis of psychopathology in children. Pond (1961) has criticized these studies on the ground that socio-economic factors were not adequately controlled. For example, though control and criterion groups appeared similar on most social variables, there was a significant excess (57% versus 36%) of socially disorganized families in the white behaviorally disturbed group. What is unclear too, is whether these complications are more validly indicative of brain damage (the frequency with which they actually cause brain damage is unknown) or of social pathology, which was shown to be highly correlated with the pre- and perinatal complications. It should also be pointed out that differences between the behaviorally disturbed and normal groups were quantitatively small. For example, the distribution of abnormalities of the pre- and perinatal period in the criterion and control groups was: white children, 39% versus 31%; nonwhite children 73% versus 54% (Rogers et al. 1955 p. 56). Thus, many normal children had complications and many behaviorally disturbed had none. Even in the most divergent hyperactive/confused-disorganized group which was contributing all the excess of complications in the white psychopathological group, the difference between the behaviorally disturbed and control groups was only 42% versus 31% frequency of complications (p. 60). In view of the unknown but likely low probability with which these complications actually result in significant brain injury, it is apparent that brain damage could at best only be a minor determinant of the behavior disorders observed.

Wolff (1967a) did a comparative study of the paranatal histories of 100 elementary school children (mean age 8.4 years) with "reactive" psychiatric disorders referred consecutively to the psychiatric outpatient department of a Scottish pediatric hospital where referral is by physicians only and mostly on parental instigation. Children with mental retardation, minimal brain damage, schizoid personality, and those in institutions and without mothers were excluded although there were no more than a few children in each category. The control group consisted of children from the same school class, matched for sex, age, and social class. Mothers were interrogated and hospital records were scrutinized for abnormalities of pregnancy, delivery, and post-natal life, all fairly objectively defined by Wolff. There were no significant differences between the two groups. The listing of the symptomatology (Wolff, 1967b) suggests that despite the emphasis on "reactive" psychiatric disorders, clinic children comprise a typical mixed population of conduct, personality disorder, and immature children. Wolff concluded that if potentially brain-damaging events are important in the predisposition to certain psychopathological disorders, they can be so only in a minority of disturbed children. It is unfortunate that Wolff did not attempt to subdivide the clinic children nosologically since Rogers et al. (1955) had shown a differential frequency of brain-damaging events in different diagnostic groups.

Kennard (1960) studied 123 adolescent children who had been admitted to a state mental hospital with more severe types of disorders, comparing their neurological status on a wide range examination and EEG's with a control group of 65 "successful" children from nearby schools. The psychopathological groups as a whole had more neurological abnormalities than the control group, being highest in the group diagnosed (apparently largely from history or behavioral observations) as having organic syndromes, intermediate in the schizophrenic group, and lowest in the neurotic and sociopathic group where the frequency was only slightly higher than in the normal children. Certain signs (extraocular weakness, tremor, reflex inequalities, athetoid movements, tics, speech difficulties, hyperactivity, and nystagmus) were more frequent in patient than in control groups, whereas many other signs failed to discriminate the two groups. Kennard postulated that, in the light of the kind of neurological signs found, the psychopathological group showed evidence of a dysfunction of subcortical parts of the brain such as the basal ganglia or brain stem rather than cortical damage. She felt that this hypothesis received some confirmation from the lack of any correlation between the EEG and neurological abnormality since the subcortical regions are largely beyond the reach of the EEG. Historical data did not appear to be particularly helpful in suggesting an etiology for these neurological signs. This study suffers from lack of statistical analyses, which makes determination of the significance of the findings rather difficult. Further, Kennard's conclusion that the discriminating neurological signs, all minor or equivocal, indicated brain damage or dysfunction because they were commoner in children in whom other organic factors were thought to be operative, is subject to the criticism that the criteria for organicity appeared dependent on history, psychological tests, and ward behavior, none of which can be considered really adequate for such a diagnosis (see above).

Lucas et al. (1965) and Rodin et al. (1963) studied 72 children referred by school authorities because of undesirable classroom behavior or poor academic progress (mostly the former). The behavioral symptoms exhibited included withdrawal, antisocial behavior, hyperactivity, and emotional immaturity. A large number of medical, historical, behavioral, and neurological variables was measured, the most frequent were intercorrelated and then subjected to a rotated factor analysis. Only three behavioral factors were extracted, namely motor incoordination, hyperactivity, and antisocial behavior. Of these, only incoordination showed any relationship with possible brain-damage variables, and most of these latter were either unreliable such as "diagnosis of encephalopathy," which is usually made behaviorally, or had very small loadings like "complications of pregnancy" (.26). The hyperactivity factor seemed simply to be a psychopathological dimension of long duration. The behavioral *symptom* (as opposed to the *factor*) or hyperactivity and poor impulse control did show correlations with certain neurological abnormalities of uncertain significance such as poor coordination, motor difficulties, and abnormal movements. The authors suggested that hyperactivity thus represented some kind of cerebral dysfunction or brain damage, or an integration deficit of developmental origin. This study, like that of Kennard (1960), illustrates the typical uncertainty of the significance of the relationship between behavioral and neurological variables (see also discussion on the hyperkinetic syndrome below).

Hertzig and Birch (1968) found the frequency of four neurological indicators (neurological signs, choreiform movements, impaired auditory-visual sensory integration and mental defect) to be much higher in a group of psychiatric adolescent inpatients at Bellevue Hospital than in a control group of Scottish school children. This study has marked shortcomings, since the control group was younger in age, of different ethnic and cultural extraction, and the psychiatric population can hardly be considered typical since there was an overrepresentation of grossly behaviorally disturbed, mentally defective children from inner city minority groups. However, in a better study (Hertzig, Bortner, & Birch, 1969) they found that children in a school for brain-injured children, as defined by learning/behavior problems plus a medical affirmation of brain-injured status, did have a higher frequency of neurological signs than did a matched normal control group. However, the frequency of hard signs in both studies was much less than soft or equivocal signs. Their conclusion that the chief value of their findings was to draw attention to the role of organic factors in psychopathology seems reasonable, although they tended to minimize the uncertain neurological significance of most of the indicators. Another finding of note was that the hyperkinetic syndrome was only one of several behavioral patterns associated with neurological impairment.

Much of the inference that organic factors are important in the psychopathology of childhood comes from the high proportion of abnormal EEG's observed in children from various psychiatric settings (Ellingson, 1954). In his review Ellingson cites 18 separate studies of children with all kinds of psychopathology, 17 of which showed an EEG abnormality rate (range 33–92%) higher than those reported for normal children (range 5–15%). Aird and Yamamoto (1966) found a 49% frequency of abnormal EEG's in 100 children with behavior disorders. Although most of the studies cited by Ellingson did not include a control group, the few that did, as well as the later study by Taterka and Katz (1955), suggest that these differences are real and substantial. Even though no relationships appear to have been established between specific psychopathological symptoms and specific EEG abnormalities, there is some evidence that nosological conditions vary in the frequency with which abnormalities are to be found, being highest in children with so-called organic brain syndromes, psychosis (see Chapter Five), or conduct disorders but lower in children with neurotic symptomatology (Ellingson, 1954; Taterka & Katz, 1955; White, DeMyer, & DeMyer, 1964). As was discussed above, the significance of these findings is obfuscated by the lack of any clear relationship between EEG patterns of the kind frequently seen in psychiatric disorders and brain structure or function, and they cannot be interpreted as necessarily reflecting a CNS disorder (Freeman, 1967).

The Bellevue group (Bender, 1959; Fish, 1961; Taterka & Katz, 1955) has long argued for the significance of organic factors in the etiology of childhood psychopathology though their diagnosis of organicity has often depended on historical, behavioral, neurological, EEG, and psychometric indices of uncertain validity discussed above. According to this group, brain damage leads to disturbances of perception and motility, which create anxiety, which is then dealt with by various psychological defense mechanisms to produce in combination with the organic deficits the final clinical picture. At the moment, since unequivocal empirical support is lacking, this can be regarded as no more than an interesting hypothesis on the mechanism whereby abnormal cerebral status might influence behavior. For example, Gallagher (1957) found no correlation between degree of perceptual motor dysfunction and behavioral status. His findings suggested that environmental reaction to organically determined poor impulse control was the crucial factor in the genesis of subsequent psychopathology.

Summary

Studies of general psychiatric populations suggest that as a group emotionally disturbed children probably exhibit an increased frequency of EEG abnormalities and "equivocal" or "soft" neurological signs. The frequency of pre- and perinatal complications is less clear. There is also some slight evidence that these findings are more common in psychopathological conditions marked by psychosis, hyperactivity, or conduct disturbances (see below). Though suggestive of brain damage or dysfunction, these findings do not preclude adverse social experience, psychophysiological effects, or normal variation as etiological factors.

Specific Behavioral Syndromes

1. The Hyperkinetic Syndrome

This clinical syndrome, which has a large number of synonyms (see Clements, 1966) such as organic behavior disorders, minimal brain damage, etc. was first described as one of the sequelae in children with pandemic lethargic encephalitis (Ebaugh, 1923; Kennedy, 1924; Strecker, 1929), but received its greatest impetus from the work of Strauss and Lehtinen (1947). Descriptions of this behavioral complex of hyperactivity, short attention span, impulsiveness, irritability, clumsiness, and poor school work show a remarkable consistency across different observers (Anderson, 1963; Bakwin, 1949; Bradley, 1955; Burks, 1960; Clements & Peters, 1962; Ingram, 1956; Laufer & Denhoff, 1957; Minde, Webb, & Sykes, 1968; Ounsted, 1955; Schrager et al., 1966; Stewart, Pitts, Craig, & Dieruf, 1966; Werry, 1968; Werry, Weiss, & Douglas, 1964; Werry, Weiss, Douglas, & Martin, 1966). Most of these studies confirm this syndrome to be associated with a high frequency of (a) history of conditions of all kinds assumed commonly to result in brain injury, (b) mild neurological abnormalities of the type described as "equivocal" or "soft," (c) mild abnormalities of cognitive and perceptual function (agnosias), (d) mild EEG abnormalities, (e) mild degrees of sensorimotor incoordination (apraxias). Thus the hyperkinetic syndrome in children of normal intelligence is now commonly described as part of a wider disorder of attention, cognition, impulse, and motor control called "minimal brain dysfunction" (m.b.d) (Clements, 1966). As the name implies, the condition is presumed to be organic although the cerebral abnormality has been "softened" from one of structure (damage) to the more elusive one of dysfunction. However, many of the studies cited above are lacking in control groups, either normal or psychopathological, often use questionable or unstated diagnostic techniques, and are anecdotal rather than methodologically exact or quantitative. Thus their findings are open to considerable criticism, particularly that of the degree of deviation from normality and the generality of their findings to all hyperkinetic children. Some of these studies require special comment. Ingram's (1956) hyperkinetic group almost all proved to have frank cerebral palsy and Ounsted's (1955) epilepsy, and hence undisputed major brain disorder. Several of the studies (Ounsted, 1955; Ingram, 1956; Sutherland, 1961) had a significant proportion of mentally retarded children where signs of organicity are to be expected. These findings of major neurological disorder are unusual since the hyperkinetic syndrome is entirely compatible with normal mental and neurological status (e.g., Burks, 1960; Clements & Peters, 1962; Laufer & Denhoff, 1957; Stewart et al., 1966; Werry, et al., 1966). The tendency for British psychiatrists to find an association between the hyperkinetic syndrome and neurological disorder is probably a consequence of the more neurological orientation of child psychiatry in that country, leading to biased sampling. It may be also due in part to differences in diagnostic criteria, notably in the degree of hyperactivity, which could only be resolved by some quantification of activity level (see Werry & Sprague, 1970) such as through direct counts by observers (Doubros & Daniels, 1966; Hutt et al., 1965; Patterson, James, Whittier, & Wright, 1965; Ounsted, 1955; Tizard, 1968; Waldrop, Pedersen, & Bell, 1968; Werry & Quay, 1969) and various devices such as mechanical (Schulman & Reisman, 1959; Bell, 1968), photoelectric (Ellis & Pryer, 1959), ballistographic (Foshee, 1958; Sprague & Toppe, 1966), ultrasonic (McFarland, Peacock, & Watson, 1966), cinematic (Lee & Hutt, 1964), or telemetric techniques (Davis, Sprague, & Werry, 1969; Herron & Ramsden, 1967). (These same techniques would incidently also afford more objective ways of evaluating treatment of hyperactivity.)

In an elegant study using the EEG photometrazol threshold, Laufer, Denhoff, and Solomons (1957) found that a small group of hyperkinetic children, presumably diagnosed according to the widely accepted clinical criteria of Laufer and Denhoff (1957), had a significantly lower mean photometrazol threshold than nonhyperkinetic emotionally disturbed controls. Also, this threshold could be raised to the level of the other group by the use of amphetamine, one of the drugs often used in the treatment of this disorder. Laufer et al. suggested that this electrophysiological abnormality results from a dysfunction of the diencephalon so that the CNS of hyperkinetic children is more readily disorganized. They speculated that this dysfunction probably resulted from early brain injury, but no evidence to this effect was offered, and it could well have been psychophysiologic or reactive, as discussed above. To date this important study has not been replicated.

Several studies (Burks, 1960; Minde et al., 1968; Stevens, Boydstun, Dykman, Peters, & Sinton, 1967; Rogers et al., 1955; Stewart et al., 1966; Werry,

1968; Werry et al., 1964, 1966) have attempted to ascertain whether the historical, neurological, perceptual, cognitive, and EEG correlates of the hyperkinetic syndrome are present to a greater degree than in normal children of similar intelligence. These studies suggest that this is indeed so, although there are some minor contradictions, especially with respect to birth history. Thus Burks (1960) found an excess of pre- and paranatal complications in the histories of hyperkinetic children as compared with a normal control group and a group of retarded readers without the hyperkinetic syndrome. The report by Pasamanick (Rogers et al., 1955) discussed in detail above, also had similar findings.

On the other hand, Stewart et al. (1966) found an excess of speech, coordination, learning, and infantile adjustment (feeding and sleeping) abnormalities in 37 hyperkinetic children (defined symptomatically), but there was no increased frequency of pre- and paranatal abnormalities as compared with a matched control group. The Montreal group (Minde et al., 1968; Werry, 1968; Werry et al., 1964) found significantly more visuomotor, minor neurological, and early infantile adjustment abnormalities, but a slight excess $(p = .10)$ of pre- and paranatal abnormalities in the history of hyperactives as obtained from mothers' histories disappeared when direct inspections were made of hospital records, suggesting that having a disturbed child may selectively influence recall. Minde et al. found significant discrepancies between mothers' histories and the case records though mostly underreporting. Although Burks did find an excess of EEG abnormalities, Werry et al. (1964) found that the only difference between hyperactives and matched normal controls lay in the *kind* of abnormality (slow dysrhythmia), which was inexplicably less serious than the abnormalities found in the normals (epileptiform tracings).

Tizard (1968) studied two groups of severely retarded children, one overactive and one not, matched for IQ. She found that although the hyperactive children had higher locomotion counts in the classroom or, in short, were validly diagnosed as hyperactive, they had few other features of the hyperkinetic syndrome, notably agressiveness, but did have an increased frequency of abnormal histories and major neurological complaints, especially epilepsy. In a good study Waldrop et al. (1968) found hyperactive-aggressive behavior to be somewhat correlated with minor physical anomalies.

Several studies have attempted to examine the relationship between behavioral and various organic indicators through the use of multivariate statistical techniques. Jenkins (1964), using the technique of cluster analysis on clinical records of 3000 children seen at the Institute for Juvenile Research, isolated a behavioral dimension which he called "brain injury" despite the fact that the only item in the cluster that was in any way indicative of brain injury was "question of encephalitis," a diagnosis most likely to be made from behavioral rather than medical examination and/or history (see above). Further, only in girls did this dimension have any features of the hyperkinetic syndrome.

Most of the extensive factor analytic studies of clinical symptomatology in normal, delinquent, and disturbed children (see Chapter One) have not succeeded in isolating a separate hyperkinetic or brain-damage syndrome factor. Instead, the symptoms of the hyperkinetic syndrome emerge as part of a conduct disorder (or, in psychiatric parlance, primary behavior or acting-out disorder).

Dreger (1964), Paine, Werry, and Quay (1968), Rodin et al. (1963), and Werry (1968), using factor analytic techniques, found behavioral, cognitive, neurological, and medical historical variables to emerge in discrete factors, suggesting that certainly as presently measured, various components of the m.b.d. syndrome show little common variance. Schulman et al. (1965) studied the relationship between a number of cognitive, neurological, EEG, and behavioral measures in a group of 37 mildly to moderately retarded boys (IQ 55 to 57). They found a very low degree of interrelatedness between (and very often low reliability in) all variables. In particular, four behavioral symptoms of the brain-damage behavior syndrome, namely hyperactivity, distractibility, inconsistency, and emotional lability, all operationally defined and measured, did not intercorrelate to form a syndrome, and with the exception of distractibility, neither were they related to other indices of brain damage. Schulman et al. concluded that any effects of brain damage are complex and probably depend on the extent and locus of the damage so that the idea of a single "brain-damage syndrome" is invalid.

Thus, empirical studies of clinical symptomatology have thrown considerable doubt on the specificity of hyperkinetic syndrome as apart from behavior disorders in general and have failed to demonstrate clear or invariant relationships between the hyperkinetic syndrome and other so-called "organic" indicators.

Prechtl (1960) has suggested a subtype of the hyperkinetic syndrome associated with a specific neurological sign—pronounced choreiform movements—much more regularly results from brain damage than the hyperkinetic syndrome in general. Since the lower motor neuron is, in Sherrington's terminology, the final common pathway for the expression of a wide variety of higher CNS activities, Prechtl's technique of attempting neurological subclassifications of the hyperkinetic syndrome is laudable. Wolff and Hurwitz (1966) surveyed over 2000 normal school children aged 10 to 15 years and 278 delinquent emotionally disturbed and blind children in the U.S. and Japan for the choreiform sign, which they found could be reliably observed (93% agreement). In confirmation of Prechtl's work they found that the abnormal group had significantly ($p = .01$) higher frequencies of the sign (as high as 47% versus about 12% normals). However, Rutter, Graham, and Birch (1966) found the choreiform sign to be of fairly low reliability and failed to observe any relationship between the choreiform sign on the one hand and behavioral status (as judged by a reliable and valid symptom checklist or standardized psychiatric examination) or complications of pregnancy on the other. Their sample consisted of approximately 250 children with a variety of neurological, educational, and psychiatric abnormalities and a contrast group of 50 normal 9-year-olds. Thus, the validity of Prechtl's subclassification remains unclear.

Graham and her group (Ernhart et al., 1963) have pointed out that it is commonly assumed not only that the hyperkinetic syndrome is necessarily a sign of brain damage, but that it is the *only* behavioral disorder resulting from brain damage (e.g., Bakwin, 1949; Bradley, 1955). This latter hypothesis is not well supported by studies which take brain damage as the independent variable (see above). Although Gallagher (1957) and Prechtl (1960) did find evidence of some specificity, the more usual finding is that when psychopathology occurs in association with brain damage, it may take many forms (e.g., Clements, 1966; Ernhart et al., 1963; Graham et al., 1962; Graham & Rutter, 1968; Harrington & Letemendia, 1958; Pond, 1961).

Summary

Studies of unequivocally brain-damaged children suggest that the hyperkinetic syndrome is neither a necessary nor very frequent occurrence after brain injury. Although there is no unanimity, the majority of studies suggest that the behavior disorder of the hyperkinetic syndrome is associated to a varying extent with certain paranatal, neurological, EEG, and cognitive abnormalities. The relationship between these variables and indeed their very significance is obscure, but they seem to be weakly suggestive of some kind of a cerebral dysfunction, the nature of which is unclear but which may reflect a variety of causes ranging from frank brain damage through normal variation to adverse socio-familial experience.

An extensive argument, based on deprivation studies in animals, for the role of maternal deprivation in producing the hyperkinetic syndrome has been advanced by Prescott (1967).

In the majority of cases where the minimal brain dysfunction syndrome exists it will be impossible to determine accurately which of the three or more etiological factors above is operative. Furthermore, the nosological distinctness of the hyperkinetic syndrome or "organic behavior" disorders from conduct and immaturity disorders has not been well demonstrated. A significant number of children who exhibit some of the behavioral components of the hyperkinetic syndrome probably have no abnormalities in any other areas of function or, in short, have no signs of cerebral dysfunction. In no sense, then, can these behavioral symptoms be taken in themselves as diagnostic of cerebral damage of dysfunction. Careful empirical subclassification of the hyperkinetic syndrome by means of associated neurological, electrophysiological, behavioral and cognitive abnormalities might prove ultimately more heuristic than the present global approach (Clements, 1966, Werry, 1968).

2. Childhood Psychosis

This is discussed in detail in Chapter Five where it is concluded that childhood psychosis appears to be increasingly widely regarded as having an organic component, a thesis that has some highly suggestive but not unequivocal empirical support. The nature of this organic defect and the mechanism whereby it produces the clinical syndrome are the subject of much speculation but at the moment remain quite obscure.

3. Personality (Neurotic) Disorders and Special Symptom Reactions

The search for organic etiologies in these conditions seems to have received much less attention than in childhood psychosis or in the hyperkinetic syndrome. There is some evidence from the EEG findings (Ellingson, 1954; White et al., 1964), neurological examinations (Kennard, 1960), and epidemiological studies (Rogers et al., 1955) that the indices of cerebral dysfunction are less frequent in children with neurotic disorders than in those with the hyperkinetic syndrome or childhood psychosis and probably no more frequent than in normal children. The studies by Eysenck and Prell (1951) on twins of school age suggest that the *predisposition* to neurosis is to a significant extent determined by heredity and hence by organic factors of a subtle nature, although they could probably be better classed as normal variations instead of frank damage or dysfunction.

On the basis of a reported increased prevalence of abnormal EEG's and deeper sleep, as well as the apparent role of heredity in at least some cases, enuresis has been attributed to delayed myelination of the CNS (*British Medical Journal*, 1960). However, when studies are properly controlled, most of the supposed indicators of higher CNS dysfunction disappear (e.g., Boyd, 1960; Vulliamy, 1956; Werry & Cohrssen, 1965) and there is reason to suppose that those which do remain reflect the biased sample of enuretics seen by a physician (Halgren, 1957). The studies by Mueller (1960) suggest that the fairly well-established hereditary influence in enuresis could be expressed in the genito-urinary tract or in the higher CNS (see Chapter Four).

Pasamanick (Pasamanick & Knobloch, 1960) found a correlation between complications of pregnancy and the subsequent development of tics in childhood. Prechtl (1960), in his follow-up studies of children who were neurologically abnormal at birth, reported that a high proportion exhibited choreiform movements, which are often mistaken for tics. However, there are elegant theories of the psychological etiology of tics, which in the case of learning theory, seem supported by the response of tics to treatment (see Chapter Four).

In general then, unequivocal evidence that organic factors are important in the genesis of the neurotic conditions of childhood is lacking though the number of studies is too few to contradict any hypothesis with any degree of certitude.

4. Conduct Disorders

It is almost impossible to discuss this type of disorder separately from the hyperkinetic syndrome since, although the distinction is common evidence that they are indeed separate clinical entities rather than reflections of similar basic behavioral or personality dimensions is lacking (see Chapter One). Indeed, the sole distinguishing criterion appears to be the amount of hyperactivity, which is seldom objectively measured. Oppositional, antisocial, and learning problems are common in both. The findings by Rogers et al. (1955, p. 66) that psychopathology in higher socio-economic groups was more likely to be hyperactive and in lower groups antisocial, suggests that the constituent behaviors in conduct disorders may be more socially than organically determined. Studies of organic factors in conduct disorders separated from the hyperkinetic syndrome appear to be practically nonexistent. EEG studies (Ellingson, 1954; Taterka & Katz, 1955) suggest that the prevalence of abnormalities in the so-called "primary behavior disorder" and the "psychopathic personalities" are high as they are in the hyperkinetic syndrome. In multivariate studies Paine et al. (1960) found no correlation between conduct problem disorder and organic indicators, while Rodin et al. (1963) found a negative relationship. In view of the nosological uncertainty it does not seem possible to make definitive statements about the relationship between conduct disorders and organic factors except that in all probability what has been said about the hyperkinetic syndrome is equally applicable.

Specific Brain-Damage Variables

1. Age of Injury

Ernhart et al. (1963) point out that it is commonly assumed that brain injury early in life is particularly likely to produce the hyperkinetic syndrome despite the fact that there is little evidence to support this contention. While clinical studies (Laufer & Denhoff, 1957; Rodin et al., 1963; Stewart et al., 1966; Werry et al., 1964) suggest that the hyperkinetic syndrome in most cases begins in infancy, it is widely assumed that this condition is negatively correlated with age (Cromwell, Baumeister, & Hawkins, 1963; Rutter, 1965), the motor psychopathology becoming translated into other forms of behavioral or social maladjustment such as rebelliousness, paranoid ideation, delinquency, etc. (Anderson & Plymate, 1962; Menkes, Rowe, & Menkes, 1967; Weiss, Minde, Werry, Douglas, & Nemeth—in press). Thus, the hyperkinetic syndrome probably reflects not so much the age of the child at the time of any brain injury as the age of the child at the time of examination. However, evidence is beginning to accumulate that, as postulated by Hebb (1949, p. 289), the type of cognitive deficit produced by brain damage is influenced by age of injury (Ernhart et al., 1963). Hence it is not unreasonable to expect that if, with improved techniques of personality and behavior measurement, brain damage should be shown unequivocally to produce psychopathology, the age at which the lesion is suffered may also be shown to influence psychopathology—quantitatively or qualitatively.

2. Site of the Lesion

Eisenberg (1957) has presented in detail the experimental neurophysiological evidence which suggests that the site of the lesion should influence consequent behavioral deviance. He notes particularly the role of the cortical suppressor areas, the reticular activating or arousing system, and the emotional expressive circuit or visceral brain involving particularly the temporal lobes. However, the empirical evidence linking particular chronic psychopathological states to cerebral topography is slender and mostly inferential. Laufer and Denhoff (1957) felt that their photometrazol studies implicated the centrencephalic region in the production of hyperkinesis. Rimland (1964) implicated somewhat the same region as the cause of autism, and Kennard (1960) felt that subcortical lesions best explained her findings in a mixed psychopathological group. The affinity of theorists for the subcortical regions may reflect the absence of cortical signs rather than presence of subcortical ones. The effect of the phenothiazine and sympathomimetic amine drugs in the management of the hyperkinetic syndrome (see Chapter Eight), even though the site of their action is subcortical, does not necessarily indicate that there is any abnormality of these regions in hyperkinesis.

Tizard (1962) states that it is widely held that temporal lobe epilepsy is associated with a higher prevalence of psychopathology and with explosive and aggressive behavior in particular, and that this belief is further buttressed by the reported decrease in these behaviors after temporal lobectomy. Most of these studies have grave methodological inadequacies except four—Aird and Yamamoto (1966) found a much higher prevalence of temporal lobe foci in the EEG's of behaviorally disturbed children than in nondisturbed peers with abnormal EEG's. Nuffield (1961) demonstrated a correlation between the location of the epileptogenic focus on the EEG in epileptic children and the frequency with which they exhibited certain behavioral symptoms. The temporal lobe epileptics had higher mean aggressive scores whereas the group with classical petit mal pattern (centrencephalic focus) had higher mean neurotic scores. Graham and Rutter (1968) found temporal lobe epileptics to have the highest prevalence of psychopathology. The study of children with temporal lobe epilepsy by Ounsted et al. (1966) discussed above found the frequency of the hyperkinetic syndrome to be higher than in other epileptics but still to occur only in a minority (24%). The longitudinal studies by Slater (Slater & Beard, 1963) in adults suggest that temporal lobe epileptics may be more prone to develop paranoid schizophrenia, but interestingly only after their seizures have ceased.

Summary

The role of site of the lesion in influencing both general and specific psychopathology seems supported more by neurophysiological theory than by sound clinical observation.

3. Etiology

Despite attempts that have been made to relate specific types of psychopathology to specific etiological conditions such as the epileptic personality (see Tizard, 1962) or postencephalitic behavior disorders (Levy, 1959; Mayer-Gross et al., 1960, p. 446) as was already discussed, there is really little evidence to support these contentions. What there is could probably be more heuristically interpreted in terms of the topographical location of the lesion instead of its etiological nature.

4. Sex

Most of the studies of "organic behavior disorders" report a significant excess of boys (e.g., Ounsted, 1955; Stewart et al., 1966; Strecker, 1929; Werry, 1968). While there is an apparently greater vulnerability of males to neonatal insults as adjudged by perinatal mortality rates (Butler & Bonham, 1963, p. 133), it remains to be demonstrated that this excess of hyperkinetic boys reflects a brain damage instead of a cultural or biological sex effect of more pronounced aggressiveness in males leading to higher referral rates. Conversely, since most of the symptoms of the hyperkinetic syndrome are of the aggressive or conduct-problem kind, boys would be more prone to receive an "organic" diagnosis. It is of interest to note that in their population study, Graham and Rutter (1968) found rates of disturbance in neurologically impaired children to be equal in the two sexes supporting the selective referral hypothesis.

5. Organic Indicators and Treatment

This is somewhat outside the main thrust of this review and so will be discussed only briefly. A diagnosis of "organicity" is often held adversely to influence treatment and outcome in psychopathological states. In one of the few careful studies of this Eisenberg (Eisenberg, 1966; Eisenberg, Gilbert, Cytryn, & Molling, 1961) found that, unlike neurotic children, hyperkinetic children were refractory to brief psychotherapy and responded better to stimulant drugs. Although this may be true of verbal techniques, recent studies in behavior therapy have shown that hyperkinetic children respond to the principles of social learning theory in the same way as do normal children (Doubros and Daniels, 1966; Hall and Broden, 1967; Patterson et al., 1965; see also Chapter Seven). In a behaviorally engineered classroom hyperactive aggressive children can be made to exhibit classroom behavior (notably attention) similar to that of normal children (Werry & Quay, 1969). This would suggest that a more pragmatic behavioral approach to so-called minimally brain-injured children is preferable to neurologically derived concepts. Long-term outcome is discussed in Chapter Eleven. Although the prognosis for hyperactivity is good, that for academic achievement and social adjustment is poor (Menkes et al., 1967; Weiss et al.—in press).

Conclusions

This discussion of clinical studies on the relationship between abnormal cerebral status and the psychopathology of childhood may now be summarized.

1. There is little evidence to suggest that brain damage or dysfunction is either necessarily, or indeed even frequently, accompanied by psychopathology. When brain damage or dysfunction is accompanied by psychopathology there is no good evidence that it necessarily or even commonly takes a specific form such as the hyperkinetic syndrome. In fact, there is reason to doubt the existence of the hyperkinetic syndrome as independent from conduct disorder and immaturity. The age of injury and site of the brain damage or dysfunction have strong *theoretical* but little *empirical* support (because of the lack of studies) as potentially important variables in determining specificity of psychopathological symptoms. In the present state of knowledge it seems that etiology of the cerebral abnormality is unlikely to have effects that cannot be more heuristically conceptualized in terms of such

variables as site, age of onset, rate of development, and constancy of the cerebral lesion or dysfunction.

2.   There is no support for the idea that all psychopathological conditions are organically determined or that certain behavioral symptom-complexes (with the exception of acute brain syndromes or dementias) always reflect brain damage or dysfunction. There is, however, some indication that certain behavioral symptoms such as hyperactivity and distractibility, or certain patterns such as the hyperkinetic syndrome, childhood psychosis, or conduct disorders tend to be associated more frequently with slight neurological, electrophysiological, perceptual, cognitive, and motor signs of impaired higher CNS integration than in normal children. There is no evidence that these concomitants are valid indices of brain damage and they may in some instances be experientially determined (Prescott, 1967). Even if physically determined they may represent normal biological variants instead of frank abnormalities of structure or function. There is some conflicting evidence to suggest that children with these symptoms or patterns may more often have a history of complications of the pre- and perinatal period than do normal children. However, these differences are small quantitatively, and the frequency with which these complications result in significant cerebral damage is probably low. Further, these complications are highly correlated with social pathology, which is itself a cause of behavior disorders. Thus, the purported excess of pre- and perinatal complications cannot be inferred to imply brain damage as an etiological agent. It is not yet clear whether these findings of cerebral dysfunction are indeed peculiar to the hyperkinetic syndrome or whether they are a feature of psychopathology per se since studies comparing the supposedly non-organic psychopathological conditions such as neurotic or conduct disorders are few and inconclusive.

3.   Most of the studies examining the relationship between brain damage and behavior in children are methodologically grossly inadequate. Little progress is likely to be made in this area until (a) more careful attention is paid to the development of reliable and valid ways of establishing the diagnosis of brain damage or dysfunction not only globally but more importantly in terms of neuroanatomical locus and neurophysiological function; (b) measures of psychopathology are greatly improved not only in terms of reliability and validity which they presently often lack, but also in their ability to be quantified and to be recast within the framework of the basic processes by which behavior is learned and unlearned. When this framework of social learning is used, subtle quantitative instead of qualitative effects of brain damage on behavior may become apparent with important therapeutic implications. Thus, for example, brain damage in certain regions may be found to increase the probability of occurrence of certain behaviors, alter the rate at which learning occurs, or the responsivity to certain types or schedules of reinforcement; (c) adequate ex-

perimental designs such as the use of quantitative analyses, inferential statistical interpretations of results, and proper control of experimental variables are more widely used; (d) proper attention is given to studies comparing diagnostically different disorders such as the hyperkinetic syndrome and neurotic disorders.

4. On the basis of present evidence, it seems most reasonable to conclude that brain damage or dysfunction is simply one of several variables such as temperamental proclivity, familial, social, and educational experiences that interact in a complex multivariate fashion in determining personality and behavior. In this interaction brain damage appears in the vast majority of instances to be a variable of relatively weak effect, the action of which is further complicated by its psychological as well as its physiological impact.

5. In the present state of knowledge, the diagnosis of brain damage appears to have little significance in the treatment situation. Techniques aimed at explicating abnormalities and deficits of behavior and their functional relationships to environmental stimuli or events are likely to prove much more fruitful in planning therapeutic programs than speculations about brain function. Certainly this will remain so until it can be shown how particular disturbances of brain function will influence the remediation of particular behavioral problems.

References

Aird, R., & Yamamoto, T. Behavior disorders of childhood. *Electroencephalography and clinical neurophysiology*, 1966, **21**, 148–156.

Anderson, C., & Plymate, H. Management of the brain-damaged adolescent. *American Journal of Orthopsychiatry*, 1962, **32**, 492–500.

Anderson, W. The hyperkinetic child: A neurological appraisal. *Neurology*, 1963, **13**, 968–973.

Bakwin, H. Cerebral damage and behavior disorders in children. *Pediatrics*, 1949, **35**, 271–382.

Bell, R. Adaptation of small wrist watches for mechanical recording of activity in infants and children. *Journal of Experimental Child Psychology*, 1968, **6**, 302–305.

Bender, L. *Psychopathology of children with organic brain diseases.* Springfield, Ill.: Charles C Thomas, 1959, pp. 114–138.

Benton, A. Behavioral indices of brain injury in school children. *Child Development*, 1962, **33**, 199–208.

Birch, H. *Brain damage in children: The biological and social aspects.* Baltimore: Williams and Wilkins Co., 1964, pp. 3–11, 134.

Blau, A. Exposure and defenses of the brain of the normal newborn infant to trauma. *Archives of Neurology and Psychiatry*, 1938, **39**, 197.

Blau, A. The psychiatric approach to posttraumatic and postencephalitic syndromes. In R. McIntosh (Ed.), "Neurology and Psychiatry in Childhood." *Proceedings of the Association for Research in Nervous & Mental Diseases.* Baltimore: Williams and Wilkins Co., 1954, Vol. 34, pp. 404–423.

Bower, E. *Early identification of emotionally handicapped children in school.* Springfield, Ill.: Charles C. Thomas, 1960, pp. 21–28.

Boyd, M. The depth of sleep in enuretic school children and in non-enuretic controls. *Journal of Psychosomatic Research*, 1960, **4**, 274–281.

Bradley, C. Organic factors in the psychopathology of childhood. In P. Hoch and J. Zubin (Eds.), *Psychopathology of Childhood.* New York: Grune and Stratton, 1955.

British Medical Journal, Enuresis (Editorial), 1960, **2**, 1416–1417.

Burks, H. The hyperkinetic child. *Exceptional Children*, 1960, **27**, 18–26.

Butler, N., & Bonham, D. *Perinatal mortality.* Edinburgh: E. & S. Livingstone, Ltd., 1963.

Caplan, H., Bibace, R., & Rabinovitch, M. Paranatal stress, cognitive organization and ego function: A controlled follow-up study of children born prematurely. *Journal of the American Academy of Child Psychiatry,* 1963, **2**, 434–450.

Chess, S., Thomas, A., Rutter, M., & Birch, H. Interaction of temperament and environment in the production of behavioral disturbances in children. *American Journal of Psychiatry,* 1963, **120**, 142–147.

Clements, S. *Minimal brain dysfunction in children.* NINDB Monograph #3. Washington, D.C.: U.S. Public Health Service, 1966.

Clements, S., & Peters, J. Minimal brain dysfunction in the school-age child. *Archives of General Psychiatry,* 1962, **6**, 185–197.

Cramblett, H., Stegmiller, H., & Spencer, C. California encephalitis virus infections in children. *Journal of the American Medical Association,* 1966, **198**, 128–132.

Cromwell, R., Baumeister, A., & Hawkins, W. Research in activity level. In N. Ellis (Ed.), *Handbook of mental deficiency.* New York: McGraw-Hill, 1963, pp. 632–663.

Cruickshank, W., & Bice, H. In W. Cruickshank, (Ed.), *Cerebral palsy: Its individual and community problems.* (2nd ed.) Syracuse, N.Y.: Syracuse University Press, 1966.

Davis, K., Sprague, R., & Werry, J. Stereotyped behavior and activity level in severe retardates: The effect of drugs. *American Journal of Mental Deficiency,* 1969, **73**, 721–727.

Demerdash, A., Eeg-Olofsson, O., & Petersen, I. The incidence of 14 and 6 per second positive spikes in a population of normal children. *Developmental Medicine and Child Neurology,* 1968, **10**, 309–316.

Dencker, S. A follow-up study of 128 closed head injuries in twins using co-twins as controls. *Acta Psychiatrica et Neurologica Scandinavica,* 1958, **33**, Supp. 123.

Doubros, S., & Daniels, G. An experimental approach to the reduction of overactive behavior. *Behaviour Research and Therapy,* 1966, **4**, 251–258.

Dreger, R. A progress report on a factor analytic approach to classification in child psychiatry. In R. Jenkins and J. Cole (Eds.), *Research Report No. 18.* Washington, D.C.: American Psychiatric Association, 1964.

Ebaugh, F. Neuropsychiatric sequelae of acute epidemic encephalitis in children. *American Journal of Diseases in Children,* 1923, **25**, 89–97.

Eisenberg, L. Psychiatric implications of brain damage in children. *Psychiatric Quarterly,* 1957, **31**, 72–92.

Eisenberg, L. The management of the hyperactive child. *Developmental Medicine and Child Neurology,* 1966, **8**, 593–598.

Eisenberg, L., Gilbert, A., Cytryn, L., & Molling, P. The effectiveness of psychotherapy alone and in conjunction with perphenazine or placebo in the treatment of neurotic and hyperkinetic children. *American Journal of Psychiatry,* 1961, **117**, 1088–1093.

Ellingson, R. The incidence of EEG abnormality among patients with mental disorders of apparently nonorganic origin: A critical review. *American Journal of Psychiatry,* 1954, **111,** 263–275.

Ellis, N., & Pryer, R. Quantification of gross bodily activity in children with severe neuropathology. *American Journal of Mental Deficiency,* 1959, **63,** 1034–1037.

Ernhart, C., Graham, F., Eichman, P., Marshall, J., & Thurston, D. Brain injury in the preschool child: Some developmental considerations: II. Comparison of brain injured and normal children. *Psychological Monographs,* 1963, **77,** 17–33.

Eysenck, H., & Prell, D. The inheritance of neuroticism: An experimental study. *Journal of Mental Science,* 1951, **98,** 441–465.

Fish, B. The study of motor development in infancy and its relationship to psychological functioning. *American Journal of Psychiatry,* 1961, **117,** 1113–1118.

Foshee, J. Studies in activity level: I. Simple and complex task performance in defectives. *American Journal of Mental Deficiency,* 1958, **62,** 882–886.

Fraser, M., & Wilks, J. The residual effects of neonatal asphyxia. *Journal of Obstetrics & Gynaecology of the British Empire,* 1959, **66,** 748–752.

Freeman, R. Special education and the EEG: Marriage of convenience. *Journal of Special Education,* 1967, **2,** 61–73.

Gallagher, J. A comparison of brain injured and non-brain injured mentally retarded children on several psychological variables. *Society for Research in Child Development,* Monograph No. 65, **22,** No. 2, 1957.

Gibbs, F., Gibbs, E., Spies, H., & Carpenter, P. Common types of childhood encephalitis. *Archives of Neurology,* 1964, **10,** 1–11.

Graham, F., & Berman, P. Current status of behavior tests for brain damage in infants and preschool children. *American Journal of Orthopsychiatry,* 1961, **4,** 713–727.

Graham, F., Ernhart, C., Thurston, D., & Craft, M. Development three years after perinatal anoxia and other potentially damaging newborn experiences. *Psychological Monographs,* 1962, **76,** 1–53.

Graham, P., & Rutter, M. Organic brain dysfunction and child psychiatric disorder. *British Medical Journal,* 1968, **3,** 695–700.

Halgren, B. Enuresis—A clinical and genetic study. *Acta Psychiatrica et Neurologica Scandinavica,* 1957, **32.** Supp. No. 114.

Hall, R., & Broden, M. Behavior changes in brain-injured children through social reinforcement. *Journal of Experimental Child Psychology,* 1967, **5,** 463–479.

Harrington, J., & Letemendia, F. Persistent psychiatric disorder after head injury in children. *Journal of Mental Science,* 1958, **104,** 1205–1218.

Hebb, D. *The Organization of behavior: A neuropsychological theory.* New York: Wiley, 1949.

Herbert, M. The concept and testing of brain-damage in children: A review. *Journal of Child Psychology and Psychiatry,* 1964, **5,** 197–216.

Herron, R., & Ramsden, R. Continuous monitoring of overt human body movement by radio telemetry: A brief review. *Perceptual Motor Skills,* 1967, **24,** 1303–1308.

Hertzig, M., & Birch, H. Neurological organization in psychiatrically disturbed adolescents. *Archives of General Psychiatry,* 1968, **19,** 528–537.

Hertzig, M., Bortner, M., & Birch, H. Neurologic findings in children educationally designated as "brain damaged." *American Journal of Orthopsychiatry,* 1969, **39**, 437–466.

Hutt, C., Hutt, S., & Ounsted, C. The behavior of children with and without upper CNS lesions. *Behavior,* 1964, **24**, 246–268.

Ingram, T. A characteristic form of overactive behaviour in brain damaged children. *Journal of Mental Science,* 1956, **102**, 550–558.

Jenkins, R. Diagnoses, dynamics and treatment in child psychiatry. *Research Report No. 18.,* R. Jenkins and J. Cole (Eds.), 1964, 91–120. Washington, D.C.: American Psychiatric Association.

Kellaway, P., Crawley, J., & Maulsby, R. The electroencephalogram in psychiatric disorders in childhood. In W. Wilson (Ed.), *Applications of Electroencephalography in Psychiatry.* Durham, N.C.: Duke University Press, 1965, pp. 30–53.

Kennard, M. Value of equivocal signs in neurologic diagnosis. *Neurology,* 1960, **10**, 753–764.

Kennedy, R. Prognosis of sequelae of epidemic encephalitis in children. *American Journal of Diseases in Children,* 1924, **28**, 158–172.

Kety, S. Biochemical theories of schizophrenia. *International Journal of Psychiatry,* 1965, **1**, 409–446.

Kløve, H. Clinical neuropsychology. *The Medical Clinics of North America,* 1963, **47**, 1647–1658.

Knights, R., & Watson, P. The use of computer test profiles in neuropsychological assessment. *Journal of Learning Disabilities,* in press.

Knobloch, H., & Pasamanick, B. The developmental behavior approach to the neurologic examination in infancy. *Child Development,* 1962, **33**, 181–198.

Laufer, M., & Denhoff, E. Hyperkinetic behavior syndrome in children. *Journal of Pediatrics,* 1957, **50**, 463–474.

Laufer, M., Denhoff, E., & Solomons, G. Hyperkinetic impulse disorder in children's behavior problems. *Psychosomatic Medicine,* 1957, **19**, 38–49.

Lee, D., & Hutt, C. A play-room designed for filming children: A note. *Journal of Child Psychology and Psychiatry,* 1964, **5**, 263–265.

Lennox, G., & Lennox, M. *Epilepsy and Related Disorders.* Boston: Little, Brown and Co., 1960. Vol. 2, pp. 659–699.

Levy, S. Post-encephalitic behavior disorder—A forgotten entity: A report of 100 cases. *American Journal of Psychiatry,* 1959, 115, 1062–1067.

Lucas, A., Rodin, E., & Simson, C. Neurological assessment of children with early school problems. *Developmental Medicine and Child Neurology,* 1965, **7**, 145–156.

Mayer-Gross, W., Slater, E., & Roth, M. *Clinical Psychiatry.* London: Cassell and Co., Ltd., 1960, p. 446.

McFarland, J., Peacock, L., & Watson, J. Mental retardation and activity level in rats and children. *American Journal of Mental Deficiency,* 1966, **71**, 381–386.

Menkes, M., Rowe, J., & Menkes, J. A twenty-five year follow-up study on the hyperkinetic child with minimal brain dysfunction. *Pediatrics,* 1967, **39**, 393–399.

Meyer, V. Psychological effects of brain damage. In H. J. Eysenck (Ed.), *Handbook of Abnormal Psychology*. New York: Basic Books, 1961.

Minde, K., Webb, G., & Sykes, D. Studies on the hyperactive child VI: Prenatal and paranatal factors associated with hyperactivity. *Developmental Medicine and Child Neurology*, 1968, **10**, 355–363.

Mueller, R. Development of urinary control in children: A new concept in cause, prevention and treatment of primary enuresis. *Journal of Urology*, 1960, **84**, 714–716.

Nuffield, E. Neuro-physiology and behaviour disorders in epileptic children. *The Journal of Mental Science*, 1961, **107**, 438–458.

Ounsted, C. The hyperkinetic syndrome in epileptic children. *Lancet*, 1955, **269**, 303–311.

Ounsted, C., Lindsay, J., & Norman, R. *Biological factors in temporal lobe epilepsy.* London: William Heinemann Medical Books, 1966.

Ozer, M. N. The neurological evaluation of school-age children. *Journal of Learning Disabilities*, 1968, **1**, 84–87.

Paine, R., Werry, J., & Quay, H. A study of "Minimal Cerebral Dysfunction." *Developmental Medicine and Child Neurology*, 1968, **10**, 505–520.

Pasamanick, B., Rogers, M., & Lilienfeld, A. Pregnancy experience and the development of behavior disorder in children. *American Journal of Psychiatry*, 1956, **112**, 613–619.

Pasamanick, B., & Knobloch, H. Brain damage and reproductive casualty. *American Journal of Orthopsychiatry*, 1960, **30**, 298–305.

Patterson, G., James, R., Whitter, J., & Wright, M. A behaviour modification technique for the hyperactive child. *Behaviour Research and Therapy*, 1965, **2**, 217–226.

Pond, D. Psychiatric aspects of epileptic and brain-damaged children. *British Medical Journal*, 1961, **2**, 1377–1382, 1454–1459.

Prechtl, H. The long term value of the neurological examination of the newborn infant. *Developmental Medicine and Child Neurology*, 1960, **2**, 69–74.

Prechtl, H., & Dijkstra, J. Neurological diagnosis of cerebral injury in the newborn. In B. tenBerge (Ed.), *Prenatal Care*. Groningen, Netherlands: Noordhoff, 1960.

Prescott, J. Central nervous system functioning in altered sensory environment. In M. Appley and R. Trumball (Eds.), *Psychological Stress*. New York: Appleton-Century-Crofts, 1967, pp. 113–120.

Quay, H., & Peterson, D. Manual for the behavior problem checklist. University of Illinois, Urbana, Illinois (mimeo), 1967.

Reitan, R. A research program on the psychological effects of brain lesions in human beings. In N. Ellis (Ed.), *International Review of Research in Mental Retardation*. New York: Academic Press, 1966.

Reitan, R., & Heineman, C. Interactions of neurological deficits and emotional disturbances in children with learning disorders: Methods for differential assessment. In J. Hellmuth, *Learning Disorders*, Vol. 3. Seattle: Special Child Publications, 1968, pp. 93–136.

Rimland, B. *Infantile Autism*. New York: Appleton-Century-Crofts, 1964.

Robinson, H., & Robinson, N. *The Mentally Retarded Child.* New York: McGraw-Hill, 1965, pp. 148–150.

Rodin, E., Lucas, A., & Simson, C. A study of behavior disorders in children by means of general purpose computers. In *Proceedings of the Conference on Data Acquisition and Processing in Biology and Medicine.* New York: Pergamon, 1963, pp. 115–124.

Rogers, M., Lilienfeld, A., & Pasamanick, B. Pre and Para-natal factors in the development of childhood behavior disorders. *Acta Neurologica et Psychiatrica Scandinavica,* 1955, 56–66. Supp. 102.

Rutter, M. The influence of organic and emotional factors on the origins, nature and outcome of childhood psychosis. *Developmental Medicine and Child Neurology,* 1965, **7**, 518–528.

Rutter, M., Graham, P., & Birch, H. Interrelations between the choreiform syndrome, reading disability and psychiatric disorder in children of 8–11 years. *Developmental Medicine and Child Neurology,* 1966, 8, 149–159.

Sabatino, D., & Cramblett, H. Behavioral sequelae of California encephalitis virus infection in children. *Developmental Medicine and Child Neurology,* 1968, **10**, 331–337.

Sarason, S. *Psychological Problems in Mental Deficiency.* New York: Harper, 1949, pp. 52–58.

Schachter, F., & Apgar, V. Perinatal asphyxia and psychological signs of brain damage in childhood, *Pediatrics,* 1959, **24**, 1016–1025.

Schrager, J., Lindy, J., Harrison, S., McDermott, J., & Killins, E. The hyperkinetic child: Some consensually validated behavioral correlates. *Exceptional Children,* 1966, *32*, 635–637.

Schulman, J., Kaspar, J., & Throne, F. *Brain damage and behavior: A Clinical-Experimental Study.* Springfield, Ill.: Charles C Thomas, 1965.

Schulman, J., & Reisman, J. An objective measure of hyperactivity. *American Journal of Mental Deficiency,* 1959, **64**, 455–456.

Slater, E., & Beard, A. The schizophrenic-like psychoses of epilepsy. *British Journal of Psychiatry,* 1963, **109**, 95–150.

Sprague, R., & Toppe, L. Relationship between activity level and delay of reinforcement in the retarded. *Journal of Experimental Child Psychology,* 1966, 3, 390–397.

Stevens, D., Boydstun, J., Dykman, R., Peters, J., & Sinton, E. Presumed minimal brain dysfunction in children. *Archives of General Psychiatry,* 1967, **16**, 281–285.

Stewart, M., Pitts, F., Craig, A., & Dieruf, W. The hyperactive child syndrome. *American Journal of Orthopsychiatry,* 1966, **36**, 861–867.

Strauss, A., & Lehtinen, L. *Psychopathology and Education of the Brain-Injured Child.* New York: Grune and Stratton, 1947.

Strecker, E. Behavior problems in encephalitis. *Archives of Neurology and Psychiatry,* 1929, **21**, 137–144.

Strecker, E., & Ebaugh, F. Neuropsychiatric sequelae of cerebral trauma in children. *Archives of Neurology and Psychiatry,* 1924, **12**, 443–453.

Sutherland, I. Study of a hyperkinetic syndrome and resultant social disability in childhood. In *Proceedings of Third World Congress of Psychiatry*, Montreal, 1961, 724–725. (Abstract)

Taterka, J., & Katz, J. Study of correlations between electroencephalographic and psychological patterns in emotionally disturbed children. *Psychosomatic Medicine*, 1955, **17**, 62–72.

Teuber, H. The premorbid personality and reaction to brain damage. *American Journal of Orthopsychiatry*, 1960, **30**, 322–327.

Tizard, B. The personality of epileptics: A discussion of the evidence. *Psychological Bulletin*, 1962, **59**, 196–210.

Tizard, B. Observations of over-active imbecile children in controlled and uncontrolled environments. I: Classroom studies. *American Journal of Mental Deficiency*, 1968, **32**, 540–546.

Ucko, L. A comparative study of asphyxiated and non-asphyxiated boys from birth to five years. *Developmental Medicine and Child Neurology*, 1965, **7**, 643–657.

Vulliamy, D. The day and night output of urine in enuresis. *Archives of Diseases in Childhood*, 1956, **31**, 439–443.

Waldrop, M., Pedersen, F., & Bell, R. Minor physical anomalies and behavior in preschool children. *Child Development*, 1968, **39**, 391–400.

Weiss, G., Minde, K., Werry, J., Douglas, V., & Nemeth, E. Studies on the hyperactive child VIII. Five year follow up. *Archives of General Psychiatry*—in press.

Wenar, C. The reliability of developmental histories: Summary and evaluation of evidence. *Psychosomatic Medicine*, 1963, **25**, 505–509.

Werry, J. Studies on the hyperactive child IV. An empirical analysis of the minimal brain dysfunction syndrome. *Archives of General Psychiatry*, 1968, **19**, 9–16.

Werry, J., & Cohrssen, J. Enuresis—An etiological and therapeutic study. *Journal of Pediatrics*, 1965, **67**, 423–431.

Werry, J., Weiss, G., & Douglas, V. Studies on the hyperactive child I. Some preliminary findings. *Canadian Psychiatric Association Journal*, 1964, **9**, 120–130.

Werry, J., Weiss, G., Douglas, V., & Martin, J. Studies on the hyperactive child III. The effect of chlorpromazine upon behavior and learning. *Journal of the American Academy of Child Psychiatry*, 1966, **5**, 292–312.

Werry, J., & Sprague, R. Hyperactivity. In C. Costello (Ed.), *Symptoms of Psychopathology*. New York: Wiley. 1970, 397–417.

Werry, J., & Quay, H. Observing the classroom behavior of elementary school children. *Exceptional Children*, 1969, **35**, 461–470.

Wiener, G. Psychologic correlates of premature birth: A review. *Journal of Nervous and Mental Disease*, 1962, **134**, 129–144.

Wiener, J., Delano, J., & Klass, D. An EEG study of delinquent and nondelinquent adolescents. *Archives of General Psychiatry*, 1966, **15**, 144–150.

White, P., deMyer, W., & deMyer, M. EEG abnormalities in early childhood schizophrenia: A double-blind study of psychiatrically disturbed and normal children during promazine sedation. *American Journal of Psychiatry*, 1964, **120**, 950–958.

Wolff, P., & Hurwitz, I. The choreiform syndrome. *Developmental Medicine and Child Neurology,* 1966, **4,** 160–165.

Wolff, S. The contribution of obstetric complications to the etiology of behaviour disorders in childhood. *Journal of Child Psychology and Psychiatry,* 1967a, **8,** 57–66.

Wolff, S. Behavioural characteristics of primary school children referred to a psychiatric department. *British Journal of Psychiatry,* 1967b, **113,** 885–893.

Chapter Four

Psychosomatic Disorders (with a note on anesthesia, surgery, and hospitalization)

John S. Werry

Introduction

Definition

Psychosomatic or psychophysiologic disorders are defined as <u>physical illnesses that are of proven or presumed psychogenic origin</u> (American Psychiatric Association, 1968).

Theories of Psychosomatic Disease

A full discussion of this complex topic is not possible here and comprehensive reviews may be found in Engel (1962), Kaplan and Kaplan (1959), Mendelson, Hirsh, and Webber (1956), Sternbach (1966), and Ullmann and Krasner (1969), the first three being concerned with more traditional points of view and the latter with the newer approaches of psychophysiology and social learning. For our purpose it is sufficient to note some of the main features of current theories.

Depending on how psychogenic variables are viewed, <u>theories may be classified as *specific* or *nonspecific*</u> (Kaplan & Kaplan, 1959). Specific theories posit that the etiological variables in the form of personality, psychodynamic conflict, or mood state are specific for that disorder and are always found in individuals with it (Alexander, 1950; Engel, 1962). Nonspecific theories (Wolff, 1950) view the psychogenic factors as varying not only from individual to individual but even in the same individual at different times, although generally all these disparate idiosyncratic factors are reducible to the common denominator of stress.

Thus, in specific theories the particular disease is determined by the psychological pattern; in nonspecific theories the disease is determined by each individual's own particular physiological vulnerability to stress, the breakdown organ or point of least resistance being a matter of heredity or sensitization through previous physical disease or autonomic conditioning (Malmo, 1957; 1959; Sternbach, 1962; Ullmann and Krasner, 1969; Wolff, 1950).

Specific theories that are mostly psychoanalytic in nature have lost ground in the past two decades as empirical tests have failed to support theoretical overelaboration (Kaplan & Kaplan, 1958; Mendelson et al., 1956; Prugh, 1963). This has resulted in a shift toward narrowing the scope of the psychogenic variables from personality to conflict to mood (Alexander, 1950; Engel, 1962) and toward decreasing emphasis on rigid specificity (e.g., Engel, 1962). However, the majority of investigations still being done with children show little evidence of this theoretical shift.

All theories assume that the psychological variables are aversive or result in unpleasant affect (which may, however, be repressed or otherwise rendered unconscious) and that tissue damage results from the inappropriate, overfrequent, or exaggerated elicitation of normally adaptive psychophysiological mechanisms. Understanding of these mechanisms continues to advance through continuation of Cannon's pioneering work on the physiology of emotion by such investigators as Selye and Engel (see Engel, 1962) and of Pavlov's studies of autonomic conditioning in the relatively new branch of psychology, psychophysiology (Sternbach, 1966). However, much remains unknown, particularly about the beginnings of the actual disease process or when psychophysiology becomes pathophysiology.

Studies in Children

Most of the studies on psychosomatic disorders in childhood have concentrated their effort first on attempting to show that psychological factors are indeed causal and second on describing the nature and source of the psychogenic agent. Techniques of demonstrating causality are mostly correlative; that is, an effort is made to show that the psychological factors are either invariably or highly probably associated with the disease. Since children are assumed to be most responsive in their formative years to the influence of their parents, proof of this association is often shifted from child to parent, especially the mother. Sometimes this association is sought in specific events presumed to be traumatic (such as coercive toilet training) rather than persons, but in the main, focus has been on demonstrating the coexistence of psychopathology in child (and/or parent) with physical disease.

Because of the predominance in child psychiatry of psychoanalytic theory with its strong emphasis on the roots of psychopathology in early life, demonstration that the psychopathology stands in an antecedent relationship to the disease is seldom considered necessary—proof of coexistence is quite incorrectly assumed to be proof of causality. Effects of the disease on the child and coincidental relationships of disease and psychopathology [which is, after all, quite common in children (Bower, 1960)] are seldom considered. This problem of establishing causal relationship between physical symptoms and psychological state has been discussed in more detail in Chapter Three.

The nature of extant studies has thus forced considerable constraint on the scope and substance of the reviews below in that they mostly devolve into an examination of whether correlation has been proven and if so, whether it is invariant as it should be if the condition is exclusively psychosomatic.

It is hoped that despite these constraints the review will have value in putting certain current mythologies to rest and pointing the way to more profitable lines of investigation. Since the studies of the individual psychosomatic disorders have a certain repetitiousness of theoretical content, execution, and errors of logic and methodology, one or two conditions such as asthma have been examined in more detail and are presented first. Other conditions such as peptic ulcer and headache have not been discussed at all largely because there were few if any studies and even fewer good enough to merit examination.

At the end of the section on psychosomatic conditions is a review of the effect of hospitalization and its associated procedures on children, since this is an important area and is not covered elsewhere. Again, coverage is not complete but the nidus of knowledge necessary to extrapolate to missing areas such as the effect of specific physical illnesses is present.

Asthma

Definition

Asthma is a disorder of the respiratory system marked by paroxysms of difficulty in breathing, particularly in expiration, resulting from an episodic narrowing of the bronchioles. It is basically a localized overreaction of the parasympathetic nervous system and is hence often treated medically by sympathomimetic drugs such as epinephrine. A recent and more detailed review of the psychosomatic aspects of asthma can be found in Purcell and Weiss (1970).

Occurrence

Asthma occurs with a frequency of about 2% in the child population (Graham, Rutter, Yule, & Pless, 1967). It is said to be more common in children than adults (Apley & McKeith, 1962, p. 29), and in boys than girls (Purcell, 1965; Graham et al., 1967).

Etiology

Asthma is usually classified with the allergic disorders, a class of diseases often regarded as strongly psychosomatic. Etiological factors in an allergic disorder may be thought of as *primary*, or those that create the pathological condition initially (and which, of course, may continue to operate), and *secondary*, or those precipitating attacks when the allergic sensitization is once established. There are three broad classes of potential primary and secondary etiological agents (Rees, 1964): (a) allergens such as dust (e.g., Carroll, 1968), (b) infection of the respiratory tract, and (c) psychological variables (Rees, 1964). They are assigned differing importance by different investigators and specialists, but only the psychological variables will be discussed in detail in this review.

Psychological etiological theories have been summarized and critically reviewed by a number of investigators (Dubo, McLean, Ching, Wright, Kauffman, & Sheldon, 1961; Herbert, 1965; Purcell, 1965; Purcell & Weiss, 1970). Specific theories posit (a) a personality type most commonly according to Herbert (1965), the anxious-dependent personality characterized additionally by an inability to express emotions, especially aggression and grief and (b) a specific conflict most notably in the hypothesis of French and Alexander (1941) that asthma symbolizes a suppressed cry for help, its roots lying in infantile suppression of separation anxiety feelings because of fear of maternal retaliation.

Nonspecific theories are represented by Rees (1964) who, in a fashion customary of such theorists (see section on tics) sees all psychological variables reducible to the common denominator of their incremental effect on the child's anxiety level. This, by some nonspecific psychophysiological concomitant, precipitates the asthmatic attack. It should be noted, however, that Rees does not believe anxiety to be the *only* or even often the primary cause of asthma. Learning theory explanations of the pathogenesis of asthma (see Ullmann & Krasner, 1969, pp. 346–347), although nonspecific, may be primary or secondary, classical or operant. Classical (Franks & Leigh, 1959) theorists see the link between the eliciting stimuli and asthma as accidental and purposeless as typified in the many anecdotal stories of attacks being precipitated by flowers and then pictures of flowers, while operant explanations (Purcell, Turnbull, & Bernstein, 1962) see stimulus and response functionally linked in an escape-avoidance situation. It is interesting to note that despite their hostility to each other, psychoanalytic and operant learning theories of asthma have a common conceptual core centering on the usefulness of the response to the child—principally relief of anxiety. Differences lie mainly in the degree to which stimuli and responses are perceived as literal or symbolic.

There are derivatives of these etiological theories that should enable some empirical testing of their validity at least in an indirect way. Thus, the specific personality theory posits that all asthmatics would have similar profiles and that these profiles should be more common in asthmatics than controls. French and Alexander's conflict theory would predict that asthmatics would be less able to express grief or anxiety (see Purcell, 1965). The nonspecific theory of Rees should demonstrate the covariance of asthma and the state of arousal independent of its source of elicitation. The learning theory explanations would predict that certain psychological stimuli peculiar to each individual asthmatic would precipitate attacks and that conditioning-extinction procedures could strengthen and weaken the power of eliciting stimuli and of the asthmatic response. Purcell (1965) and Purcell and Weiss (1970) point out that there have been remarkably few systematic attempts to test these postulates, but we shall now discuss what exists.

Miller and Baruch (1950) compared 90 allergic (including asthmatic) children with 53 nonallergic matched normal controls by means of interviews and observations. They found that the allergic group had more difficulty expressing hostility than the nonallergic group although their methods of evaluating this were extremely subjective and crude. Neuhaus (1958) studied 34 asthmatics aged 8 to 14, 34 children with cardiac disorders requiring restricted activity, 25 sibling controls, and 24 normal children matched for IQ, sex, socioeconomic status, religion, and number of sibs. Using a measure of neuroticism and some projective tests including the Rorschach, Neuhaus found no significant differences between asthmatics, cardiacs, and sibs. However, significant differences were found between normals on the one hand and asthmatics, cardiacs and, interestingly, sibs on the other. This study is important because it illustrates clearly that children with physical disorders represent a more appropriate contrast group than normals since there is some control for both the effect of the illness on the child and for the sampling bias in studying children seen by doctors or professionals. Some of the most significant research on asthma has perhaps not surprisingly come from the Children's Asthma Hospital and Research Institute in Denver under the direction of Purcell. In the first of a series of papers (Purcell, Bernstein, & Buckantz, 1961), the Denver group, using response to hospitalization as criterion, subdivided asthmatics into two broad groups—the rapidly remitting type (RR) who became free of all attacks within three months of hospitalization without steroid therapy, and the steroid-dependent (SD) type who could not be maintained free of attacks without steroid therapy. In subsequent papers, they showed that although the RR group were perceived by their parents to have a higher frequency of neurotic symptoms (Purcell et al., 1961) a battery of personality tests failed to discriminate the two groups (Purcell, Turnbull, & Bernstein, 1962). However, the RR group perceived the origin of their attacks to be most closely related to emotional arousal, particularly when of negative affect. Both groups, however, stated that they tried to avoid states of excitement of any kind and certain responses associated with increased respiration such as coughing, laughing, and crying (Purcell, 1963). This led Purcell et al. to hypothesize that if, as was suggested by French and Alexander, it were true that asthmatics suppress crying, that this may be a learned mechanism for preventing attacks, rather than of psychopathological import. As in other psychosomatic conditions (see ulcerative colitis section), Purcell et al. observed that children given psychotherapy improved behaviorally but that this improvement did not correlate with changes in their asthma. In another study, Dubo et al. (1961) also failed to show any correspondence between severity of asthma and severity of psychopathology. Purcell (1965) concluded that studies of personality in asthma are not fruitful ways of studying asthma and that attention should be focused on the individual asthmatic attack and immediately antecedent psychological events which is, of course, a learning theory approach. In a study along these lines from the Denver Hospital, Weiss (1966) investigated the mood states of SD children during and between attacks using an adjective checklist. He found negative mood to be significantly more frequently associated with attacks than asthma-free periods, which is perhaps hardly surprising, but he also found that in both situations indices of positive mood far overshadowed negative, suggesting that asthmatic children are far from anxious or unhappy most of the time. This study suffers from the weakness of using projective test which are highly inferential (See Chapter Six), of excluding the psychologically most vulnerable group (RR), and an absence of normative data by which to evaluate the significance of the positive/negative mood ratio.

In what appears to be an independent but parallel strategy to the Denver group, Block (Block, 1968; Block, Jennings, Harvey, & Simpson, 1964) divided 67 asthmatic children seen in a pediatric clinic into two groups by a median split using a highly objective "allergic potential score" (APS). The high and low APS groups were then compared with each other and with a matched contrast group of 30 children suffering from physical illnesses of indisputably congenital etiology. A 100-item Q sort by mothers and the Children's Apperception Test were used as measures of maladjustment. All too infrequently found features of this study were the use of blind testers and of four independent raters to evaluate the Q sort and CAT scores. Although the asthmatic group as a whole was not significantly different from the physically disabled group, when the asthmatic group was subdivided on the basis of high and low Allergic Potential Scores, significant differences in emotional immaturity emerged between the low group on the one hand and the high APS and disability groups on the other. The latter, however, did not differ from each other. Since the severity of the asthma was similar in the two groups, Block argued that the psychopathology could not be reactive to the disease as others have hypothesized. Like the Denver group (Purcell, 1965), Block also stressed the futility of continuing to study asthmatics as a homogeneous group.

Rees (1964) studied 383 asthmatics (not subcategorized) seen at an asthma clinic in a Welsh hospital and contrasted them with a group of children seen in the accident unit of the same hospital at the same time and matched as closely as possible for age, sex, and socioeconomic status. Children were evaluated in a psychiatric examination (all done by Rees) under blind conditions, although how he was able to prevent at least a significant proportion of the children or parents talking about their asthma in the course of the interview is not clear. He also studied social history information obtained by social workers who, however, were presumably not blind. He found that the asthmatic children had significantly more neurotic symptomatology (anxiety, depression, tension, and psychophysiological symptoms). After case conferencing in the allergy clinic and observation over a period of several months, the dominant, subsidiary, and unimportant causes of asthmatic attacks were assessed for each child. Children were further grouped as maladjusted or not. Psychological precipitants were more important in maladjusted children, but the differences were not very great, and infections ranked first as the dominant cause in both groups. Rees interpreted his data to suggest that multiple causation is the rule in asthma and infective, allergic, and psychological factors are of varying importance in different individuals and in different attacks in the same individual. He felt that the common denominator to psychological variables precipitating attacks was their generation of anxiety. Rees appears one of the few to draw a distinction between the primary and the secondary causes, the latter of which he felt were always heterogeneous whatever the primary etiology. Unfortunately, like Rees' study of attitudes in parents of asthmatic children (Rees, 1963), this careful and thoughtful study stands or falls on his ability as a diagnostician, which was not formally tested as, for example, Graham et al. (1967) did.

Beech and Nace (1965) studied the expression of aggression in 13 asthmatic boys aged 7 to 15 in an attempt to replicate the study by Miller and

Baruch (1950) but using a "more objective" and quantifiable assessment of aggression, namely a specially derived sentence completion test. They validated the test by comparing a group of psychiatric clinic children subdivided into aggressive and nonaggressive groups by their psychiatrists. The asthmatics proved to have a mean score not significantly different from the aggressive group but substantially higher than that of the nonaggressive group. These findings thus contradict those of the original study by Miller and Baruch, although it is impossible to tell which is the more valid since while Beech and Nace used more careful methodology their group was small and their measures were restricted.

Herbert (1965) did a cross-cultural study of 32 asthmatic South African Indian children attending the hospital clinic. His two contrast groups consisted of stammerers and normals matched for IQ, sex, age, social class, and school achievement. Measures used were the common projective tests, social history, and a standard interview of the child in which he was asked a series of questions relating to his daily life. Herbert confessed to great difficulty in interpreting the projective tests, but generally found more indices of maladjustment and dependency among the asthmatics and stammerers than among the normals; but no common personality or conflict profile emerged. Like Purcell (1965), Herbert concluded that the study of personality variables is not likely to be heuristic and that better hypotheses centered on psychophysiological relationships instead of on personality structure are needed.

Graham et al. (1967) pointed out that the typical study of the asthmatic child samples only a highly selective portion of the total asthmatic population, which is biased toward overinclusion of the emotionally disturbed child. In their epidemiological investigation of the physical health, behavioral, and educational adjustment of all children aged 9 to 11 years on the Isle of Wight, they studied (a) the behavioral status as judged by teachers' and parents' symptom checklists and psychiatric examination, all of demonstrated reliability, and (b) the demographic backgrounds of the 76 asthmatic children in the sample. These data were then compared both with the population norms and the scores of contrast groups of normals, maladjusted, and physically handicapped children. There was no significant difference between asthmatics and normals in the frequency of psychopathology as judged by teachers and psychiatrists. Interestingly, Purcell (Purcell et al., 1961, 1962) notes that parents of asthmatics reported their children to have more symptoms than did parents of normals. In this respect they resembled parents of physically handicapped children. The psychiatric examination revealed no differences between the physically handicapped and the asthmatics in their ability to express emotion, although it is doubtful that this could be adequately tested in such a short interview. There was some relationship between the severity of emotional disorder and of the asthma, a finding contradictory to that of

Block (1968), Dubo et al. (1961), and Purcell (1965). According to parents, both negative and positive excitement (fear, anxiety, anticipation, and anger) were important in precipitation. The asthmatic children were slightly under-achieving and slightly more commonly from the higher socio-economic classes. Graham et al. concluded that previous studies finding a marked excess of emotional disturbance in asthmatic children resulted from faulty sampling. Graham also concluded that because of the similarities with physically handicapped children, the disturbance that occurs is the result not the cause of the illness. In assessing this latter conclusion it has to be borne in mind that Graham et al. did not subdivide their asthmatics into the two subcategories suggested by Block (1968) and Purcell (1965).

Parents of Asthmatic Children

There are numerous studies of the parents of asthmatic children which attempt to demonstrate an increased disturbance in parents or their child-rearing attitudes and thus confirm a psychosomatic basis to asthma in children. However, Fitzelle (1959) has pointed out that if parental disorder and asthma in the child coexist, it is impossible on a retrospective basis to determine if they are causally related or which came first. This has not, however, deterred many investigators, including himself. Using psychological tests, he studied the personality characteristics and child-rearing attitudes of parents of 100 asthmatic children seen in a hospital clinic and the parents of 100 physically disabled children matched along a wide variety of demographic and other variables. No differences were found. Dubo et al. (1961) studied the parents of 71 asthmatic children undergoing desensitization with allergists to see if the severity of disturbance in the home varied with the severity of the asthma as might be suspected if they were causally related. Determination of severity was carefully delineated, and assessment of parent's and child's psychopathology was determined by a two-hour clinical interview. A total of 71 variables, some relating to the asthma, some to the child, and some to the parents, were measured and compared statistically. The only relationships that emerged were within the various measures of severity and between the child's and the parent's level of adjustment. Dubo et al. concluded that past finding of correlations between parental disturbance and asthma must be attributed to poor methodology and naive concepts of causality. Although criticism may be levelled at the method used in their study to evaluate psychopathology and the method's nonblind nature, there appears to be some indirect indication of validity in the finding of the correlation between child and parental psychopathology. An incidental finding was that the child's anxiety seemed most closely related to reality issues (the availability and efficacy of medical treatments) instead of to unconscious conflicts.

The Denver group found the rapidly remitting (RR) group generally to

have more punitive and authoritarian parents (Purcell and Metz, 1962) as adjudged by the Parent Attitude Research Instrument, than the steroid dependent group; the RR group to view their fathers as weak and passive as judged
by a semantic differential test and a laboratory test of perceptual preference;
and the SD group to not differ in any way from a normal control group matched
for sex, age, school grade (Baraff & Cunningham, 1965; Purcell & Clifford,
1966b). Mothers, however, were similarly regarded by all children within a
more passive-affectional role.

Block (Block et al., 1964; Block, 1968) using her high and low Allergic
Potential Score (APS) as a diagnostic criterion, and evaluative techniques and
control methods already outlined above, found that although there were no
differences between mothers of asthmatic and physically handicapped children, there were significantly more indices of unhealthy attitudes (overprotection, ambivalence about motherhood) and more marital conflicts in the
mothers of the low APS group as compared to the high APS and physically
handicapped groups. Block's studies generally are methodologically sound
and can be faulted only on the grounds of her dependent variable measures, a
criticism from which few studies can escape and which to a certain extent
reflect the state of the art of evaluating parental attitudes (see Chapter Two).

In an ingenious and unusual study, Block, Harvey, Jennings, and Simpson
(1966), impressed by the disparity in descriptions of the typology of the "Asthmatogenic" mother by various investigators, used a forced-choice, 100-item,
Q-sort technique to get 14 clinicians interested in asthma to describe the attributes of the asthmatogenic mother. There proved to be a very low degree
of agreement between clinicians with the average coefficient being .29 ranging
from a high of .63 to a low of −.29. A factor analysis revealed three distinct
concepts of the asthmatogenic mother, only one of which proved to discriminate, on subsequent validation, between a group of mothers of asthmatic
children and a group of mothers of chronically disabled children. The discriminating concept was termed the deprived mother—one who was preoccupied with her own adequacy, overprotective, sensitive, guilty, and
controlling. Again, these differences were most pronounced in the low APS
group.

Using basically the same technique outlined above in his study of the
adjustment of asthmatic children except that it would seem to have been nonblind, Rees (1963) also studied parental attitudes. Ignoring the complexity of
assessment and classification of maternal attitudes, Rees categorized mothers
as rejecting, perfectionistic, overprotective, and satisfactory. There was a
significant difference between mothers of asthmatics (44%) and mothers of
accident cases (88%) in the frequency of satisfactory mothering. Of the
unsatisfactory mothers in the asthmatic group, 45% were overprotective, 10%
overtly or covertly rejecting, and 6% perfectionistic. The relative distribution,
but not the absolute frequency of the three types in the two groups of mothers,

was basically similar. The value of Rees' classifications is somewhat dubious, especially in view of Kendell's (1968) clear demonstration that what clinicians see is greatly influenced by their particular views of nosology and etiology. There proved to be a statistically significant relationship between unsatisfactory parenting and both neurotic traits and a dominantly psychological precipitation of attacks in the asthmatic child, although both these differences were small in degree. As with Rees' study of the children (1964), this study is entirely dependent on his competence as a diagnostician, since unlike Block's studies, objective techniques were not used, nor were blind conditions maintained. Additional discussion of parental factors may be found in Chapter Two.

Psychophysiological Studies

As was pointed out by Purcell (1965) and Herbert (1965), studies that attempt to link closely antecedent events with the child's asthmatic attacks or respiratory function are likely to be of greater value than the more typical correlational studies of asthma and child or parental psychopathology discussed above. In an ingenious and carefully controlled study Owen and Williams (1961) showed that abnormal respiratory responses in asthmatics could be related specifically to the mother's voice independent of content. Apley and MacKeith (1962, pp. 30–32) cite a study by Neale and Harris showing a 26% reduction in maximal expiration in an 11-year-old boy as a result of the stress of an impending examination. The Denver group (Hahn, 1966) studied the psychophysiological responses of asthmatics and normals and showed that asthmatics have abnormal autonomic responses suggestive of homeostatic dysfunction and tend to overreact with negative mood as judged by an adjective checklist to stress such as a loud noise, shock, or problem-solving tasks.

Franks and Leigh (1959), arguing from animal studies of conditioned abnormal respiratory responses that asthma in man was a conditioned response, tested the conditionability of asthmatics but found no difference between them and normals and neurotics. However, Purcell (1965) in reviewing the animal and human studies, concluded that although certain abnormal respiratory responses have been conditioned particularly in animals, there is as yet no successful conditioning of asthma in animal or man.

In a somewhat esoteric study, Epstein (1964), of the Denver group, studied the ability of asthmatic children to increase their emission of hostile verbalizations through operant techniques, since asthmatic children are posited to be unable to express hostility and this thus might prove to have some application in treatment. While the rate of hostile verbalization in the base-line state was low, it could be readily increased in some of the asthmatic children, namely those who showed a need for approval.

With the exception of the study by Owen and Williams (1961) and that cited by Apley and MacKeith (1962, pp. 30–32), these studies are all rather reified and closer attention to the relationship between the asthmatic response and naturally occurring psychological variables both immediately before and after would seem to be necessary if this type of study is to fulfill its enormous potential.

Treatment

Physical treatments such as corticosteroids and sympathomimetic amines that form the cornerstone of the treatment of asthma will not be discussed here, their value, particularly in the management of the acute attack and status asthmatics, being assumed. Rather this discussion will be confined to psychological or psychotropic treatments. It is obvious that if certain states such as anxiety are important in asthma, treatments aimed at relieving such states could be predicted to be useful in asthma insofar as they are effective in their purported aims. Unfortunately, we are dealing with two as yet undemonstrated classes of assumption, and it is therefore necessary to look at treatment studies specific to asthma.

These studies have been reviewed by Purcell and Weiss (1970) who point out that practically every psychotherapeutic procedure from psychoanalysis to hypnosis has been claimed to be of value in asthma, but that such claims are based on studies replete with the kind of methodological errors that have been repeatedly noted in this chapter and this book. There are, in effect, no acceptable studies of the effect of psychotherapy on asthma in children and few in adults to offer any possibility of extrapolation to children.

Behavior therapy can offer one controlled study—that by Moore (1965) in which reciprocal inhibition was found to be superior to relaxation and suggestive procedures in its effect on respiratory function in asthma, although not on subjective improvement.

Despite the fact that psychotropic drugs are frequently described as useful (Purcell and Weiss, 1970), evaluation of their true usefulness is difficult since good studies are lacking.

Hospitalization itself is claimed to be useful in cases refractory to outpatient care, particularly for the rapidly remitting asthmatic, with improvement persisting after discharge (Purcell and Weiss, 1970). It should be remembered, however, that these studies were done in a special hospital for asthmatic children where they received an unusually high quality of care.

Conclusions

There is no evidence that all asthmatic children have significant psychopathology or abnormal parenting. Indeed, as with enuretic children, when all asthmatic children in the population are studied, differences from normal children become statistically imperceptible. Thus there is no good evidence that asthma is necessarily a psychosomatic disease.

However, again as with enuresis, asthmatic children seen in hospitals and clinics do show evidence of increased psychopathology and abnormal parenting though there is little convincing evidence to show that this is greater in degree or different in kind from that seen in other physically handicapped children. Further, as in ulcerative colitis, the severity of the physical disease is not correlated with the severity of the emotional disorder or the response to psychotherapies, as might be expected if the relationship between the two was strong and meaningful.

There is no good evidence of a specific personality conflict in asthmatic children or their parents. The evidence that anxiety and other states of arousal can have precipitating and modifying effects in individual children and on individual attacks in the same child is plausible, but has only circumstantial support.

That asthma, like enuresis, is a phenotype with differing and multifactorial etiologies seems highly probable. When asthmatic children are divided into subcategories on the basis of severity (as determined by source of the sample) and on response to nonspecific procedures or estimates of the contribution of the allergic etiological component, a distinct group that has many of the hallmarks of a psychosomatic one emerges. But it is doubtful, even in this group, that psychological factors are of primary etiological significance instead of being grafted onto an abnormal respiratory response pattern produced initially by physical means (allergy or infection).

Correlational studies between asthma and either child or parental psychopathology have been remarkably unfruitful except perhaps for delineating typological subgroups in which the role of psychological variables might profitably be explored in more detail. What is needed are psychophysiological studies that seek to relate naturally occurring antecedent stimuli and contingent environmental events to the asthmatic attack, employing the precision of subject selection, definition, measurement, and experimental control that has characterized laboratory studies in experimental psychology.

Tics

Definition

Tics are defined by Kanner (1957, pp. 422–423) as muscular movements that are sudden, repetitive, involuntary, apparently purposeless, and restricted to some circumscribed muscle group. They are distinguished from hyperkinetic and choreiform movements (see p. 105 and Yates, 1970) by the invariability of their expression and by their <u>restriction in most cases to a small group of muscles, most conspicuously those of the head and neck.</u> When the tics are widespread and include vocal tics often but not necessarily of coprolalic content, a diagnostic subcategorization of Gilles de la Tourette syndrome is made (see review by Kelman, 1965). Though Gilles de la Tourette believed that this constituted a distinct disorder (in keeping with the mood of the times —1885—leading to an inevitable degeneration), Kelman suggests that the sex distribution, age on onset, initial locus in head and neck, and prognosis (Kelman, 1965; Lucas, Kauffman, & Morris, 1967) indicate that this syndrome is simply a more severe variant of children's tics.

In one of the most extensive, most cited, and least emulated studies of children's tics, Olson (1929) offered an extensive regional classification of tics, and proposed ways of measuring them, although his definition was considered by Kanner (1957) to have been overliberal.

Occurrence

The few studies of children's tics in the general population show widely varying frequencies ranging from 23% (see Kanner, 1957; and Torup, 1962) to 4.5% in boys and 2.6% in girls (see Torup, 1962). In one of the few studies that is available and able to be evaluated, Lapouse and Monk (1958, 1964) found the frequency of tics to be 12% between the ages of 6–12 years, slightly commoner in boys in the 9–12 age group, and in black children, even when socioeconomic status was controlled. Lapouse and Monk's sampling techniques and reliability of measurement were reasonably satisfactory and, thus, their results are worthy of note.

Studies of pediatric (Torup, 1962) and psychiatric clinic populations (Kelman, 1965; Lucas et al., 1967; Mahler, 1949; Ritvo, 1945; Torup, 1962; Zausmer, 1954) show that, consistent with general intake patterns, males predominate especially in the psychiatric groups, and that tics are ordinarily of over a year's duration before referral. Both epidemiological and clinical studies suggest that although the peak prevalence is between 9 and 12 years of age, many cases are of earlier onset, and that the course is typically benign, most cases not being seen by pediatricians and even less so by psychiatrists (Torup, 1962).

Etiology

<u>Suggestions that tics may reflect an organic brain disorder have always</u> had strong proponents especially for Gilles de la Tourette syndrome (Kelman, 1965). In her exhaustive review, Kelman came to the conclusion that birth history, EEG, neurological, and autopsy data offered no support for this theory. Lucas et al. (1967) found signs of minimal brain dysfunction (mostly learning

and visuomotor disorders) in two thirds of their cases, but these findings are not uncommon in boys seen at psychiatric clinics (see section on organic disorders) and are of uncertain implication. Pasamanick and Kawi (1956) studied birth records of 83 children with tics from Kanner's clinic and compared them with those of a contrast group matched for sex, race, maternal age, place of birth, and proximity on the birth register. They found that complications of delivery were more common in the group with tics (33.3% versus 17.6%), but there was no difference in the frequency of prenatal complications such as prematurity. It is of interest to note that Mahler (1949), one of the leading exponents of the psychoanalytic theory of etiology, has argued for a constitutional predisposition in the form of "motor urgency" and explains the preponderance of boys (at least in clinic cases) as a result of the differing biological function of the neuromuscular apparatus in the two sexes. Despite this, the evidence for an organic etiology of most tics is at best rather rudimentary.

Psychoanalytic theories have received their greatest elaboration in the study by Mahler (1949). She classifies children with tics into five groups (1) transient tics indicating simple tension, (2) tic as a sign of a reactive behavior disorder on verge of internalization, (3) psychoneurotic tic in which the tic is only one symptom, together with many others, of a neurosis, (4) as part of a character disorder (especially Gilles de la Tourette syndrome), (5) psychosomatic tic disease in which there is an organ neurosis of the neuromuscular system. In all these, but to a lesser degree in the tension tic, psychoanalytic theory is distinguished by its emphasis on the symbolic value of the tic in expressing the particular conflict or character organization of the child.

As in other conditions, nonspecific theories vary in sophistication from seeing tics as a simple physiological concomitant of anxiety (Bakwin & Bakwin, 1966; Kanner, 1957) to a learned pattern of behavior by imitation of other children, the consolidation of some physiological response such as the blink reflex (Bakwin & Bakwin, 1966), or the adventitious association of anxiety reduction with a tension response (Walton, 1961; Yates, 1970). The process by which this learning purportedly occurs and operates has been made explicit by Walton (1961) and Yates (1958, 1970) who use Hullian drive reduction theory. The uniqueness of this approach is that certain predictions useful and testable in treatment can be made (see Yates, 1970)—a rare enough phenomenon in the therapy of the psychopathological disorders of childhood.

Yates (1970) notes that since rhythmic and repetitive movements are very common in childhood, it is entirely possible that tics are simply exaggerated forms of these movements. Yet in the prevalence and etiological studies discussed it is unusual to find anything but an assumption that tics are necessarily abnormal phenomena right from their inception. The alternative suggested by Yates (1970), that tics are normal movements that have become overlearned, could prove a more profitable line of study, particularly for prevention and early intervention.

Psychopathology in Tiqueurs and Their Families

Specific theorists such as Mahler (1949) expect and find specific personalities or conflicts in tiqueurs though the methodology of determining this (psychiatric interviews) is highly suspect. She found tiqueurs to fall into a hyper- and a hypokinetic group, each with particular conflict patterns. On the other hand, Kanner (1957, p. 422), while equating tics with the presence of psychopathology, sees this only as a nonspecific product of any kind of emotional stress. In his study of 96 children with tics, Zausmer (1954) found the majority of children to be suffering from a variety of tension symptoms such as restlessness, irritability, phobias, and excitability. Torup (1962), in a detailed psychological evaluation of 72 children using projective tests, found that although no specific personality or conflict profile emerged, restlessness and sensitivity were the most commonly reported symptoms supporting the nonspecific anxiety-related view of tics. In her review of Gilles de la Tourette syndrome, Kelman (1965) does not go into the area of psychopathology, but Lucas et al. (1967) found that only some of their children exhibited psychoneurotic mechanisms while two thirds had signs of minimal cerebral dysfunction.

Kanner (1957, p. 422) considers the primary cause of tics to lie in rigid and overdemanding parents—but this is characteristic of Kanner's view of psychopathogenesis in general. Zausmer (1954) found most of the parents of his patients to be anxious, restrictive, rigid, and the source of major anxiety for the child. Torup (1962) claimed that the onset of tics in her group of 237 children was commonly associated with some dramatic and sudden home conflict, but she found the frequency of disturbed families to be highest in children referred to the psychiatric clinic. Mahler (1949) noted that because of sickness in the children, mothers had had to supply an unusual amount of motor restriction during the motor impulsive stage of development. Also, she claimed that mothers tended to be overprotective, prolonged the symbiotic period, were intolerant of aggression, and set overly high standards for their children. Like Kanner's view, this one appears more characteristic of the author than the subject. Lucas et al. (1967) found that there were three types of families —those in which aggression was freely and overly expressed at home, those in which aggression was excessively inhibited, and normal families (2 out of 15). Both Zausmer (1954) and Torup (1962) found a significant family history of tics, which is interpretable within either a hereditary or psychogenic etiological framework.

Despite the fact that tics are considered anxiety-related there are few psychophysiological studies of tics, which is all the more surprising in view of the ease with which tics can be measured. Connell, Corbett, Horne, and Matthews (1967), Feldman and Werry (1966), Walton (1961), and Yates (1958) did take systematic measures of tics in the course of treatment and found tics to obey Hullian learning theory, which predicts a close relationship between tics and anxiety. Connell et al. and Feldman and Werry also found some direct empirical evidence of this relationship. However, this area is virtually unexplored and could be one of the more profitable fields of investigation of tics.

In summary, it can be said that while the notion that tics are reflections of an increased anxiety level is credible clinically and theoretically, it awaits better demonstration.

Treatment

There is no doubt that psychotherapy of various kinds is frequently given to children with tics, but there are no adequate studies by which to evaluate its effectiveness. Reliable dependent measures are seldom taken and sampling bias is routine, with psychotherapy being given only to the most severely disturbed tiqueurs (e.g., Zausmer, 1954). Mahler (1949) does mention psychoanalytic-type psychotherapy to be very difficult with Gilles de la Tourette syndrome. Zausmer (1954) found that the prognosis of tics was not influenced by the particular treatment a child had been given; but this was a poorly designed study, since only severer cases received psychiatric treatment. In her review, Kelman (1965) summarized the treatments given for the 44 reported cases of Gilles de la Tourette syndrome. In 11 cases psychotherapy had been given with two-thirds improving. Phenothiazine or buyterophenone drug treatment was given in 15 cases, and the improvement rate in these was 83%. Lucas et al. (1967) obtained varying degrees of improvement in 6 of 8 children treated with the same drugs.

Although drugs are used in the treatment of tics, few studies including the above are satisfactory since they lack double blind controls, quantitative and reliable measures of the tics, and the effect of drugs is confounded with that of other treatments. Only the study by Connell et al. (1967) can be considered adequate. In a double-blind crossover study with counting of tics under standard conditions, Connell et al. found diazepam and placebo to be statistically not different, while haloperidol significantly decreased the frequency of tics. They also found a decrease in the frequency of tics as a function of time, which they interpreted as resulting from persistence of the drug, but which seemed more probably an artifact of habituation to the measurement situation.

Yates (1958) was the first to reapply the treatment technique of massed or negative practice developed by Dunlap (1932) in which the tic is voluntarily practiced. However, unlike Dunlap, Yates offered a theoretical rationale in Hullian learning theory and then tested some of the predictions of the theory in an adult patient. Walton (1961) was the first to apply this technique in a child but, unfortunately, the treatment was confounded by simultaneous administration of chlorpromazine and no control such as measuring one of the child's untreated tics was used. Furthermore, though Walton did measure the frequency of the tic, he did so only during the times that the patient was practicing the tic and relied on vague reports of improvement as his criterion of success. Feldman and Werry (1966) obtained base-line rates of tiquing in a pubescent boy with multiple tics. They then treated one by massed practice and used another as a no-treatment control. All tics were increased in frequency by treatment and one previously present reappeared. Feldman and Werry concluded that their subject was made so anxious by the treatment, which he and his father thought harmful, that treatment was vitiated. Clark (1966) successfully treated a 17-year-old boy having Gilles de la Tourette syndrome with massed practice and found him to be symptom-free four years later. Other forms of behavior therapy such as operant techniques for the treatment of tics have not yet been applied in children even though they have been used in adults.

Outcome

There are two follow-up studies of large groups of children with tics— that by Zausmer of 96 children seen in a psychiatric clinic and that by Torup of 220 children seen in a pediatric and child psychiatry clinic. Using fairly objective and stringent criteria of improvement, Zausmer found that 1 to 5 years after referral about 25% were virtually free of tics and another 50% greatly improved. Improvement was not related to treatment (see above), there was more improvement with longer follow-up periods, and there was more improvement in girls than in boys. Torup interviewed children and families in the majority of cases in their homes, and the follow-up interval, which ranged from 2 to 15 years, with the mean age of the subject at follow-up being 18. For more than a year, 50% had had no tics, 46% were greatly improved with only blinking and slight grimacing persisting, and only 6% had shown no change. The average age at cessation was 12 to 13 and most tics had lasted 4 to 6 years before disappearance. Where tics were persistent there tended to be associated mental retardation, epilepsy, severe home difficulty, or parents with persistent tics. In her review of Gilles de la Tourette syndrome, Kelman (1965) concluded that although the data did not permit firm conclusions, it was obvious that the prognosis was not always poor. Lucas et al. (1967) found that 6 cases showed almost no tics, 6 great improvement, and only 3 (the most recent) no change at follow-up after 2 to 15 years (mean 6).

Summary

Tics are a common childhood problem and only a small minority of tiqueurs find their way to clinics. The age of incidence is most commonly between 6 and 12 years, with the peak prevalence between 9 and 12 years.

There appears to be a spontaneous remission in most tics at or before puberty though mild residua in the face may persist. In clinics, boys with tics are seen more frequently than girls but there is reason to suppose that this is no more so than for most psychopathological disorders. The separateness of Gilles de la Tourette syndrome as a clinical entity is questionable. There is some evidence to suggest that tics are related to anxiety, but their exact origin and relationship to common rhythmic and repetitive movements of childhood remains obscure. There is a strong clinical belief, theoretical prediction, and some weak empirical evidence that children with tics seen in clinics have an anxiety disorder and live in anxiogenic families. There is some evidence that drugs such as buyterophenones may reduce tiquing, but better studies like those by Connell et al. (1967) are needed before definitive statements can be made. The usefulness of psychotherapy, parental counselling, and behavior therapy cannot yet be assessed; only behavior therapy has shown signs that it may ultimately produce the data necessary to evaluate it.

The studies on tics are amongst the most sparse and poorest in the field of psychosomatic conditions, and practically any study that obeys presently acceptable standards of methodology should yield valuable information.

Stereotypies, Rhythmic Motor Behaviors, and Self-Mutilation

Definition

This group of behaviors will be discussed together since, although they are by no means synonymous, there is a great deal of overlap. Thus, many stereotypies are rhythmic, and much self-mutilation results from stereotypies, perhaps the best example of this communality being seen in headbanging (Green, 1967). Stereotypies are repetitive, relatively invariant movements of head, body, and/or hands (Berkson, 1967; Kaufman & Levitt, 1965) which, unlike tics, involve at least a region of the body instead of a single muscle group. They take such forms as rhythmic movements of head or trunk, self-manipulations, flapping of the hands, posturing, picking at or biting oneself (Berkson & Davenport, 1962).

Occurrence

Stereotypies, notably headbanging and rocking, are common in normal infants, especially males, estimates of frequency ranging from 15–20% in better studies (De Lissovoy, 1961; Lourie, 1949) to 3.6% in less meticulous ones (Kravitz, Rosenthal, Teplitz, Murphy, & Lesser, 1960). However, such stereotypies are ordinarily short-lived, rarely persisting beyond the age of two or three years (De Lissovoy, 1962; Kravitz et al., 1960; Lourie, 1949).

After this age, rhythmic stereotypies tend to be replaced by irregular manipulations of the self, clothes, and environment (Hutt, Hutt, Lee, & Ounsted, 1965; Lebowitz, Colbert, & Palmer, 1961). Although thumbsucking is perhaps not strictly a stereotypy, it does follow the same pattern except that its frequency is much higher in infancy and also in childhood (10%) and the sexes are equally represented (Davidson, 1970; Lapouse & Monk, 1964).

While common in normal infants and toddlers, stereotypies occur more commonly and persist longer in certain abnormal populations—retarded, blind, psychotic, and institutionalized children. Other differences are that whereas in normal children the stereotypies occur in highly specific situations and states such as social isolation, in the crib, when fatigued or inactive, in abnormal populations they are usually persistent, relatively independent of environmental situation, and take exaggerated or bizarre forms such as twirling, handflapping, plunging, and self-mutilation. As a general rule, it seems that the less stimulation the child can or does receive (blind, profoundly retarded, psychotic, institutionalized) the more obstinate, the more exaggerated, and the more bizarre the stereotypy (Berkson, 1967; De Lissovoy, 1962; Green, 1967, 1968; Hutt et al., 1965; Lebowitz et al., 1961; Litrownik, 1969; Ritvo, Ornitz, & La Franchi, 1968; Rutter & Lockyer, 1967; Sorosky, Ornitz, Brown, & Ritvo, 1968; Wolf & Chess, 1964).

Etiology

Etiological hypotheses fall into four broad groups.

1. Stereotypies result from understimulation of the organism and represent an effort to restore optimal level of arousal (see Berkson, 1967). This underarousal may be because of a deficiency of stimulation in the environment as in institutionalization or an inability to utilize environmental stimulation through sensory, intellectual, or interpersonal deficits.
2. Conversely, the stereotypies are a consequence of overstimulation and are homeostatic mechanisms to cut down responsiveness to impinging stimuli (Hutt et al., 1965).
3. They are neurogenic, that is, the direct result of a neurological lesion (Ritvo et al., 1968).
4. They are operant behaviors that reward the organism either through internal proprioceptive stimulation or favorable response of the external environment (Green, 1968; Greenberg, 1964; Lovaas, Freitag, Gold, Kassorla, 1955a; Schaefer, 1970).

Although each of these hypotheses is theoretically testable by the response of stereotypies to variations in amount and kind of external stimuli, the results of studies in animals and humans are generally contradictory, suggesting that the etiological hypotheses are neither mutually exclusive nor valid in every case (Baroff & Tate, 1968; Berkson, 1965; Berkson & Mason, 1964a & b; Davis, 1970; Davis et al., 1969; Hutt et al., 1965; Kaufman & Levitt, 1965; Litrownik, 1969; Lovaas & Simmons, 1962; Lovaas, Schaeffer, & Simmons, 1965b; Lovaas et al., 1965a; KcKinney, 1962; McKinney & Keele, 1963; Ritvo et al., 1968; Sorosky et al., 1968).

What does seem clear is that many abnormal stereotypies have a high degree of autonomy, but that they can be both produced (Schaefer, 1970) and influenced (at least transitorily) by strong stimuli within an operant learning paradigm (Berkson, 1967; Davis, 1970; Lovaas & Simmons, 1962; Lovaas et al., 1965a & b). Further, since stereotypies are common in animals reared in isolation (Berkson & Mason, 1964; Harlow, 1962; Mason & Sponholz, 1963), in children reared in institutions (Freud & Burlingham, 1944; Levy, 1944; Spitz & Wolf, 1946), and in multihandicapped children, all of whom are characterized by an impaired capacity to utilize normal environmental stimulation, it seems most likely that the refractoriness of stereotypies to external stimuli is less a reflection of some neurogenic periodicity (Ritvo et al., 1968; Ornitz et al., 1968) than it is of the difficulty of finding a reinforcer that can compete with this aboriginal self-generated one.

Treatment and Prognosis

Despite the significant amount of experimental work on stereotypies, there have been few studies of treatment or outcome in normal children where the prognosis without treatment is good. Lourie (1949) claimed complete success in treating rhythmic stereotypies in four normal infants by setting a metronome to the periodicity, but in the only attempt to replicate this, De Lissovoy (1962) found that it was ineffective except in modifying the basic rhythm in a few cases.

In abnormal populations, nonspecific environmental enrichment can be effective in reducing stereotypies in certain deprived institutionalized retardates (Berkson, 1967; Berkson & Mason, 1964a), but in severely emotionally, physically, or intellectually handicapped children stereotypies are highly resistant to modification. Self-destructive behavior has been the subject of more study and appears to be amenable at least in the short run to aversive and, less commonly, nonaversive operant procedures (Hutt et al., 1965; Lovaas & Simmons, 1962; Lovaas et al., 1965a & b; Tate & Baroff, 1966; see also Chapter Seven).

Summary

Despite the fact that the exact etiology of stereotypies and self-mutilating behavior is unknown, there is good reason to suppose that they have their roots in certain transitory behaviors of early life which become highly indurated as a result of deficiencies of the supply, reception, or utilization of complex environmental stimuli, which prevent the learning of higher more satisfying patterns of behavior. There is little information on treatment, although there is reason to believe that better attention to experimental control, particularly using the operant learning paradigm, could prove fruitful.

Obesity

Introduction

Although it is customary to stress the impact of obesity on physical health as a major reason for its importance as a field of study and therapeutic intervention, it is likely that the psychological disability accompanying obesity is of equal importance (Mayer, 1966a & b).

Definition

It is now generally recognized that except perhaps in the grossly overweight, the use of weight alone as a criterion of obesity is invalid, since obesity implies an excess of adipose tissue, and the source of excess weight may lie entirely in skeletal and muscular tissues (e.g., football players). This distinction is not trivial since it is likely that the mortality rates may be quite different in the two groups.

The most commonly used scales employ a two-dimensional index for the definition of obesity, namely height and weight (sometimes as in the life insurance tables with a third, a crude estimate of the skeletal size added as well). For children, the practice seems to be to relate the height and weight to developmental tables such as the Wetzel grid.

Dissatisfaction with the height–weight method has led to efforts to measure adipose tissue directly using certain skin folds as representative of the whole (Mayer, 1966b).

When height–weight data are related to existing developmental tables, the prevalence of obesity is found empirically to vary with age (Rauh, Schumsky, & Witt, 1967). Mayer (1966b), on the other hand, has proposed a statistical definition of obesity (using the thickness of the triceps skin fold as an estimate of adipose tissue), namely, one standard deviation from the logarithmic mean in all age groups under 30. Thus, for any age group the prevalence of the obesity is necessarily always 16%. (After the age of 30 the use of 30-year-old norms is proposed so that the prevalence of obesity increases sharply in the next decade.) While this Mayerian definition has the virtue of simplicity, it has a number of defects. First, it equates the mean with the norm when, for example, in New Zealand children, even though height (and hence presumably optimal nutrition) has been stable for 15 years, weight has continued to increase suggesting incipient obesity on a population basis. Finally, it suffers from the improbable assumption either that obesity is a chronic, lifelong disease, or if not always so, that the incidence rate (number of new cases in unit time) always equals the remittance rate. However, this need not be a handicap to the growth of knowledge, since three important groups, as demonstrated by Grant (1966), should be easily discernible from longitudinal (though not from the simpler cross-sectional) studies: (a) the chronically obese child, (b) the becoming obese child, and (c) the remitting obese child.

Hypothetical reasons and empirical data, sketchy as they are, suggest that these three groups are prognostically and probably etiologically different (Asher, 1966; Grant, 1966; Heald, 1966), and the potential yield of knowledge from researching each group is different.

Given the unsatisfactory and often arbitrary definition of obesity epidemiological data is at best of limited value. Obesity in children may be bimodal in age incidence (early and middle childhood) (American Academy of Pediatrics, 1967; Asher, 1966; Heald, 1966; Rauh et al., 1967); it is influenced by gender, but in a complex way (Rauh et al., 1967), and by ethnic and socioeconomic group. These demographic features tend to become much clearer in adulthood where socially and sexually disadvantaged groups show higher prevalences of obesity (Mayer, 1966b). However, in childhood, these tendencies are often actually reversed (Rauh et al., 1967). A most important concomitant of obesity, at least in the adolescent and adult female, is somato-type obesity being correlated with a complex somatotype of mesomorphy with endomorphy and ectopenia; that is, muscularity, robusticity, and large skeletal size (Mayer, 1966a). It is also more common in natural than adoptive children of obese parents (see Mayer, 1966b) suggesting possible genetic influences in etiology.

Etiology

It is easy enough to see that to *become* obese, intake must exceed expenditure of energy. There are, however, numerous complexities in this deceptively simple equation, since environmental and biological influences on intake and especially output of energy are myriad (Mayer, 1966b). These complexities are seldom recognized and obesity is usually regarded, especially in psychiatric literature, as etiologically simple and homogeneous.

A further, almost always ignored, complication is to assume that original etiology must still be present. Studies in animals in which energy intake or output are altered experimentally show that obesity develops over a period of time but that ultimately a steady (obese) state is achieved. The only difference in this new steady state may be the now greatly increased adipose tissue. An etiological study done at this phase could conceivably show no disturbance of either energy intake or output. How true this steady state (excluding normal growth needs) is of human beings and of children in particular, is not clear at the moment except that while it is certainly not true of all obese children, it is characteristic of some (Grant, 1966).

Mayer (1966b) has exhaustively reviewed both the homeostatic mechanisms that maintain balance between energy intake and energy output, and the disturbances that may occur. For present purposes it may be assumed that very few cases of obesity in children have demonstrable organic causes. This leaves two possible causes: eating too much or exercising too little. The first Mayer (1966b) calls the Fundamentalist view since it has its roots in the Puritanical aversion to gluttony. Considering the Puritanical roots of Anglo-Saxon culture, it is not surprising to find that the etiological notions of obesity in both medical and psychiatric literature in English have been dominated by the gluttony hypothesis. Yet, Mayer's reviews of his own work and others' studies have revealed the rather disquieting fact that obese children and adolescents seldom seem to eat more or different food than their peers. This would suggest either that studies are usually done in the steady state or that the cause lies primarily in inadequate consumption of energy rather than gluttony. This impairment could be some yet undiscovered metabolic differences or insufficient physical activity. Mayer (1966b) claims that the empirical data support the latter as an important cause in our increasingly sedentary society. A complication here, of course, is that the reduction in physical activity could be, at least in part, secondary—obesity leads to difficulty in moving, clumsiness, rejection by peers and, hence, for children, reduction in opportunities for activity (Mayer, 1966b). The etiological link between the observed somatotypic differences and obesity is not clear and could involve a variety of gustatory, metabolic, temperamental, and activity factors (American Academy of Pediatrics, *British Medical Journal*, 1966; Mayer, 1966b).

Psychopathological Studies of Obese Children and Their Parents

It is apparent that social and psychological variables could operate causatively at one or many points: on feeding (amount, quality, frequency), appetite, satiety point, metabolism, and activity (opportunity and motivation for), so that their potential role is not in question. Their relative importance and locus of action, however, has not been established despite voluminous literature. As was discussed above, little profit comes from speculation of this kind, and clearer empirical demonstrations of correlation of psychopathology with and its clear functional relation to obesity is a prerequisite.

As in so many other conditions, there are virtually no studies that are not based on single or small numbers of highly selected children, using poor diagnostic methods in poor experimental designs. Unfortunately, this criticism applies to the best known worker in this area, Hilda Bruch. She (Bruch, 1963a & b) considers obesity to result from a hyperphagia embedded in a matrix of severe disturbance of body concept similar to schizophrenia. This disorder is hypothesized to result from impaired communication within the family, particularly between mother and child with the former smothering the child and the latter passively compliant. In the eating situation, this means that mother's needs dominate over the child's own hunger and satiety sensations. Bruch seems to make it clear that obesity is not necessarily associated with severe psychopathology, but the basic mechanism is etiologically similar in all severe cases.

Mayer (1966b) strongly supports any psychopathology being the consequence of obesity (i.e., somatopsychic), principally from the severe rejection by peers and adults. He points out that many of the psychological phenomena said to be associated with obese children are characteristic of discriminated-against minority groups, which could support such an hypothesis.

At this point, the frequency and kinds of psychopathology associated with obesity in children appear to be unknown and, when present, their relationship to the etiology of the obesity is quite unclear.

Treatment and Prognosis

There seem to be few controlled studies of treatment of obesity in children and none using psychotherapeutic methods. Bruch (1963a) has emphasized the difficulty of treating obesity by psychoanalytic psychotherapy. Controlled studies, mostly with anorectic drugs, suggest that while almost anything, including placebo, works somewhat in the short run, long term results are disappointing especially in amount of weight lost (Christakis, Sajecki, Hillman, Miller, Blumenthal, & Archer, 1966; Lancet, 1966; Lloyd, Wolff, & Whelan, 1961; Shutter & Garell, 1966).

While undoubtedly some fat children do grow up to be physically normal adults, most do not, and further, the more overweight the child or the earlier the onset of obesity the worse the ultimate prognosis (American Academy of Pediatrics, 1967; Asher, 1966; British Medical Journal, 1966; Grant, 1966; Lloyd et al., 1961; Mayer, 1966b).

In the end, the best treatment for obesity would seem to lie in its prevention, which implies the need for much better studies of the eating habits and activity patterns of the becoming obese child at all ages. The importance of the mental health sciences is in their application to the study of any antecedents of increased eating or reduced physical activity where these have been revealed to be causal. The treatment of obesity, involving as it probably must in most severe cases, the reduction of caloric intake to deplete fat stores or the development of greater physical activity, requires the development of better techniques derived from the application of motivation and learning theories.

Summary

To cite the Committee of the American Academy of Pediatrics (1967): "despite an imposing body of information derived from research, our ignorance concerning the etiology, pathogenesis and treatment of obesity is remarkable." In light of the discussion above, certain signposts for research should, however, be clear.

Enuresis

Definition

Enuresis is ordinarily defined as involuntary urinary incontinence in the absence of any organic abnormality after some age at which bladder control is ordinarily attained, usually the fourth birthday. It is a problem of great antiquity, its history having been illuminatingly described by Glicklich (1951).

Enuresis occurs in several forms. Nocturnal enuresis or bed-wetting refers to incontinence during sleep, diurnal enuresis to that occurring in the waking state, primary enuresis to incontinence since birth, and secondary or onset enuresis to loss of previously acquired continence.

Occurrence

Recent epidemiological studies (summarized in Jones, 1960; Oppel, Harper, & Rowland, 1968a) have revealed that the frequency of bed-wetting is much higher than previously suspected, rising as high as 20% at the age of six years depending on the thoroughness of survey of the population, the definition of dryness, and the country studied. Although absolute figures may differ, prevalence curves for enuresis show a characteristic sharp fall between the ages of one and four years with a gradual flattening out of the gradient of decline from four through to adolescence. One of the better studies, that by Oppel et al., (1968a) further suggests that continence is a parlous condition for over 25% of children nocturnally and for 10% diurnally. These relapses have a median duration of 2.5 years in the case of bed-wetting and 1.2 years for diurnal enuresis. Epidemiological studies also generally demonstrate that enuresis is more prevalent in boys except perhaps after the age of ten (Oppel et al., 1968a); in lower socioeconomic or disadvantaged groups (Blomfield &

Douglas, 1956; Hallgren, 1956a & b; Oppel et al., 1968a); in certain cultures (Stein & Susser, 1967); and in neurologically handicapped and children of lower I.Q. (Oppel, Harper, & Rider, 1968b).

The studies by Stein and Susser (1967) suggest that the acquisition of bladder control is part of an orderly sequence of control of elimination proceeding from control of bowel at night to bowel by day, then bladder by day and, finally, after a period of several months, of bladder by night. Stein and Susser therefore hypothesized that bladder control is part of an overall pattern of physical maturation; but they could offer no direct evidence to support this.

Family factors correlated with enuresis are both a positive family history of enuresis and indicators of social disorganization, such as broken homes, mother-child separations, maternal incompetence (Bakwin, 1961; Hallgren, 1956a, b, 1957; Oppel et al., 1968a & b; Stein & Susser, 1966, 1967).

Despite common and apparently authoritative statements to the contrary (e.g., Nelson, Vaughan, & McKay, 1969) the relationship of enuresis to child-rearing practices is unclear. For example, Klackenberg (1955), and McGraw (1940) in her twin study, failed to find any influence of time of toilet training. On the other hand, Dimson (1959) did find a relationship between enuresis and resistance to toileting by the child, while Stein and Susser (1967) suggested that their observed differences in acquisition of continence between English and American children (later) was due to greater permissiveness about toileting in the American parents.

Etiological Theories

In their excellent review, Lovibond and Coote (1969) consider that etiological theories are reducible to two—psychodynamic and physiological behavioristic. The former consider enuresis necessarily to be the symptom of an underlying emotional disturbance and have been elaborated by such persons as Gerard (1939), Michaels (1955), and Sperling (1965). It should be noted that most of the psychodynamic theories have been developed from studies of very small numbers of children who have a high probability of being emotionally disturbed, seen in psychoanalytically oriented psychotherapy under nonblind conditions using observational techniques of unknown reliability (Werry, 1967a). Such scientific shortcomings scarcely enhance the credibility of such theories.

Psychological behavioristic theories consider enuresis as a simple deficit in function, a failure to develop cortical control over the subcortical micturition reflex instead of as a positive symptom meaningful in the psychodynamic economy of the child. According to Lovibond and Coote (1969), individual theories within this physiological behavioristic category differ in the extent to which they locate the failure primarily in the physical systems or in the psychological process of acquisition of the conditioned reflexes necessary for bladder control.

Not surprisingly, psychologists (Jones, 1960; Lovibond & Coote, 1969; Mowrer & Mowrer, 1938; Eysenck, 1959) tend to focus on the learning process, while physicians (Bakwin, 1961; British Medical Journal, 1960; Broughton, 1968; Muellner, 1960; Stein & Susser, 1967) emphasize physical abnormalities and dysfunctions usually of the urinary tract or nervous system. Discussion of the learning etiological theories can be found in Chapter Seven).

Points suggested in evidence of some mild developmental neurological disorder are the purported association of enuresis with EEG abnormalities (British Medical Journal, 1960; Lovibond & Coote, 1969), a positive family history (Bakwin, 1961; Hallgren, 1957), and sleep abnormalities. EEG studies have shown that enuresis most typically occurs in deep sleep in children, but it can in fact occur at any stage (Broughton, 1968; Ditman & Blinn, 1955; Ritvo, Ornitz, Gottlieb, Poussaint, Maron, Ditman, & Blinn, 1969; Boyd, 1960). Boyd (1960), in the only controlled study, was unable to demonstrate that enuretics were less rousable than normal children. In elegant studies Broughton (1968) has shown that a more probable explanation is that the developmental disorder is reflected in more extreme psychophysiological reactions (including larger and more frequent bladder contractions) to the arousal episodes from deep sleep, which normally recur irregularly throughout the night.

Hallgren (1957), Lovibond and Coote (1969), and Muellner (1960) have shown that diurnal frequency, urgency, and reduced bladder capacity are very often correlated with nocturnal enuresis and influence its prognosis. Muellner (1960) has elaborated these findings into an "overreactive bladder" etiological hypothesis. It is also obvious that often cited but seldom demonstrated abnormalities of the urinary system, such as malformations and infections, could make the acquisition of nocturnal continence more difficult.

Psychopathology and the Enuretic Child

In keeping with the main emphasis of this chapter, namely examining the evidence for the correlation of somatic condition and psychopathology, an attempt will now be made to summarize this area. There are a large number of studies which purport to show that enuretic children have a significantly increased prevalence of psychopathology. These range all the way from extreme positions such as that of Anderson (1930), Gerard (1939), Lickorish (1964) and Sperling (1965) which claim or imply a practically invariant correlation between enuresis and psychopathology to more recent and generally better controlled studies such as those by Hallgren (1957), Oppel et al.

(1968b), Stein, Susser, and Wilson (1965) and Werry and Cohrssen (1965) which, while confirming a somewhat higher frequency of psychopathology in enuretic children, show that this correlation is by no means absolute or even very sizable. One cause of some of the overestimation of the size of this correlation is biased sampling, no doubt most extreme in psychiatric samples. Hallgren (1957) found that enuretic children who were not seen by a physician tended to have a lower frequency of psychopathology than those seen medically and, in fact, were scarcely distinguishable from normal children. To this error are added very often small sample size, lack of proper double-blind conditions, and vague and probably unreliable measurement techniques (Werry, 1967a).

Now it seems best to conclude that there is a significant but small and infrequent correlation between enuresis and psychopathology. This means that the majority of enuretics in the population (as opposed to those seen by physicians and especially those referred to psychiatrists) do not have any apparent emotional disturbance. Furthermore, in those that do, the causal relationship to the symptom of enuresis is unestablished and in some cases, at least, it may be either coincidental or secondary to the enuresis.

Also unestablished at this point is that there is any specific kind of psychopathology correlated with enuresis. Although it is commonly assumed that enuresis is correlated particularly with anxious, hypersensitive personalities, most studies beginning with those by Michaels and Goodman (1934) and supported by Hallgren (1957), Oppel et al. (1968), and Stein and Susser (1968) suggest that it is associated at least equally frequently with the conduct or acting out disorders.

Treatment and Prognosis

(a) Placebo. There is strong evidence to show that enuresis is often responsive to a wide variety of nonspecific procedures (see summary in Werry & Cohrssen, 1965). No doubt, in some cases, particularly in younger age groups, this is part of the normal spontaneous remission-relapse cycle (Forrester, Stein, & Susser, 1964; Oppel et al., 1968a) instead of a true placebo response.

(b) Psychotherapy. Because of the wide acceptance by mental health professionals, doctors, and lay public of the psychodynamic etiological theory of enuresis, psychotherapy is one of the most often recommended treatments for enuresis for the North American middle class child (Nelson, Vaughan, & McKay, 1969). Despite this, there is little data on the effectiveness of this treatment technique, especially by the protagonists. Two controlled studies (De Leon & Mandell, 1966; Werry & Cohrssen, 1965) did not find six to twelve sessions of psychotherapy to be superior to no formal treatment.

Although these two studies do not definitively exclude psychotherapy as a useful treatment in certain kinds of enuresis, it must be concluded that firm evidence of the usefulness of this technique is presently lacking.

(c) *Drug Treatment.* A variety of drugs has been used ranging from pituitary snuff (for its antidiuretic effect), amphetamines (for their sleep lightening effect), anxiolytic drugs such as meprobamate and hydroxyzine (Breger, 1961, 1962a & b), the tricyclic-antidepressants such as imipramine and amitryptyline (Alderton, 1967; Kardash, Hillman, & Werry, 1968; Poussaint & Ditman, 1965; Ritvo et al., 1969). However, with the exception of the antidepressant drugs, medication has not earned a significant place in the treatment of enuresis. Controlled studies have shown repeatedly that the antidepressants, probably by virtue of their direct action on the bladder reflex instead of their antidepressant effect, are superior to placebo, but the number of children who are cured rather than simply improved is usually under 30%. Furthermore, dosages recommended (up to 75 milligrams per child at night) must be considered fairly high. Despite this and though cure rates are inferior to those reported for the bed buzzer (see Chapter Seven), simplicity, economy, and convenience make the antidepressants like placebo well worth a trial.

Conditioning Treatment

Originally introduced by the German pediatrician, Pfaundler in 1904, and rediscovered by Mowrer and Mowrer in 1938, the bed buzzer has recently undergone a great increase in popularity concomitant with the development of behavior therapy which has given the treatment a respectability and rationale it previously lacked. Reviews of the effectiveness and rationale of the conditioning apparatus may be found in Chapter Seven of this book as well as in Jones (1960), Lovibond and Coote (1969), and Werry (1967b), the latter two of which give detailed instructions on how to implement treatment programs. There is now compelling evidence, notably in carefully controlled studies by De Leon and Mandell (1966), Forrester et al. (1964), and Werry and Cohrssen (1965), that the conditioning treatment is superior to no treatment as well as to psychotherapy and to amphetamine.

The bladder training method of Muellner (1960) is also basically a learning technique aimed at increasing the functional capacity of the bladder by successive approximation (postponing the act of micturition for increasing periods). However, the effectiveness is unknown since no controlled studies have yet been executed.

Prevalence studies suggest that the prognosis for untreated enuresis is benign. By the age of 14, all but about 2% of enuretic children will have undergone spontaneous remission (Lovibond & Coote, 1969). Nevertheless, as

Lovibond and Coote point out, the unpredictability of the time of spontaneous cure and the general inconvenience of the symptom suggest that a "nonheroic" trial of treatment in willing and suitable patients should be undertaken probably beginning with a placebo, then an antidepressant, and finally the conditioning treatment. Other promising avenues to explore in resistant cases are combinations of drugs and conditioning treatments (Young & Turner, 1965).

Summary

Enuresis appears to be a multifactorially determined condition or, in short, a phenotype in which a multiplicity of physiological, psychological, and social factors can be etiological either singly or in combination. In the majority of instances, however, enuresis is probably not a psychosomatic disorder (Kanner, 1960).

Encopresis

Definition

Even though some (Anthony, 1957; Coekin & Gairdner, 1960) restrict the term encopresis to the deliberate deposition of feces in a place other than the toilet, it is ordinarily used to include any kind of fecal incontinence occurring in the absence of physical disease or abnormality. Since all children are born incontinent it is customary, as with enuresis, to specify a minimum age, set by Bakwin and Bakwin (1966), at the second birthday. However, Stein and Susser (1967), in their studies of the development of bowel and bladder control in 600 English preschool children, found as did Bellman (1966) in 8500 Swedish children that only about 50% of the children had achieved bowel control by two years whereas almost 100% had by the age of four years, suggesting that the latter is a more realistic point of abnormality.

Stein and Susser (1967) found that not only is bowel control typically completely achieved before any bladder control, but also that the sequence (nocturnal first, diurnal second) is exactly opposite from that of the attainment of urinary continence. As with urinary continence, however, girls usually achieve bowel control earlier than boys.

Occurrence

Bellman (1966), in his study of 8500 Swedish children, found the prevalence of encopresis to decrease slowly as a function of age reaching practically zero at 16. The prevalence in boys at 8 years was 2.3% as against

0.7% for girls. This higher frequency in boys has been observed consistently (Anthony, 1957; Bellman, 1966; Davidson, Kugler, & Bauer, 1963; McTaggart & Scott, 1959; Richmond, Eddy, & Garrard, 1954; Shirley, 1938).

In a study of about 200 hospital and clinic cases, Bellman (1966) found half had had an interval of bowel control of about one year; no physical or psychiatric differences could be discerned in this group.

Etiological Theories

As pointed out by Anthony (1957), Coekin and Gairdner (1960), and Woodmansey (1967), in discussing etiology it seems important to distinguish between two kinds of encopretic children—those who produce a fully formed, soft stool (whom we shall call nonretentive) and those in whom the encopreses consist principally of constant leaking of fecal-stained fluid from the rectum (retentive). The latter, upon physical examination, are found to have a rectum distended by hard feces. According to Coekin and Gairdner (1960), the retentive kind of encopresis is further distinguished in being of equal frequency in both sexes, though this was so only in private practice cases in Davidson et al.'s (1963) large pediatric series. There seems little doubt that this kind of encopresis is caused by retention of feces by the child to the point of extinction of the normal defecatory reflex. The cause of the retention of feces could have a number of possible causes and as with enuresis it is not surprising to find that pediatricians tend to argue more for physical factors, notably constipation developing in infancy causing pain on defecation (Coekin & Gairdner, 1960; Davidson et al., 1963) while psychiatrists have emphasized distortion of the normal anal-retentive phase of psychosexual development or disturbance of parent-child relationships (Anthony, 1957; McTaggart & Scott, 1959; Richmond et al., 1954; Shirley, 1938).

In the nonretentive kind of encopresis, Anthony (1957) has suggested that there are at least two etiological possibilities. In the first, because of coercive toilet training, the child may have developed anxiety surrounding the toileting situation which should be apparent from the child's refusal to sit on the toilet. In the second, the child has simply never learned or been taught the toileting sequence or received reward, actual or fantasied, from depositing his feces in the toilet. Woodmansey (1967) added a third, a psychophysiological kind "fear-induced diarrhea." These two possibilities are discussed in more detail in Chapter Seven and in Bellman (1966).

Coexistence of Psychopathology and Encopresis

Pediatricians, who see large numbers of unselected children (Bakwin & Bakwin, 1966; Coekin & Gairdner, 1960; Davidson et al., 1963), argue that the majority of retentive encopretics have no associated psychopathology, whereas the nonretentive encopretics, who constitute a small minority, often have. On the other hand, child psychiatrists (without making the distinction between the different groups) argue that most, if not all, encopretics have significant psychopathology (McTaggart & Scott, 1959; Richmond et al., 1954; Shirley, 1938; Warson, Caldwell, Warinner, Kirk, & Jensen, 1954).

In one of the few controlled and otherwise methodologically reasonable studies, Bellman (1966) found that his (pediatric) clinic and hospital cases differed from matched normal controls in personality (anxious, unassertive, and passive-aggressive), social skills (less peer contact), and family background (more punitive-authoritarian parents, coercive and early toilet training, more separations from mothers). Bellman (1966) was careful to notice that he was unable to tell whether these features were primary or secondary to the encopresis, although he thought the balance of evidence suggested they were primarily etiological.

The picture is thus unclear and while encopretic children may as a group be more disturbed than continent children, the possibility that this is often secondary to this extremely socially distressing condition and that its importance differs in the two kinds of encopresis is highly probable.

Treatment and Prognosis

Bellman (1966), in a two-year follow-up study of 200 clinic cases, found that about 50% of the children had remitted spontaneously and practically all had remitted by the age of 16. In view of this and since no controlled treatment trials could be found, it is difficult to evaluate the effectiveness of the various treatments available. In a large series, Coekin & Gairdner (1960) and Davidson et al. (1963) claim 80–90% success rate in the retentive kind of encopresis with enemas and laxatives. There appear to be no good studies of the effect of psychotherapy on encopresis though success appears to be under 50% (McTaggart & Scott, 1959, and Shirley, 1938) in what are probably highly selected samples.

Behavior modification techniques, currently increasing in vogue and sophistication, are summarized in Chapter Seven, but seem to consist principally still of single case studies.

Consideration of the possible etiological factors discussed above suggests that each child requires a careful assessment to see first whether he falls into the retentive group requiring primarily medical treatment probably combined with some behavior modification incentive system for going to the toilet. If he does not have the retentive kind, a program either to extinguish anxiety about the toileting situation or to make it rewarding to go to the toilet should be developed (see Chapter Seven).

Ulcerative Colitis

Definition

Ulcerative colitis is a serious disease of the colon and rectum characterized by bloody diarrhea, typical ulceration of the bowel, and the absence of pathogenic microorganisms. The first two features differentiate it from simple nervous diarrhea and the latter two from infective kinds.

The onset is usually insidious, although in about 10% of children it is fulminating and life-threatening. Even though the course of the disease in most instances is that of a low-grade chronicity with intermittent exacerbations, serious long-term complications such as anemia and cancer are common. (Broberger & Lagercrantz, 1966).

Occurrence

Good epidemiological data on ulcerative colitis in children is scanty, since most of it is derived from small and selected (hospitalized) samples. The age of onset is variable ranging from infancy to old age, but the majority of childhood cases occur from the age of 9 on. "Children and adolescents constitute about 10% of hospital admissions for the disease. In this age group the sexes appear equally represented and although the distribution as a function of socioeconomic class is unknown all classes appear represented. However, the prevalence is said to vary in different ethnic groups and nationalities and to be increasing in Western countries, but this may be an artifact of better hospital services (Broberger & Lagercrantz, 1966; Canby & Mehlhop, 1964; McDermott & Finch, 1967).

Etiology

Feldman, Cantor, Soll, and Bachrach (1967) have drawn attention to the split between nonpsychiatric physicians who favor physical etiological theories and psychiatrists who espouse psychogenesis. Principal physical theories are infective, biochemical, and immunological. With the discovery of an anticolonic antibody in ulcerative colitis patients, the latter seems currently the most popular (Broberger & Lagercrantz, 1966; McDermott & Finch, 1967).

While psychiatrists have increasingly recognized the primary etiological importance of constitutional factors, Feldman et al. (1967) point out that they still discuss the condition as if it were a true psychosomatic (psychogenic) disease. Even when proponents admit the importance of physical factors (Engel, 1962; Jackson & Yalom, 1966; Josselyn, Littner, & Spurlock, 1966; McDermott & Finch, 1967), psychosomatic theories are characterized by a set of common beliefs, namely that practically all ulcerative colitis patients (and their parents) have severe abnormality of personality, unconscious conflict, mood, or family interaction that long predated the onset of the illness. Further, that this abnormality is specific enough for patients to be recognized as a distinctive group (Askevold, 1964; Feldman et al., 1967). The kinds of disturbance reported are obsessive-compulsive and dependent personalities, depressive conflict, anxiety about being overwhelmed, controlling, controlled, inadequate sexually, and humorless (Askevold, 1964; Feldman et al., 1967). A glance at this list will immediately raise questions about specificity in ulcerative colitis.

One important pediatric source did find a high prevalence of psychopathology in the children (Broberger & Lagercrantz, 1966), but they did not confirm the abnormality of the parents whose overprotective controlling behavior was found to dissipate when the children's physical condition improved. How both these determinations were made is not described.

Feldman et al. (1967) have been sharply critical of the assumptions and methodological shortcomings of most psychiatric studies of ulcerative colitis citing deficiencies repeatedly emphasized throughout this and other chapters, namely small and highly selected samples of children, no controls, reliance on retrospective data, uncertain or poor evaluative techniques, and ignoring of the somatopsychic effects of what is a dangerous, painful, and socially embarrassing illness. It is remarkable in this latter respect that there are virtually no studies which have employed the logically necessary control group of chronically physically handicapped children as was done in the case of childhood psychosis (see Chapter Five).

The study by Feldman et al. (1967) is a remarkable exception from the usual study both conceptually and methodologically. By means of a standardized, carefully detailed checklist completed after several psychiatric interviews, they examined 34 patients, of whom 25% were under 20 years of age, and a matched group of patients with gastrointestinal disease (excluding colitis). Using normative and control data, Feldman et al. failed to find any apparent importance in ulcerative colitis of psychopathology whether general or specific, of psychological precipitation or aggravation, of nuclear conflicts, or of symptom shifts between depression and colitis.

Feldman et al. were themselves at pains to point out the study has some serious methodological shortcomings such as limited contact, nonblind observers, committee evaluations and psychiatric interviews as data base, but the study's clear superiority to most others gives it an unusual credibility strongly sustained by the observations of most nonpsychiatric physicians.

Treatment and Prognosis

Despite the fact that the mortality rate in children with ulcerative colitis has been greatly reduced in the last decade and that a drug dependent improvement can now be obtained in many cases with corticosteroids, a significant and ever-increasing number (over 40%) of patients ultimately require surgery (Broberger & Lagercrantz, 1966; McDermott & Finch, 1967).

The efficacy of psychotherapeutic techniques is unknown except that there appears to be little correlation between psychological and physical improvement (Feldman et al., 1967; McDermott & Finch, 1967) casting further doubt on the functional relationship between psychological variables and ulcerative colitis. The role of psychotherapy in children appears to have shifted among its protagonists from a primary to a supportive role in the disease (McDermott & Finch, 1967).

Conclusions

Ulcerative colitis resembles many other psychosomatic diseases in children in the fundamental failure to date to establish the importance and exact role of psychological factors in the etiology and treatment of the disease. Thus, as Feldman et al. (1967) point out, it cannot be regarded as a proven psychosomatic disease.

Conclusions

This review of certain physical disorders of childhood commonly called psychosomatic has revealed the following.

1. There is no evidence in any disorder that all children or their parents show current or past indications of psychopathology or pathogenic environment and thus that the disorder is *necessarily* psychosomatic.

2. There is evidence that in some disorders such as asthma, enuresis, and obesity several different etiological factors (including psychological ones) singly or in varying combinations can be operative. Thus, these disorders can be subdivided into physical, psychosomatic, and mixed etiological subgroups. In other conditions such as ulcerative colitis, any primary role of psychogenic factors seems highly dubious. None of the above considerations precludes aggravating effects of psychological variables once the disease process is established, but that is not the meaning of psychosomatic disorder as currently used (American Psychiatric Association, 1968).

3. When psychopathology of child or parent is associated with the disease, the evidence that it takes the form of a personality-type conflict or mood specific to that disorder is unconvincing. The most plausible theory of psychosomatic relationships is that advanced by Sternbach (1966); the psychosomatic disorder is perceived as the result of three interacting components (a) the psychogenic stimuli partly unconditioned and hence universal and partly conditioned or idiosyncratic but always aversive, frequent, and strongly elicitive of (b) the physiological-biochemical response involving one particular vulnerable organ or system to a greater extent than others (response stereotypy), (c) a failure of normal homeostatic damping mechanisms so that the response is exaggerated and results ultimately in tissue damage.

How this combination of response stereotypy and homeostatic failure develops is obscure but heredity, constitution, injury, prior disease, or conditioning may all be involved. Thus individuals with the same psychosomatic disease are much more likely to have similar physiological responses than psychological patterns.

4. The focus of studies needs to shift from abtruse and often untestable theory and from correlational methods to a study of the functional relationships between objectively defined and measured psychological stimuli or states, on the one hand, and the physiological response both in high risk populations and in children with the disease, on the other. While correlational studies can point to psychogenic stimuli or states of possible importance and to useful taxonomies, their value in the forseeable future is likely to be limited. To overcome the unbalanced nature of past studies, the study of functional relationships requires that experimental psychologists, physiologists, and clinical investigators work together or at least consult with each other.

5. Simplistic and reductionist notions of etiology need to be abandoned. For example, individual disorders should not be viewed as homogeneous, but rather as in all probability phenotypes in which different kinds of variables may be etiological either singly, or more likely, in varying combinations. The study of asthma for example has shown that progress is more likely to be made when some subcategorization is used. Physiological variables need to be given far greater recognition and study. The absence of a known physical etiology does not imply that a condition is psychosomatic.

6. This review has revealed a set of methodological errors in most studies that must be corrected if our knowledge about psychosomatic conditions in children is to advance.

(a) Since there is abundant evidence to show that such populations are biased toward the overinclusion of emotionally disturbed children, sampling must extend beyond psychiatric and clinic populations to include particularly children who are never seen by a doctor for the disorder but also those handled by nonpsychiatric physicians such as pediatricians or community physicians.

(b) Measures of psychological states and variables must not be assumed to be reliable and valid; they must be of previously demonstrated precision or shown in the study to possess it. This does not preclude the clinical history and interview since with proper attention they can attain acceptable scientific standards (Graham & Rutter, 1968; Rutter & Graham, 1968).

(c) Acceptable standards of experimental control such as double-blind techniques and contrast groups and of quantification and statistical interpretation of data must be applied.

Hospitalization, Anesthesia, and Surgery as Pathogenic Agents[1]

In their comprehensive view of the literature on the psychological responses of children to hospitalization and illness, Vernon, Foley, Sipowicz and Schulman (1965) delineated four variables most often cited as determinants of psychological upset: (a) unfamiliarity of the hospital setting, (b) separation from parents, (c) age, and (d) pre-hospitalization personality. They concluded that there was considerable evidence that unfamiliarity and separation could be implicated in the etiology of psychological disturbances in the *post-hospital* period while the effect of age was unclear. Separation and age were the two variables most important to the etiology of upsets *during* hospitalization, the relationship with age being curvilinear, with children between the ages of six months and three to four years appearing to be particularly susceptible. The role of the fourth variable, pre-hospitalization personality, was judged not proven though there was some evidence that poor adjustment prior to hospitalization was likely to result in more frequent and more severe upsets in the intra- and post-hospital periods.

Some additional variables examined by Vernon et al. (1965) were (a) previous hospitalization (insufficient data to make a conclusion; while most authors seem to assume that this would necessarily increase the likelihood of disturbance, Vernon et al. (1965) suggest that by reduction of unfamiliarity it may, in at least a significant number of cases, actually reduce the incidence of upset); (b) sex (nonconsistent relationship); (c) characteristics of the

[1] This section is based on portions of an article (Davenport & Werry, 1970) appearing in the *American Journal of Orthopsychiatry*, copyright, The American Orthopsychiatric Association and reproduced by permission.

illness and treatment (no relationship established thus far but the reviewers considered all studies to date have grave shortcomings); (d) pre-operative sedation (few studies but they suggest that the efficacy of pre-operative sedation as judged by status during induction of anesthesia, is an important variable).

In addressing themselves to the general thesis "Is hospitalization upsetting?" Vernon et al. (1965) concluded that this question is difficult to answer, first because of the variability of the crucial etiological factors discussed above from child to child, from illness to illness and from hospital to hospital. Further, the absence of appropriate norms for the prevalence and incidence of psychological upsets in the general population, notably in children who have never been hospitalized, makes a control group mandatory. Though several authors have used control groups in studying the effect of specific treatment procedures designed to reduce the frequency of psychological upset during hospitalization, the use of non-hospitalized control groups has been rare. Two studies which did, namely those by Woodward (1959) and by Stott (1959) both found that hospitalization and illness were traumatic experiences for children, but both were retrospective and long-term (two to five years) and as Vernon et al. (1965) point out, both may now be invalid since hospital procedures with children have changed dramatically in the past ten to fifteen years.

Cassell (1965) states that though most of the recent studies support the widely held view that hospitalization and its procedures are likely to have a serious effect on later psychological adjustment in a significant number of children (she reports a range of 20–36% prevalence of upset) she cautions against accepting these findings as necessarily valid because of generally poor methodology. Vernon et al. (1965) also felt that any conclusions about the effects of hospitalization on children should be considered tentative because of "the paucity of quantitative systematic research" (p. 156). They delineated seven weaknesses characteristic of research in the area: (a) inadequate description of procedures used to measure the child's response to hospitalization (b) failure to control observer bias, blind ratings and multiple observers being employed infrequently, (c) very little use of statistical tests to interpret the findings, (d) the failure to control or examine the crucial pathogenic variables involved in hospitalization outlined above. In the typical study these variables were hopelessly intermixed, (e) failure to measure the direct effects of experimental conditions, notably failure to assess the extent to which psychological procedures aimed at increasing the child's knowledge about forthcoming surgical procedures actually achieved this informational goal, (f) failure to establish the reliability and validity of the measures of the child's behavioral or emotional states, (g) disregard of potential psychological benefit from hospitalization; most authors anticipating psychological upset have failed altogether to study the possibility that some children may be benefited from hospitalization (pp. 162–164).

In an effort to improve methodology in the area, Vernon and Schulman (1964) developed a parental questionnaire of 27 behavioral symptoms comprising those most frequently cited in the literature as occurring in children *following hospitalization*. In commenting on the reliability of the questionnaire in a later study, Vernon, Schulman and Foley (1966) cited a study by Cassell (1965) in which the correlation between total symptom scores 3 and 30 days after discharge in 37 children undergoing cardiac catheterization was $r = .65$ which suggests acceptable though modest reliability in the mothers' reporting. Some moderate support for the validity of the questionnaire came from a well-designed study by Vernon et al. (1966) in which the findings on the questionnaire were compared with those of a psychiatric interview with 20 children who had been hospitalized for tonsillectomy ($r = .47$). Further evidence of the construct validity of the questionnaire comes from its detection of changes as predicted in studies by Vernon et al. (1966), Vernon, Foley and Schulman (1967), and Kay (1966).

In an effort to reduce the 27 symptoms to a conceptually manageable small number of symptom clusters or sub-syndromes, Vernon et al. (1966) factor analyzed the questionnaire and discovered that six independent factors emerged. (I) general anxiety and regression; (II) separation anxiety; (III) anxiety about sleep; (IV) eating disturbance; (V) aggression towards authority; (VI) apathy-withdrawal.

Vernon et al. (1966) used the questionnaire to study the effect of hospitalization and illness on post-hospital adjustment in children aged 1 month to 9 years, employing a mail inquiry sent out one week after discharge. They found that while, in confirmation of the widely held opinion, illness/hospitalization "is an upsetting experience for children in general, resulting in increased separation anxiety, sleep anxiety, and aggression towards authority" (Vernon et al., 1965, p. 593) these changes were of minimal nature and 25% of the children (largely from the lower socio-economic classes) actually showed improvement. They found that age (6 months to 3 years 11 months), length of hospitalization (2 weeks or more) and socio-economic class (high) increased the susceptibility to post-hospitalization upset while sex, prior hospitalization, degree of pain experienced during hospitalization and birth order appeared without any such systematic efforts.

On the other hand, Cassell (1965) found the majority of her group of 40 children undergoing cardiac catheterization to be actually slightly improved at follow-up as adjudged by the same questionnaire. These differences may be explicable by the generally better methodology of Cassell, thus making her findings probably more valid—she administered the questionnaire both before and after hospitalization and retained 100% of her sample whereas the reply rate of Vernon et al.'s (1966) single post-hospitalization mailing of the questionnaire was only 48%. Another difference possibly of significance in the two studies, is the longer mean duration of hospital stay in the group studied by Vernon et al. (8.8 days versus 3 days).

Since the time of the review by Vernon et al. (1965) studies have shown a laudable improvement in methodology. An interesting development has been an increasing concern with testing specific manipulations of hospital procedures as Cassell had done in 1965. Vernon, Foley and Schulman (1967) and Kay (1966) again using (in addition to using some intra-hospital measures) a single mailing of the same questionnaire six days after discharge as their measure of post-hospitalization upset, demonstrated that variations in anesthetic technique [principally presence of the mother at induction, type of induction (concealed, painless intravenous induction versus routine intravenous or inhalation induction) and certain anesthesiologists] have slightly mitigating effects. In a substantial construct validation of their questionnaire and its factors, Vernon et al. (1965) found, as in their first study (1967), that the factors showing change were again factor II (separation anxiety—effected by presence of mother), factor III (sleep anxiety—by age), and factor V (aggression towards authority—by anesthesiologist).

In a well designed study Minde and Maler (1968) succeeded in reducing children's anxiety in hospital and expediting their discharge through a counselling procedure. They also demonstrated that the crucial therapeutic variable was not due to cognitive factors (explanations about hospital, illness, etc.) but simply to being visited regularly by an adult. Brain and Maclay (1968) found that the hospitalization of mothers with their children reduced both intra and post hospitalization disturbance particularly in younger children. Brain and Maclay used rather crude measures of disturbance and like most others did not control for observer bias.

In a less rigorous study, particularly as far as the measurement and definition of behavioral upsets were concerned McKee (1963) found no difference in the frequency of behavioral upset in operated and non-operated (and presumably thus unhospitalized) children with tonsil and adenoid disorders.

Davenport and Werry (1970) in a carefully controlled study, including "blind" observers used Vernon and Schulman's questionnaire to study the change in preoperative behavioral adjustment two weeks after discharge in 145 children undergoing general anesthesia, ENT and dental surgery in two hospitals compared with 145 non hospitalized controls. No differences were found in the two groups though there was some evidence that children upset at the time of induction of anesthesia were more likely to be more disturbed both before and by hospitalization.

In summary then, it may be said that the data supporting the widely held view that hospitalization and its concomitant procedures, such as surgery and anesthesia cause psychological upset in a significant number of children following hospitalization has some empirical support which is, however, far from unanimous. Furthermore, the evidence suggests that despite the findings of earlier studies, the degree of any disturbance is slight. Variables which appear possibly to affect the frequency of disturbance and probably its degree also are age, socioeconomic status, length of hospitalization, anesthetic and hospital procedures. This is not to say that other variables as yet untested are not also influential, that individual children may not be severely traumatized or that many children do not suffer temporary and avoidable upset *during hospitalization.* There is a great need for studies which adhere to the methodological prerequisites outlined by Vernon et al. (1965) notably (a) the use of reliable valid, adequately described measures of psychological adjustment, (b) minimization of confounding of important etiological variables (discussed above) either through careful control or preferably through their systematic manipulation within the experimental design, (c) the use of a non-hospitalized control group, and (d) the use of statistical methods as an aid to the analysis and interpretation of the findings.

References

Alderton, H. Imipramine in childhood nocturnal enuresis: Relationship of time of administration to effect. *Canadian Psychiatric Association Journal,* 1967, **12**, 197–203.

Alexander, F. *Psychosomatic Medicine.* New York: Norton & Co., 1950.

American Academy of Pediatrics. Obesity in childhood. *Pediatrics,* 1967, **40**, 455–467.

American Psychiatric Association. *Diagnostic and Statistical Manual of Mental Disorders.* (2nd ed.). Washington, D.C., 1968.

Anderson, F. The psychiatric aspects of enuresis. *American Journal of Diseases of Children,* 1930, **40**, 591, 818.

Anthony, E. An experimental approach to the psychopathology of childhood— encopresis. *British Journal of Medical Psychology,* 1957, **30**, 146–175.

Apley, J., & McKeith, R. *The Child and His Symptoms: A Psychosomatic Approach.* Philadelphia: Davis, 1962.

Asher, P. Fat babies and fat children. The prognosis of obesity in the very young. *Archives of Diseases in Childhood,* 1966, **41**, 672–673.

Askevold, F. Studies in ulcerative colitis. *Journal of Psychosomatic Research,* 1964, **8**, 89–100.

Bakwin, H. Enuresis in children. *Journal of Pediatrics,* 1961, **58**, 806–819.

Bakwin, H., & Bakwin, R. *Clinical Management of Behavior Disorders in Children.* Philadelphia: Saunders, 1966.

Baraff, A., & Cunningham, A. Asthmatic and normal children. *Journal of the American Medical Association,* 1965, **192**, 99–101.

Baroff, S., & Tate, B. The use of aversive stimulation in the treatment of chronic self-injurious behavior. *Journal of American Academy of Child Psychiatry,* 1968, **7**, 454–470.

Beech, H., & Nace, E. Asthma and aggression: The investigation of a hypothetical relationship employing a new procedure. *British Journal of Social and Clinical Psychology,* 1965, **4**, 124–130.

Bellman, M. Studies on encopresis. *Acta Pediatrica Scandinavica,* 1966, **170** (Supp.).

Berkson, G. Stereotyped movements of mental defectives. VI. No effect of amphetamine or a barbiturate. *Perceptual Motor Skills,* 1965, **21**, 698.

Berkson, G. Abnormal stereotyped motor acts. In J. Zubin & H. Hunt (Eds.), *Comparative Psychopathology*. New York: Grune & Stratton, 1967, 76–94.

Berkson, G., & Davenport, R. Stereotyped movements of mental defectives. I. Initial survey. *American Journal of Mental Deficiency*, 1962, **66**, 849–852.

Berkson, G., & Mason, W. Stereotyped movements of mental defectives. IV. The effects of toys and the character of the acts. *American Journal of Mental Deficiency*, 1964a, **68**, 511–524.

Berkson, G., & Mason, W. Stereotyped behaviors of chimpanzees: Relation to general arousal and alternative activities. *Perceptual Motor Skills*, 1964b, **19**, 635–652.

Block, J. Further considerations of psychosomatic predisposing factors in allergy. *Psychosomatic Medicine*, 1968, **30**, 202–208.

Block, J., Harvey, E., Jennings, P., & Simpson, E. Clinicians' conceptions of the asthmatogenic mother. *Archives of General Psychiatry*, 1966, **15**, 610.

Block, J., Jennings, P., Harvey, E., & Simpson, E. Interaction between allergic potential and psychopathology in childhood. *Psychosomatic Medicine*, 1964, **26**, 307–320.

Blomfield, J., & Douglas, J. Bedwetting prevalence among children aged 4–7 years. *Lancet*, 1956, **1**, 850–852.

Bower, E. *Early Identification of Emotionally Handicapped Children in School*. Springfield, Ill.: Charles C Thomas, 1960.

Boyd, M. The depth of sleep in enuretic school children and in non-enuretic controls. *Journal of Psychosomatic Research*, 1960, **4**, 274–281.

Brain, D., & Maclay, I. Controlled study of mothers and children in hospital. *British Medical Journal*, 1968, **1**, 278–280.

Breger, E. Meprobamate in the management of enuresis. *Journal of Pediatrics*, 1961, **59**, 571–576.

Breger, E. Hydroxyzine hydrochloride and methylphenidate hydrochloride in the management of enuresis. *Journal of Pediatrics*, 1962a, **61**, 443–447.

Breger, E. The maintenance of therapeutic effect in children with enuresis. *Journal of Pediatrics*, 1962b, **61**, 723–725.

British Medical Journal, Enuresis, (Editorial), 1960, **1**, 1416–1417.

British Medical Journal, Management of the fat child (Editorial), 1966, **2**, 961–962.

Broberger, O., & Lagercrantz, R. Ulcerative colitis in childhood and adolescence. *Advances in Pediatrics*, 1966, **14**, 9–54.

Broughton, R. Sleep disorders: Disorders of arousal? *Science*, 1968, **159**, 1070–1078.

Bruch, H. Psychotherapeutic problems in eating disorders. *Psychoanalytic Review*, 1963a, **50**, 43–57.

Bruch, H. Disturbed communication in eating disorders. *American Journal of Orthopsychiatry*, 1963b, **33**, 99–104.

Canby, J., & Mehlhop, F. Ulcerative colitis in children. *American Journal of Gastroenterology*, 1964, **42**, 66–76.

Carroll, R. Epidemiology of New Orleans epidemic asthma. *American Journal of Public Health*, 1968, **58**, 1677–1683.

Cassell, S. Effect of brief puppet therapy upon the emotional responses of children undergoing cardiac catheterisation. *Journal of Consulting Psychology*, 1965, **29**, 1–8.

Christakis, G., Sajecki, S., Hillman, R., Miller, E., Blumenthal, S., & Archer, M. Effect of a combined nutrition education and physical fitness program on the weight status of obese high school boys. *Federation Proceedings*, 1966, **25**, 15–19.

Clark, D. Behaviour therapy of Gilles de la Tourette's syndrome. *British Journal of Psychiatry*, 1966, **112**, 771–778.

Coekin, M., & Gairdner, D. Faecal incontinence in children. *British Medical Journal*, 1960, **2**, 1175–1180.

Connell, P., Corbett, J., Horne, D., & Mathews, A. Drug treatment of adolescent tiqueurs. *British Journal of Psychiatry*, 1967, **113**, 375–381.

Davenport, H., & Werry, J. The effect of general anesthesia surgery and hospitalization upon the behavior of children. *American Journal of Orthopsychiatry*, 1970, **40**, 806–824.

Davidson, M., Kugler, M., & Bauer, C. Diagnosis and management in children with severe and protracted constipation and obstipation. *Journal of Pediatrics*, 1963, **62**, 261–275.

Davidson, P. Thumbsucking. In C. Costello (Ed.), *Symptoms of Psychopathology*. New York: Wiley, 1970, 359–372.

Davis, K. The effect of drugs on stereotyped and nonstereotyped operant behaviors in retardates. Unpublished doctoral dissertation, University of Illinois at Urbana, 1970.

Davis, K., Sprague, R., & Werry, J. Stereotyped behavior and activity level in severe retardates: The effect of drugs. *American Journal of Mental Deficiency*, 1969, **73**, 721–727.

De Leon, G., & Mandell, W. A comparison of conditioning and psychotherapy in the treatment of functional enuresis. *Journal of Clinical Psychology*, 1966, **22**, 326–330.

De Lissovoy, V. Head banging in early childhood. *Child Development*, 1962, **33**, 43–56.

De Lissovoy, V. Head banging in early childhood: A study of incidence. *Journal of Pediatrics*, 1961, **58**, 803–805.

Dimson, S. Toilet training and enuresis. *British Medical Journal*, 1959, **2**, 666–670.

Ditman, K., & Blinn, K. Sleep levels in enuresis. *American Journal of Psychiatry*, 1955, **111**, 913–920.

Dubo, S., McLean, J., Ching, A., Wright, H., Kauffman, P., & Sheldon, J. A study of relationships between family situation, bronchial asthma, and personal adjustment in children. *Journal of Pediatrics*, 1961, **59**, 402–414.

Dunlap, K. *Habits, Their Making and Unmaking*. New York: Liveright, 1932.

Engel, G. *Psychological Development in Health and Disease*. Philadelphia: Saunders, 1962.

Epstein, R. Need for approval and the conditioning of verbal hostility in asthmatic children. *Journal of Abnormal and Social Psychology*, 1964, **69**, 105–109.

Eysenck, H. Learning theory and behaviour therapy. *Journal of Mental Science*, 1959, **105**, 61–75.

Feldman, F., Cantor, D., Soll, S., & Bachrach, W. Psychiatric study of a consecutive series of 34 patients with ulcerative colitis. *British Medical Journal*, 1967, **3**, 14–17.

Feldman, R., & Werry, J. An unsuccessful attempt to treat a tiqueur by massed practice. *Behaviour Research and Therapy*, 1966, **4**, 111–117.

Fitzelle, G. Personality factors and certain attitudes toward child rearing among parents of asthmatic children. *Psychosomatic Medicine*, 1959, **21**, 208–217.

Forrester, R., Stein, Z., & Susser, M. A trial of conditioning therapy in nocturnal enuresis. *Developmental Medicine and Child Neurology*, 1964, **6**, 158–166.

Franks, C., & Leigh, D. The conditioned eyeblink response in asthmatic and non-asthmatic subjects. *Journal of Psychosomatic Research*, 1959, **4**, 88–98.

French, T., & Alexander, F. Psychogenic factors in bronchial asthma. *Psychosomatic Medicine Monographs*, 1941, **4**(1).

Freud, A., & Burlingham, D. *Infants Without Families*. New York: International Universities Press, 1944.

Gerard, M. Enuresis: a study in etiology. *American Journal of Orthopsychiatry*, 1939, **9**, 45–58.

Glicklich, L. An historical account of enuresis. *Journal of Pediatrics*, 1951, **8**, 859–876.

Graham, P., & Rutter, M. The reliability and validity of the psychiatric assessment of the child: II. Interview with the parent. *British Journal of Psychiatry*, 1968, **114**, 581–592.

Graham, P., Rutter, M., Yule, W., & Pless, I. Childhood asthma: A psychosomatic disorder? Some epidemiological considerations. *British Journal of Preventive and Social Medicine*, 1967, **21**, 78–85.

Grant, M. Juvenile obesity—chronic, progressive, and transient. *Medical Officer*, 1966, **115**, 331–335.

Green, A. Self-mutilation in schizophrenic children. *Archives of General Psychiatry*, 1967, **17**, 234–244.

Green, A. Self-destructive behavior in physically abused schizophrenic children. *Archives of General Psychiatry*, 1968, **19**, 171–179.

Greenberg, N. Origins of head-rolling (spasmus nutans) during early infancy. *Psychosomatic Medicine*, 1964, **26**, 162–171.

Hahn, W. Autonomic responses of asthmatic children. *Psychosomatic Medicine*, 1966, **28**, 323–332.

Hallgren, B. Enuresis. I. A study with reference to the morbidity risk and symptomatology. *Acta Psychiatrica et Neurologica Scandinavica*, 1956a, **31**, 379–403.

Hallgren, B. Enuresis. II. A study with reference to certain physical, mental, and social factors possibly associated with enuresis. *Acta Psychiatrica et Neurologica Scandinavica*, 1956b, **31**, 405–436.

Hallgren, B. Enuresis: A clinical and genetic study. *Acta Psychiatrica et Neurologica Scandinavica*, 1957, **32**, 114, (Supp.).

Harlow, H. The heterosexual affectional system in monkeys. *American Psychologist*, 1962, **17**, 1–9.

Heald, F. Natural history and physiological basis of adolescent obesity. *Federation Proceedings*, 1966, **25**, 1–3.

Herbert, M. Personality factors and bronchial asthma: a study of South African Indian children. *Journal of Psychosomatic Research*, 1965, **8**, 353–364.

Hutt, S., Hutt, C., Lee, D., & Ounsted, C. A behavioral and electroencephalographic study of autistic children. *Journal of Psychiatric Research*, 1965, **3**, 181–197.

Jackson, D., & Yalom, I. Family research on the problem of ulcerative colitis. *Archives of General Psychiatry*, 1966, **15**, 410–418.

Jones, H. The behavioural treatment of enuresis nocturna. In H. Eysenck (Ed.), *Behaviour Therapy and the Neuroses*. Oxford: Pergamon, 1960, 377–403.

Josselyn, I., Littner, N., & Spurlock, J. Psychologic aspects of ulcerative colitis in children. *Journal of American Medical Women's Association*, 1966, **21**, 303–306.

Kanner, L. *Child Psychiatry*. Springfield: Charles C Thomas, 1957.

Kanner, L. Do behavior symptoms always indicate psychopathology? *Journal of Child Psychology and Psychiatry*, 1960, **1**, 17–25.

Kaplan, H., & Kaplan, H. Current theoretical concepts in psychosomatic medicine. *American Journal of Psychiatry*, 1959, **117**, 1091–1096.

Kardash, S., Hillman, E., & Werry, J. Efficacy of imipramine in childhood enuresis. *Canadian Medical Association Journal*, 1968, **99**, 263–266.

Kaufman, M., & Levitt, H. A study of three stereotyped behaviors in institutionalized mental defectives. *American Journal of Mental Deficiency*, 1965, **69**, 467–473.

Kay, B. Paediatric anaesthesia without tears. Paper presented at meeting of Association of Anaesthetists of Great Britain, November, 1966.

Kelman, D. Gilles de la Tourette's disease in children: A review of the literature. *Journal of Child Psychology and Psychiatry*, 1965, **6**, 219–226.

Kendell, R. An important source of bias affecting ratings made by psychiatrists. *Journal of Psychiatric Research*, 1968, **6**, 135–141.

Klackenberg, G. Primary enuresis: When is a child dry at night? *Acta Paediatrica*, 1955, **44**, 513–517.

Kravitz, H., Rosenthal, V., Teplitz, Z., Murphy, J., & Lesser, R. A study of head-banging in infants and children. *Diseases of the Nervous System*, 1960, **21**, 203–208.

Lancet, Obesity in childhood (Annotation), 1966, **2**, 327.

Lapouse, R., & Monk, M. An epidemiologic study of behavior characteristics in children. *American Journal of Public Health*, 1958, **48**, 1134–1144.

Lapouse, R., & Monk, M. Behavior deviations in a representative sample of children: variation by sex, age, race, social class, and family size. *American Journal of Orthopsychiatry*, 1964, **34**, 436–446.

Lebowitz, N., Colbert, E., & Palmer, J. Schizophrenia in children. *American Journal of Diseases of Children*, 1961, **102**, 25–27.

Levy, D. On the problem of movement restraint (tics, stereotyped movements, hyperactivity). *American Journal of Orthopsychiatry*, 1944, **14**, 644–671.

Lickorish, J. One hundred enuretics. *Journal of Psychosomatic Research*, 1964, **7**, 263–267.

Litrownik, A. The relationship of self-stimulatory behavior in autistic children to the intensity and complexity of environmental stimulation. Unpublished master's dissertation, University of Illinois at Urbana, 1969.

Lloyd, J., Wolff, O., & Whelen, W. Childhood obesity. A long term study of height and weight. *British Medical Journal,* 1961, **2**, 145–148.

Lourie, R. The role of rhythmic patterns in childhood. *American Journal of Psychiatry,* 1949, **105**, 653–660.

Lovaas, O., Freitag, G., Gold, V., & Kassorla, I. Experimental studies in childhood schizophrenia: Analysis of self-destructive behavior. *Journal of Experimental Child Psychology,* 1965a, **2**, 67–84.

Lovaas, O., Schaeffer, B., & Simmons, J. Building social behavior in autistic children by use of electric shock. *Journal of Experimental Research in Personality,* 1965b, **1**, 99–109.

Lovaas, O., & Simmons, J. Manipulation of self-destruction in three retarded children. *Journal of Applied Behavior Analysis,* 1962, **2**, 143–157.

Lovibond, S., & Coote, M. Enuresis. In C. Costello (Ed.), *Symptoms of Psychopathology,* New York: Wiley, 1969, 373–396.

Lucas, A., Kauffman, P., & Morris, E. Gilles de la Tourette's disease: a clinical study of fifteen cases. *Journal of American Academy of Child Psychiatry,* 1967, **6**, 700–722.

Mahler, M. A psychoanalytic evaluation of tic in psychopathology of children. *Psychoanalytic Study of the Child,* 1949, **3/4**, 279–310.

Malmo, R. Activation: a neuropsychological dimension. *Psychological Review,* 1959, **66**, 367–386.

Malmo, R. Anxiety and behavioral arousal. *Journal of Psychological Review,* 1957, **64**, 276–287.

Mason, W., & Sponholz, R. Behavior of Rhesus monkeys raised in isolation. *Journal of Psychiatric Research,* 1963, **1**, 299–306.

Mayer, J. Physical activity and anthropometric measurements of obese adolescents. *Federation Proceedings,* 1966a, **25**, 11–14.

Mayer, J. Some aspects of the problem of regulation of food intake and obesity. *New England Journal of Medicine,* 1966b, **274**, 610–616, 662–673, 722–731.

McDermott, J., & Finch, S. Ulcerative colitis in children: reassessment of a dilemma. *Journal of the American Academy of Child Psychiatry,* 1967, **6**, 512–525.

McGraw, M. Neurological maturation as exemplified by the achievement of bladder control. *Journal of Pediatrics,* 1940, **16**, 580–590.

McKee, W. A controlled study of the effects of tonsillectomy and adenoidectomy in children. *British Journal of Preventive and Social Medicine,* 1963, **17**, 49–69.

McKinney, J. A multidimensional study of the behavior of severely retarded boys. *Child Development,* 1962, **33**, 923–938.

McKinney, J., & Keele, T. Effects of increased mothering on the behavior of severely retarded boys. *American Journal of Mental Deficiency,* 1963, **67**, 556–562.

McTaggart, A., & Scott, M. A review of twelve cases of encopresis. *Journal of Pediatrics,* 1959, **54**, 762–768.

Mendelson, M., Hirsch, S., & Webber, C. A critical examination of some recent theoretical models in psychosomatic medicine. *Psychosomatic Medicine,* 1956, **18**, 363–373.

Michaels, J. *Disorders of Character: Persistent Enuresis, Juvenile Delinquency and Psychopathic Personality.* Springfield, Ill.: Charles C Thomas, 1955.

Michaels, J., & Goodman, S. Incidence and intercorrelations of enuresis and other neuropathic traits in so-called normal children. *American Journal of Orthopsychiatry*, 1934, **4**, 79–106.

Miller, H., & Baruch, D. A study of hostility in allergic children. *American Journal of Orthopsychiatry*, 1950, **20**, 506–519.

Minde, K., & Maler, L. Psychiatric counseling on a pediatric medical ward: A controlled evaluation. *Journal of Pediatrics*, 1968, **72**, 452–460.

Moore, N. Behavior therapy in bronchial asthma: A controlled study. *Journal of Psychosomatic Research*, 1965, **9**, 257–276.

Mowrer, O., & Mowrer, W. Enuresis: A method for its study and treatment. *American Journal of Orthopsychiatry*, 1938, **8**, 436–447.

Muellner, S. Development of urinary control in children: A new concept in cause, prevention and treatment of primary enuresis. *Journal of Urology*, 1960, **84**, 714–716.

Nelson, W., Vaughan, V., & McKay, R. *Textbook of Pediatrics*. Philadelphia: Saunders, 1969.

Neuhaus, E. A personality study of asthmatic and cardiac children. *Psychosomatic Medicine*, 1958, **20**, 181–186.

Olson, W. *The Measurement of Nervous Habits in Normal Children*. Minneapolis: University Press, 1929.

Oppel, W., Harper, P., & Rowland, V. The age of attaining bladder control. *Journal of Pediatrics*, 1968a, **42**, 614–626.

Oppel, W., Harper, P., & Rider, R. Social, psychological, and neurological factors associated with nocturnal enuresis. *Journal of Pediatrics*, 1968b, **42**, 627–641.

Ornitz, E., & Ritvo, E. Perceptual inconstancy in early infantile autism. *Archives of General Psychiatry*, 1968, **18**, 76–98.

Owen, F., & Williams, G. Patterns of respiratory disturbance in asthmatic children evoked by the stimulus of the mother's voice. *American Journal of Diseases of Children*, 1961, **102**, 133–134.

Pasamanick, B., & Kawi, A. A study of the association of prenatal and paranatal factors with the development of tics in children: A preliminary investigation. *Journal of Pediatrics*, 1956, **48**, 596–601.

Poussaint, A., & Ditman, K. A controlled study of imipramine (tofranil) in the treatment of childhood enuresis. *Journal of Pediatrics*, 1965, **67**, 283–290.

Prugh, D. Toward an understanding of psychosomatic concepts in relation to illness in children. In A. Solnit & S. Provence (Eds.), *Modern Perspectives in Child Development*. New York: International Universities Press, 1963, 246–367.

Purcell, K. Distinctions between subgroups of asthmatic children: Children's perceptions of events associated with asthma. *Journal of Pediatrics*, 1963, **31**, 486–494.

Purcell, K. Critical appraisal of psychosomatic studies of asthma. *New York State Journal of Medicine*, 1965, **65**, 2103–2109.

Purcell, K., Bernstein, L., & Bukantz, S. A preliminary comparison of rapidly remitting and persistently "steroid-dependent" asthmatic children. *Psychosomatic Medicine*, 1961, **23**, 305–310.

Purcell, K., & Clifford, E. Binocular rivalry and the study of identification in asthmatic and nonasthmatic boys. *Journal of Consulting Psychology*, 1966, **30**, 388–394.

Purcell, K., & Metz, J. Distinctions between subgroups of asthmatic children: Some parent attitude variables related to age of onset of asthma. *Journal of Psychosomatic Research*, 1962, **6**, 251–258.

Purcell, K., Turnbull, J., & Bernstein, L. Distinctions between subgroups of asthmatic children: Psychological test and behavior rating comparisons. *Journal of Psychosomatic Research*, 1962, **6**, 283–291.

Purcell, K., & Weiss, J. Asthma. In C. Costello (Ed.), *Symptoms of Psychopathology*. New York: Wiley, 1970, 597–693.

Rauh, J., Schumsky, D., & Witt, M. Heights, weights, and obesity in urban school children. *Child Development*, 1967, **38**, 515–530.

Rees, L. The importance of psychological, allergic, and infective factors in childhood asthma. *Journal of Psychosomatic Research*, 1964, **7**, 253–262.

Rees, L. The significance of parental attitudes in childhood asthma. *Journal of Psychosomatic Research*, 1963, **7**, 181–190.

Richmond, J., Eddy, E., & Garrard, S. The syndrome of fecal soiling and megacolon. *American Journal of Orthopsychiatry*, 1954, **24**, 391–401.

Ritvo, S. Survey of the recent literature of tics in children. *Nervous Child*, 1945, **4**, 308–312.

Ritvo, E., Ornitz, E., & La Franchi, S. Frequency of repetitive behaviors in early infantile autism and its variants. *Archives of General Psychiatry*, 1968, **19**, 341–347.

Ritvo, E., Ornitz, E., Gottlieb, F., Poussaint, A., Maron, B., Ditman, K., & Blinn, K. Arousal and nonarousal enuretic events. *American Journal of Psychiatry*, 1969, **126**, 115–122.

Rutter, M., & Graham, P. The reliability and validity of the psychiatric assessment of the child: I. Interview with the child. *British Journal of Psychiatry*, 1968, **114**, 563–579.

Rutter, M., & Lockyer, L. A five to fifteen year follow-up study of infantile psychosis: I. Description of sample. *British Journal of Psychiatry*, 1967, **113**, 1169–1182.

Schaefer, H. Self-injurious behavior: Shaping "headbanging" in monkeys. *Journal of Applied Behavior Analysis*, 1970, **3**, 111–116.

Shirley, H. Encopresis in children. *Journal of Pediatrics*, 1938, **12**, 367–380.

Shutter, L., & Garell, D. Obesity in children and adolescents: a double-blind study with cross-over. *The Journal of School Health*, 1966, **36**, 273–275.

Sorosky, A., Ornitz, E., Brown, M., & Ritvo, E. Systematic observations of autistic behavior. *Archives of General Psychiatry*, 1968, **18**, 439–449.

Sperling, M. Dynamic considerations and treatment of enuresis. *Journal of the American Academy of Child Psychiatry*, 1965, **4**, 19–31.

Spitz, R., & Wolf, K. Anaclitic depression. *Psychoanalytic Study of Children*, 1946, **2**, 313–342.

Stein, Z., & Susser, M. Nocturnal enuresis as a phenomenon of institutions. *Developmental Medicine and Child Neurology*, 1966, **8**, 677–685.

Stein, Z., & Susser, M. Social factors in the development of sphincter control. *Developmental Medicine and Child Neurology*, 1967, **9**, 692–706.

Stein, Z., Susser, M., & Wilson, A. Families of enuretic children. *Developmental Medicine and Child Neurology*, 1965, **7**, 658.

Sternbach, R. *Principles of Psychophysiology*. New York: Academic Press, 1966.

Stott, D. Infantile illness and subsequent mental and emotional development. *Journal of Genetic Psychology*, 1959, **94**, 233–251.

Tate, B., & Baroff, G. Aversive control of self-injurious behaviour in a psychotic boy. *Behaviour Research and Therapy*, 1966, **4**, 281–287.

Torup, E. A follow-up study of children with tics. *Acta Paediatrica*, 1962, **51**, 261–268.

Ullmann, L., & Krasner, L. *A Psychological Approach to Abnormal Behavior*. Englewood Cliffs, N.J.: Prentice Hall, 1969.

Vernon, D., Foley, J., & Schulman, J. Effect of mother-child separation and birth order on young children's responses to two potentially stressful experiences. *Journal of Personality and Social Psychology*, 1967, **5**, 162–174.

Vernon, D., Foley, J., Sipowicz, R., & Schulman, J. *The Psychological Responses of Children to Hospitalisation and Illness*. Springfield, Ill.: Charles C Thomas, 1965.

Vernon, D., & Schulman, J. Hospitalisation as a source of psychological benefit to children. *Pediatrics*, 1964, **34**, 694–696.

Vernon, D., Schulman, J., & Foley, J. Changes in children's behavior after hospitalisation. *American Journal of Diseases in Children*, 1966, **111**, 581–593.

Walton, D. Experimental psychology and the treatment of a tiqueur. *Journal of Child Psychology and Psychiatry*, 1961, **2**, 148–155.

Warson, S., Caldwell, M., Warinner, A., Kirk, A., & Jensen, R. The dynamics of encopresis. *American Journal of Orthopsychiatry*, 1954, **24**, 402–415.

Weiss, J. Mood states associated with asthma in children. *Journal of Psychosomatic Research*, 1966, **10**, 267–273.

Werry, J. Enuresis—a psychosomatic entity? *The Canadian Medical Association Journal*, 1967a, **97**, 319–327.

Werry, J. Enuresis nocturna. *Medical Times*, 1967b, **95**, 985.

Werry, J., & Cohrssen, J. Enuresis—an etiologic and therapeutic study. *Journal of Pediatrics*, 1965, **67**, 423–431.

Wolff, H. Life stress and bodily disease—a formulation. *Research Publications of the Association for Research in Nervous and Mental Disease*, 1950, **29**, 1059–1094.

Wolff, S., & Chess, S. A behavioural study of schizophrenic children. *Acta Psychiatrica Scandinavica*, 1964, **40**, 438–466.

Woodmansey, A. Emotion and the motion: an inquiry into the causes and prevention of functional disorders of defecation. *British Journal of Medical Psychology*, 1967, **40**, 207–223.

Woodward, J. Emotional disturbances of burned children. *British Medical Journal*, 1959, **1**, 1009–1013.

Yates, A. The application of learning theory to the treatment of tics. *Journal of Abnormal and Social Psychology*, 1958, **56**, 175–182.

Yates, A. Tics. In C. Costello (Ed.), *Symptoms of Psychopathology*. New York: Wiley, 1970, 320–335.

Young, G., & Turner, R. CNS stimulant drugs and conditioning treatment of nocturnal enuresis. *Behaviour Research and Therapy*, 1965, **3**, 93–101.

Zausmer, D. Treatment of tics in childhood. *Archives of Disease in Childhood*, 1954, **29**, 537–542.

Chapter Five

Childhood Psychosis
John S. Werry

Introduction

The term childhood psychosis will be used here as a generic one to include all the psychotic disorders occurring before adolescence excluding acute and chronic brain syndromes such as deliria or amnestic states. No definition of childhood psychosis will be given at this point except that it is a condition found in children from birth to puberty which is marked by serious and extensive impairment of personosocial and, often also, intellectual functioning.

In their annotated bibliography on childhood schizophrenia, Tilton, DeMyer, and Loew (1966) cited a similar work by Goldfarb and Dorsen (1956) listing 584 English language publications which had appeared from 1812 to 1954. Tilton et al. added another 346 citations covering the years 1955 to 1964 which, with those appearing since 1964, would bring the total number of English language references to more than 1000. Obviously, it is impossible for any reviewer to attempt to cover more than a fraction of these. Nevertheless, I am fairly confident that the voluminous size of the literature is more a reflection of our ignorance and verbosity than of anything more substantial, and it is unlikely that pearls of wisdom have been missed. Generally speaking, the main criticisms that can be made of practically any area of investigation in child psychopathology apply with equal cogency to the area of childhood psychosis. The literature is largely a series of tedious case studies, inadequate and biased sampling, extraordinary concatenation of confounding

173

variables, illegitimate inferences, and sweeping generalizations. Scientifically well-designed studies are a rarity. Thus, the task of any reviewer in drawing conclusions is hazardous. Dogma about childhood psychosis desperately needs to yield to empirically derived data and thus relieve the plight of the child and his beleaguered parents who are the chief victims of our ignorance (see Kysar, 1968 for a parent's view of the state of knowledge).

Because of the central importance of this condition, despite its relative infrequency, the literature has been reviewed in detail. In this way those who wish to find coverage of a specific topic such as diagnosis or treatment can go to that section and read it in its entirety to see what is known about that area. On the other hand, those interested in an overview need only read the summary statements or the closing lines in each section, then proceed to the conclusions at the end.

History

The history of childhood psychosis has been discussed by several authors (Bradley, 1954; Eisenberg, 1957; Hunt, 1958; Kanner, 1958; Potter, 1933). Kraepelin, who first described dementia praecox in 1896, believed that the condition in a small but significant proportion of his patients had begun during childhood, as did Bleuler, who introduced the term schizophrenia. Both, however, made the diagnosis of onset in childhood retrospectively from the history of adult patients. Eisenberg (1957, 1966) stated that the first description of childhood psychosis as a specific entity appeared attributable to DeSanctis who, in the first decade of this century, coined the term "dementia praecocissima." Among the first papers based on the actual study of psychotic children to appear in the English language was that by Potter (1933), who used the term schizophrenia and utilized Bleulerian diagnostic criteria. Other significant historical landmarks are the appearance of the first of a long series of papers on schizophrenia by Bender in 1942, the delineation of the syndromes of early infantile autism by Kanner in 1943, of the atypical child by Rank in 1949, of symbiotic psychosis by Mahler in 1952, and Ferster's attempt in 1961 to apply modern learning theory, derived from animal experimentation, to the clinical syndrome of psychosis as seen in children.

The study of childhood psychosis has been marked by progressions and regressions. After a brilliant start with Potter (1933), Bradley and Bowen (1941), and Kanner (1943), precise clinical description was increasingly abandoned until severity of disorder became the sole diagnostic criterion (e.g., Szurek, 1956), and reasonable objectivity was replaced by wordy prose yielding in Wing's (1968) words, more "insights into the author's mind rather than into the child's" (p. 790). There have been recurring but, until recently, largely unheeded pleas for concerted efforts to sharpen and agree on diagnostic criteria. The infrequency of the disorder in most populations has prohibited it from being subject to the types of multivariate statistical studies described in Chapter One. Anecdotal case studies have been the rule, though happily in the last decade a small but ever-increasing amount of adequately experimental work with psychotic children has begun to appear, culminating in the elegant studies by the behaviorists who, whatever the merits of their approach, have certainly exposed the gross methodological inadequacies of most other studies.

Clinical Symptomatology, Syndromes, and Diagnosis

The concept of childhood psychosis is essentially that of a "medical" or "disease" model implying discrete clinical symptomatology, predictable outcome, etiology, and response to treatment, all of which differentiate psychotic from nonpsychotic children. Proponents of the medical model, such as Eisenberg (1966) have argued that the history of medicine suggests that careful clinical description and diagnosis should be elemental to advancing knowledge of childhood psychosis. Although such an assumption is not without its critics (e.g., Szaz, 1960; Ullmann and Krasner, 1965, pp. 1–15) and alternatives (see Chapter One), those who work with disturbed children generally agree that there are certain children called psychotic who are differentiable from other disturbed children, particularly by the severity and extensiveness of the disorder and its often poor prognosis and, thus, that the diagnostic label has some usefulness. However, beyond this there is little agreement, particularly on delimiting criteria, subgroups, etiology, and proper treatment.

Clinical description and nosology of childhood psychosis have undergone a slow evolution as increasingly younger children have been brought within the aegis of the mental health field. Originally, as is indeed true of many other areas involving the child, attempts were made to apply findings made in adults, unmodified. Thus Kraepelin and Bleuler considered psychosis in children identical to schizophrenia in adults.

Potter and Bradley

In one of the first papers to appear in the American literature, Potter (1933) took as his diagnostic frame of reference the schizophrenic symptoms

TABLE 1
Clinical Symptomatology of Childhood Psychosis

Porter (1933)	Bender†	British Working Party Creak et al., (1961) (after Goldberg & Soper (1963))
1. Generalized retraction of interests from environment	1. Vasovegetative disorder (instability of functions)*	1. Gross and sustained impairment of emotional relationships with people*
2. Dereistic thinking, feeling and acting	2. Disorders of motility (espec. anti-gravity reflexes)*	2. Apparent unawareness of his own personal identity to a degree inappropriate to his age
3. Disturbances of thought through blocking, symbolization, condensation, perseveration, incoherence, diminution mutism	3. Disorders of perception (espec. body image)	3. Pathological preoccupation with particular objects or certain characteristics of them, without regard to their accepted functions
4. Defect in emotional rapport	4. Intellectual disorder	
5. Diminution, rigidity and distortion of affect	5. Emotional disorder (espec. pervasive anxiety)	4. Sustained resistance to change in the environment and a striving to maintain or restore sameness
6. Alterations of behavior with either an increase of motility leading to complete immobility or bizarre behavior with a tendency to perseveration or stereotypy	6. Social disorder	5. Abnormal perceptual experience (in the absence of discernible organic abnormality)
	7. Disorders of developmentally integrated patterns of behavior	6. Acute, excessive and seemingly illogical anxiety as a frequent phenomenon
	Eisenberg and Kanner (1956)	7. Speech either lost, or never acquired, or showing failure to develop beyond a level appropriate to an earlier age
	1. Inability to relate to people, situations manifest from first or second year (self-isolation)*	
Bradley and Bowen (1941)	2. Failure to use language for purposes of communication	8. Distortion in motility patterns
1. Seclusiveness*	3. Anxiously obsessive desire for sameness*	9. A background of serious retardation in which islets of normal, near normal, or exceptional intellectual function or skill may appear*
2. Irritability*	4. Preoccupation with objects	
3. Daydreaming	5. Good cognitive potential	
4. Bizarre behavior		
5. Diminution of interests		
6. Regressive interests		
7. Sensitivity		
8. Physical inactivity		

* Necessary or Primary

† Abstracted by the author

of adults. He noticed that because of the immaturity of the central nervous system (CNS) in children, psychological and behavioral phenomena were bound to be less differentiated and, accordingly, he somewhat modified the symptomatology.

Potter outlined six diagnostic points (see Table 1) of which items 2 (dereistic thinking) and 3 (disturbances of thought) show clear evidence of adult derivation and are inapplicable to young mute children. The others generally presuppose a period of normality, which again would be inapplicable to many of the younger psychotic children. Like most of his successors, Potter failed to specify which symptoms were necessary or sufficient to make a diagnosis of psychosis and whether there were any delimiting criteria, notably coexistent disorders such as mental retardation or frank CNS disease.

Bradley and Bowen (1941), in what is one of the most careful (and, unfortunately, least emulated) studies of diagnosis in childhood psychosis, used an essentially empirical approach in which the symptomatology of twelve children (seven to ten years of age) in a residential treatment setting, who were agreed by several clinicians to be schizophrenic or severely schizoid, was delineated. In a statement reminiscent of the behaviorists of the 1960s, Bradley wrote about his formulation of the symptomatology: "Attention has been focussed on such overt activity of children as can be observed, described and recorded from an objective point of view." (p. 298). Symptoms were then checked by two independent raters against the symptomatology of the 130 or so nonpsychotic children in the institution and those which failed to discriminate the two groups of children were discarded. This left eight symptoms (Table 1), which Bradley and Bowen thus considered to characterize childhood schizophrenia, and which they then carefully tried to define. The definitions leave much to be desired from an operational point of view—e.g., seclusiveness is defined as "a tendency frequently pathological of an individual to cut himself off from social intercourse"—but the attempt was laudable. Using the case material, the eight symptoms were divided into primary or universally present and all apparently necessary to the diagnosis (seclusiveness, bizarre behavior, regressive nature of personal interests, and sensitivity to comments and criticisms) and secondary or nonessential. In another pioneering distinction between *necessary* and *sufficient* symptoms, Bradley and Bowen pointed out that the primary signs were necessary for the diagnosis of schizophrenia, but that they were sufficient only for the diagnosis of schizoid personality. To make a diagnosis of schizophrenia there had to be, in addition, general impairment of social functioning. Thus, a severity or *quantitative* as well as a *qualitative* dimension was necessary to diagnosis, but the severity was left undefined as was the significance of coexistent intellectual and physical handicap. This paper must be considered one of the classics in the nosology of child psychiatry and had Bradley and Bowen's careful empiricism been followed, a great deal of confusion in the literature on childhood psychosis stemming from the "autistic" nature of each investigator's definition of psychosis might have been obviated.

Bender and Fish

One of the first of Bender's long series of papers on Childhood schizophrenia appeared in 1942 in a new journal (*The Nervous Child*), which significantly devoted its complete second and third issues to a discussion of the apparently by then well-recognized condition of childhood schizophrenia. Bender, greatly influenced by Gesell and by Gestalt psychology, enunciated her concept of the schizophrenic child (which appears to have remained basically unchanged) as one who "reveals pathology at every level and in every field of integration within the functioning of the central nervous system, be this vegetative, motor, perceptive, intellectual, emotional or social" (pp. 138–40). She emphasized two other fundamental aspects, namely the disturbance of the integrated patterning of behavior (later called plasticity) and the necessity of evaluating the child within a developmental dimension. Unlike most other investigators in the area, in addition to personosocial function, Bender and her pupils (most notably Fish) have greatly emphasized (1) developmental neurological diagnosis derived from Gesell, notably a search for the persistence of islands of primitive levels of CNS organization and (2) certain cognitive abnormalities, especially disorders of perception and body image. In later articles, Bender (1947) also stressed the importance of pervasive anxiety as central to the symptomatology of childhood schizophrenia.

Bender's essential diagnostic criteria are not easy to grasp since they have been described mostly in global, almost expansive terms. From time to time more specific symptoms are alluded to. In Table 1 Bender's symptomatology of childhood schizophrenia has been abstracted from her articles (Bender, 1942, 1947, 1956; Bender & Helm, 1953). Enumeration and interpretation of the necessary presence of certain symptoms has not been made explicit by Bender herself, but is attributable to the author.

The *disturbances of vasovegetative functioning* include extremes and irregularities of (1) vasomotor function (flushing, perspiring, pallor, acrocyanosis, (2) reaction to febrile illnesses, (3) physiological rhythms (sleeping, eating, and elimination habits), and (4) growth and maturation. *Disorders of motility and other aspects of neurological organization* are found in (1) abnormal electroencephalograms (EEG), (2) awkwardness, (3) anxiety in acquiring new motor patterns such as walking or climbing stairs, (4) persistence of early or primitive reflexes, particularly choreiform activities in the hands (leading later to stereotypies and self-mutilative behavior), the tonic neck reflex, whirling, and poor motor tone resulting in hyperactivity, waxy

flexibility, and clinging to adults (which Bender, unlike Mahler, 1965, interpreted as a sign of inability to cope with gravity). The perceptual disorders
can be seen in abnormal visual motor function and disorders of body image,
typified in the child's drawings of the human form. *Disorders of intellectual
function* are: Absent or distorted language development, difficulty with the
use of pronouns, disorders of thinking such as fragmentation, dissociation, and
bizarre symbolism. The most conspicuous feature of the emotional disorder,
and a nuclear symptom, is a *pervasive anxiety* believed to result primarily
from the disintegrative effects of the schizophrenic process on the ego, a concept rather similar to the psychoanalytic one, to which is added anxiety
occasioned by the child's frustrated attempts to cope with his environment
despite his multiple handicaps. The *social disorder* is manifest in gross disturbances of interpersonal relationships such as withdrawal or clinging, which
Bender apparently sees as secondary to the child's various other handicaps,
particularly of perception.

Bender also emphasized the importance of age of onset on the manifestations of the clinical syndrome delineating three basic developmental
subtypes of childhood schizophrenia: (a) *pseudodefective*, appearing within
the first two or three years of life where the clinical symptomatology is dominated by an apparent severe mental retardation; (b) *pseudoneurotic*, appearing in early and middle childhood, marked by pan-anxiety and neurotic
defenses against it, particularly phobias and obsessions, and (c) *pseudopsychopathic*, appearing in the preadolescent child around the age of 10 to 11
years with paranoid symptomatology and consequent aimless antisocial behavior predominant.

Even though Bender is one of the major contributors to the literature on
childhood psychosis, she nevertheless appears to have no significant following
outside Bellevue Hospital. The most commonly articulated reason relates to
the large number of cases seen by Bender (over 1000) which have been
thought to reflect promiscuity in diagnosis (Kanner, 1958, p. 737). Nevertheless, the frequency of schizophrenia (8%) in her total patient population seen
over a period of 20 years (Bender, 1956), although higher than most clinics
(*vide infra.*), is not substantially different from those with a particular interest in psychotic children (e.g., Reiser, 1963). Longitudinal studies (Bender,
1953), which have shown that the majority of the schizophrenic children grow
up to be schizophrenic adults, have been cited by Bender as evidence of the
validity of her diagnostic procedures. But, as Eisenberg (1957) has pointed
out, childhood diagnosis may well influence the adult diagnosis. The most
probable reasons for the rejection of Bender's approach lie in her persistent
espousal of the unpopular organic hypothesis of etiology, her often uncritical
utilization of physical treatment such as shock treatment in young children,
which many regard as distasteful (e.g., Wing, 1966, p. 24), her obfuscating

statement that not all schizophrenic children are psychotic, and the elusive diffuseness of her diagnostic criteria. That these latter have substance has been argued by Bender and Helm (1953) in a somewhat obtuse study of case records. It was found that the symptomatology of schizophrenic children differed from that of matched nonpsychotic emotionally disturbed controls in the areas of function outlined in Table 1, whereas other symptomatology was found to be common to both groups.

In a series of generally careful papers (Fish, 1957, 1960; Fish & Shapiro, 1965; Fish, Shapiro, Campbell & Wile, 1968), Bender's diagnostic criteria were made more specific and her classification of the three basic developmental areas were elaborated. Fish used a standard 45-minute psychiatric examination of apparently satisfactory interobserver reliability focused on relation to examiner, relation to peers, relation to environment, speech, affect, motility, and adaptive function evaluated within a developmental context in which extensive use is made of Gesell-type tests, especially in younger children. Of special importance were irregularities of development marked by areas of retardation and precocity. In classification, Fish used a two-dimensional system; the first dimension, *type*, a qualitative one, was basically similar to Bender's three categories of pseudodefective, pseudoneurotic, and pseudopsychopathic except that it applied to all disturbed children. The second dimension, *severity*, was quantitative, yet appeared to be the psychotic one. Fish demonstrated the practical validity of her classificatory systems of childhood psychosis by the differences within the subtypes in the frequency of organic indicators, in intellectual level, in response to different kinds of treatment, and in prognosis (Fish & Shapiro, 1965; Fish, Shapiro, & Campbell, 1966; Fish, Shapiro, Halpern, & Wile, 1965, 1967).

Wolff and Chess (1964) also have espoused a view of childhood psychosis somewhat similar to Bender's as a maturational disorder in which islands of fixated primitive behavior persist in a matrix of reactive behavior patterns.

Kanner, Eisenberg, and Rimland

Bender believed that her three subcategories simply resulted from a differing time of onset of basically the same schizophrenic process. Beginning a still unresolved controversy, Kanner, in 1943, described what he considered to be a *qualitatively* different clinical syndrome, now generally referred to as infantile autism, marked by (1) inability to relate to people and situations from the beginning of life, (2) failure to use language for communicative purposes, and (3) an anxiously obsessive desire for the maintenance of sameness. This condition was differentiated from mental deficiency by good intellectual potential seen in performance tests or unusual feats of memory, musical ability, etc. and from childhood schizophrenia by the fact that the child had never been normal. Because they felt the diagnosis was being made too indiscriminately, Eisenberg and Kanner (1956), in a later paper, delineated two symptoms as necessary: *extreme self-isolation* (autism) and the *obsessive insistence on the preservation of sameness.* The language disturbances (see Rutter, 1965a) were felt to be secondary to the disturbance of human relatedness and hence not essential. Good intellectual potential and age of onset remained as delineating criteria although the permissible age within which the abnormality could develop was expanded to the first two years of life. Coexistent CNS disease did not appear to be a delimiting criterion though Kanner's cases appear to have on a *post hoc* basis been largely healthy in this respect. In later writings Eisenberg (1966) specifically excluded CNS disease. Eisenberg and Kanner maintained that autism was an etiologically distinct condition from childhood schizophrenia as demonstrated by differing parental psychopathology and frequency of psychosis in parents, and the failure of autistic children to develop typical schizophrenic symptoms, particularly hallucinations and delusions in later life. With the notable exception of Bender (1953), there has been increasing acceptance of Kanner's differentiation between autism and childhood schizophrenia (Rimland, 1964; Wing, 1966, pp. 22–24), the best known being Rimland's extensive and scholarly, but not always objective, review of the literature on early infantile autism through 1962. Rutter (1965b) pointed out that Rimland was sometimes somewhat selective in his citation of the literature, preferring articles or portions thereof that supported his particular hypotheses. Of particular importance from the diagnostic point of view is Rimland's development of the checklist by Polan and Spencer (1959), comprised of items not only of clinical symptomatology, but also demographic, prenatal, medical and developmental history, and parental and familial data. The checklist represented a substantial advance in the diagnosis of childhood psychosis or at least one of its subcategories, since it very clearly set out a technology by which the diagnosis of psychosis in preschool children may be researched in a systematic manner. For example, it should be possible, by the use of the same research techniques that have led to the empirical establishment of the patterns of aggression, withdrawal, and immaturity, to determine the discriminative value of items or clusters of items. Rimland's offer to coordinate the gathering of the necessary preliminary data should not be neglected since, if anything is apparent from the history of childhood psychosis in the past 50 years, it is that the time for some serious and empirically based investigation of the clinical syndromes is long overdue.

Mahler and Rank

In 1952 Mahler described a third subtype of childhood psychosis—*symbiotic psychosis*—in addition to infantile autism and childhood schizophrenia occurring in the 2 to 5 year age group (see Mahler, 1965). The characteristic clinical feature in symbiotic psychosis was the failure of the child to detach himself from his mother and become increasingly independent of her as is ordinarily the case in this age group. Although Kanner (1958) felt that this differentiation was valuable, Eisenberg (1966) concluded that there was some doubt whether symbiotic psychosis was really an entity, since reports of its occurrence appear to be very infrequent.

Over the years, a fourth diagnostic subcategory, the child of atypical development (Rank, 1949), espoused particularly by the group at the Putnam Center, has apparently become increasingly indistinguishable from early infantile autism (see Reiser, 1963).

Goldfarb

After several years' intensive and comprehensive investigation of about 30 psychotic children in a residential setting, Goldfarb (1961, 1964) concluded, on the basis of an empirical analysis of physical neurological, behavioral, sensory, cognitive, and psychomotor measures, that psychotic children were divisible into two subcategories—one organic and the other nonorganic. The differentiation on this empirical basis agreed fairly well with that made clinically by neurologists. Furthermore, though both groups were clearly inferior to normal children on most of the functional tests, the nonorganic group was superior to the organic group, while the reverse was true concerning family functioning. This latter finding was not substantiated by Gittelman and Birch (1967) though their data were less carefully obtained. Goldfarb's work then, which is among the more careful investigations of childhood psychosis, suggested that there were at least two subcategories of childhood psychosis, clinically discernible, which appear to have definite implications for treatment and for prognosis. Goldfarb's children were a highly selected group being all of school age and of extreme severity and largely from intact families, so that the generality of these findings is presently unclear. Since this subcategorizing was done *after* the diagnosis of psychosis had been made, Goldfarb had general diagnostic criteria (which obviously owe much to Kanner and Bender), namely, impaired relationships, disturbances in personal identity, resistance to change, marked anxiety, perceptual difficulties, communicative defects, bizarre motility, unusual preoccupations and sometimes, severe intellectual retardation (Goldfarb, 1964). However, Goldfarb did not specify which, if any, of these symptoms were necessary for the diagnosis or how exactly they would be defined.

British Studies

In 1961 a small group or "working party" of British pediatricians and child psychiatrists with token representation of other mental health professionals issued a memorandum outlining nine diagnostic points (see Table 1) to promote clarification of the diagnosis of childhood psychosis (Creak, Cameron, Cowie, Ini, Mackeith, Mitchell, O'Gorman, Orford, Rogers, Shapiro, Stone, Stroh, & Yudkin, 1961). Of these, the first, *gross and sustained impairment of emotional relationships with people*, and possibly also the ninth, *a background of serious retardation in which islets of normal, near normal, or exceptional intellectual function or skill may appear*, were regarded as primary or necessary symptoms. Although the nine points are most strongly derived from Kanner's description of infantile autism, they are comprehensive enough to encompass all forms of childhood psychosis so that the choice by the British working party of the term "schizophrenic syndrome of childhood" as the preferred diagnostic terms appears to be unfortunate and antithetical to current thinking. However, the nine points have become increasingly accepted as a basis for the diagnosis of childhood psychosis as demonstrated by their incorporation, virtually unchanged, into the proposed classification of children's psychiatric disorders by the prestigious (American) Group for the Advancement of Psychiatry (1966). Rutter (1966a) offered some criticism of the nine points, principally the highly inferential and overlapping nature of some of the items and the failure to specify exactly how many of the nine points are sufficient for the diagnosis.

In one of the few studies similar to Bradley and Bowen's (1941) empirical analysis of the power of individual symptoms to discriminate between unequivocally psychotic and nonpsychotic disturbed children, Rutter (Rutter, 1966a; Rutter & Lockyer, 1967) retrospectively compared the case records of a group of 63 psychotic children (most of whom were autistic) with those of a contrast group of children exhibiting other kinds of emotional and behavioral difficulties who had been seen at the same clinic at the same time and who were matched for sex, age and IQ. (This latter criterion of necessity means that most of the contrast children were retarded, with one-third organic and many epileptic).

Rutter used a checklist covering the areas of relationships, speech, compulsions, motor phenomena, concentration, self-injury, response to pain, and behavior problems comprised of symptoms commonly described as characteristic of psychotic children (as well as including items found in other kinds of emotional and behavioral disorders). Generally speaking, these items are vague, undefined and global and of apparently unchecked reliability. Though they differ in certain details from the nine points, all of the latter were covered in one way or another. Rutter found that although 22 of 34 items significantly distinguished the psychotic from the nonpsychotic children at the .05 level of confidence, no symptom occurred exclusively in the psychotic children and only two (abnormal relationship with people and speech retardation) occurred in all the psychotic children. The picture of psychosis that emerged was more in the patterning and severity of symptoms than their specificity. This finding is thus more consonant with the views of Fish (Fish & Shapiro, 1965) and Szurek (1956) than those of Eisenberg (1966) or Sorosky, Ornitz, Brown, and Ritvo (1968) and is supported (though by no means unequivocably) by direct observations of behavior discussed below which find differences of degree rather than type as characteristic of psychotic children. Rutter's study has important weaknesses (retrospective nature, use of records, questionably suitable control group, unreliable symptoms) and tells most about what two particular psychiatrists, K. Cameron and E. J. Anthony, considered to be psychosis; but it is nevertheless one of the more important studies on symptomatology.

The "nine points" approach is clinical instead of etiological and does not exclude children with coexistent physical disease from the diagnosis of childhood psychosis, which is in keeping with the British view that childhood psychosis is a phentotype with different or multiple possible causes (Creak, 1963).

Recent American Classifications

In contrast to the phenotypic British position, Eisenberg (1966) proposed a classification that is primarily etiological (psychoses associated with and psychoses without impairment of brain tissue). The first group is further subdivided on an etiological basis (e.g., psychosis associated with intoxication, psychosis associated with neoplasm, etc.), while only the second depends on clinical features for its subdivisions into autistic psychoses, the schizophrenic psychoses associated with maturation failure, *folie à deux* and manic depressive psychoses. Eisenberg felt the dysmaturational group to be of dubious value and probably to contain many children belonging in the organic group.

A system of diagnosis and classification of childhood psychosis that probably reflects a reasonably accurate distillate of current modes—at least in the United States—has recently been presented by the Group for the Advancement of psychiatry (1966). The basic symtomatology is essentially defined as the "nine points" though the more generic diagnostic term of psychosis has been preferred to schizophrenic syndrome. Despite the problems associated with the methods whereby this system was developed, already discussed in Chapter One, it offers a significant improvement over the British effort in an attempt to classify the psychotic disorders within a developmental context, namely, the psychotic disorders of infancy and early childhood and the psychoses of later childhood, though the age at which this division is to occur is not specified. The disorders of infancy and early childhood are further subdivided into (1) early infantile autism, corresponding to Kanner's syndrome, (2) interactional psychosis, incorporating Mahler's symbiotic psychosis, and

(3) other psychoses, which allow for pictures that do not fit precisely into the first two. The psychoses of later childhood are divided into two groups: (1) schizophreniform disorders (a term apparently to indicate parallels and yet to emphasize differences between this and the adult form of schizophrenia), in which more classical schizophrenic symptoms begin to make their appearance; this group corresponds with the earlier descriptions of childhood schizophrenia by Potter (1933) and Bradley and Bowen (1941) and would also include Goldfarb's (1961, 1964) sample; and (2) other psychoses of later childhood, which would include those in which affective disorders play a prominent part, schizoaffective psychosis, and manic depressive psychosis, which is extremely rare before puberty (Anthony & Scott, 1960).

Also of significance in the GAP classification are the specific exclusions of such dubious diagnostic categories as prepsychotic, borderline, latent psychotic, or pseudoneurotic conditions, all of which have done much to obfuscate and elasticize the diagnosis of psychosis. In contrast to the British point of view, but consistent with Eisenberg's view, chronic brain syndrome or mental retardation preclude a primary diagnosis of childhood psychosis though it may be included as a secondary description as for example "mental retardation with psychosis." However, the role of a past history suggestive of a chronic brain syndrome, notably seizures in early life, is not made explicit (see Schain & Yannet, 1960).

Behavioral Diagnostic Methods

Recently, there has been a commendable tendency to replace the typical inexact anecdotal description of clinical symptomatology in childhood psychosis with direct observation either in a structured situation (e.g., Haworth & Menolascino, 1967; Hutt, Hutt, Lee, & Ounsted, 1965; Jahoda & Goldfarb, 1957; Lebowitz, Colbert, & Palmer, 1961; Lovaas, Freitag, Gold, & Kassorla, 1965a; O'Connor, 1967; Simmons, Leiken, Lovaas, Schaeffer, & Perloff, 1966; Sorosky et al., 1968; Tilton & Ottinger, 1964) or in a portion of the child's normal environment (Ruttenberg, Dratman, Fraknoi, & Wenar, 1966; Wolff & Chess, 1964; Wolf, Risley, & Mees, 1964). These studies vary in quality and too few as yet use nonpsychotic contrast groups but, with the exception of O'Connor's studies, their findings generally confirm the basic symptomatology as reported in the typical clinical study especially (relative) unresponsiveness to environmental stimuli, a high level of self-stimulatory behavior, or stereotyped behavior (see Chapter Four), abnormalities of eye contact and communicative patterns. However, these studies have also emphasized the great heterogeneity and varying severity of symptomatology, and importantly that few psychotic children are totally unresponsive to environmental stimuli, including persons.

Though few of these methods are yet developed to the stage of diagnostic instruments they have established their utility as dependent variable measures for studying psychopathological processes and treatment techniques.

Summary of Clinical Symptomatology, Syndromes, and Diagnosis

Agreement and precision in the description and diagnosis of childhood psychosis and its various subcategories and obviously basic prerequisites for the study of frequency, etiology, treatment, and prognosis of the disorder in a nomothetic context. Yet this review, while by no means sampling the totality of the area, has revealed several outstanding problems requiring urgent attention if the study of childhood psychosis is to advance. (1) There has to be some general consensus about terminology and classification. In the absence of systematic multivariate statistical studies the present state of knowledge must necessarily be somewhat arbitrary, and there would seem to be merit in accepting the suggested classification by the Group for the Advancement of Psychiatry (1966), at least as an initial working basis since it appears to be the most comprehensive and generally acceptable. (2) There is need for agreement on delimiting criteria, both general for psychosis as a whole and specific for the various subcategories. Some of these, namely the coexistence of physical disease (particularly of the central nervous system) and mental retardation, are spelled out in the GAP classification, but others, notably age and history of seizures in early life, are not. (3) The descriptions of the basic clinical symptoms must be operationalized and their reliability demonstrated by means of research of the type described in Chapter One. The nine points suggested by the British working party and adopted by the GAP Committee are apparently widely acceptable, but their present crude state and lack of discriminative power (Rutter & Lockyer, 1967) indicate that they can only serve as a point of departure. (4) On the basis of preceding analyses, the identification of the pattern of behaviors identifying childhood psychosis and its possible subcategories should be made explicit. (5) Finally, when reliable diagnostic indices have been developed, their validity should be further investigated by experimental study of both psychotic and nonpsychotic children to demonstrate differences in psychological functioning beyond that implied by the behaviors defining the disorder.

Frequency of Occurrence

Considering the basic unreliability of the measures used and the absence of a well-differentiated set of diagnostic criteria, statements about the frequency of occurrence of childhood psychosis are necessarily of uncertain value. As we have already seen, there are few epidemiological studies on the frequency of empirically defined childhood disorders. In the case of childhood psychosis it may be argued that because of the severity of the disorder and the consequent high probability of referral figures reported from clinics are reasonably representative of the prevalence rate of childhood psychosis in the population as a whole. However, not only is the catchment area of a given clinic often unknown and thus prevalence rates unable to be estimated, but it seems highly probable that a significant proportion of psychotic children are not seen in child guidance or psychiatric clinics, but instead find their way to facilities for the retarded where they go unrecognized. Thus, Goldberg and Soper (1963) found a frequency of psychosis (primary and secondary to chronic brain syndrome) of 5.1% and Menolascino (1965) 5.2% in two clinics for the retarded. 3.1% of Goldberg and Soper's and 1.5% of Menolascino's cases were primary. Nicol and MacKay (1968) found that the prevalence was very much influenced by the number of child psychiatrists in a given area.

Wing (1966), citing three unpublished English studies on the prevalence of childhood psychosis in the general population by Wilson, by Lotter, and by Rutter, states that the frequency is about 2 per 10,000 (.02%). Andrews and Cappon (1957), extrapolating from their clinic statistics, estimated the base rate in the population in a Canadian urban area to be about .06%. Nicol and MacKay (1968), using medical records to confirm diagnosis, surveyed the number of psychotic children under the age of 15 referred to psychiatrists and psychiatric institutions in British Columbia each year between 1954 and 1964 (i.e., a crude incidence rate). Their most accurate estimate was a rate of 7–8 per 100,000 (.008%).

The rate in clinic referrals varies but, not surprisingly, is much higher than expected from the above figures if all psychopathological conditions had a similar probability of referral: Bradley and Bowen (1941) found 3% in 140 children over the age of six in a residential treatment center; Bender (1955), 8% in 7000 referrals of children of all ages to Bellevue Hospital; Andrews and Cappon (1957), 5.1% in the case load of an urban child-psychiatric clinic; Goldberg and Soper (1963), 5.1% in 1216 and Menolascino, 5.2% in 616 referrals to a clinic for the retarded, while Reiser (1963) reports the highest frequency of 9% in about 3000 children of preschool age. These figures are obviously influenced not only by the elasticity of diagnosis at a given clinic but also its reputation for, and interest in, childhood psychosis.

Summary

It is difficult to make meaningful statements about the frequency of childhood psychosis, except that the condition is probably rare in the general population and, despite a high likelihood of referral, it constitutes under 10%

of referrals to most clinics. The inordinate amount of attention given childhood psychosis as witnessed by the number of special facilities devoted to the care of such children and the voluminous writings on the disorder are a reflection more of its severity and obdurateness than its actual frequency.

Sex Ratio

An excess of boys is reported in all studies. Ratios reported are Hinton (1963), 1.7:1; Goldfarb (1961), 2.3:1; Nicol and MacKay (1968), 2.5:1; Bender (1953), 2.7:1; Brown (1960), 3.5:1; Kanner (1954) and Gittelman and Birch (1967), 4:1; Rutter and Lockyer (1967), 4.25:1; Annell (1963), 4.5:1; Wolff and Chess (1964), 7:1; and Andrews and Cappon (1957), 9.5:1. There is normally an excess of boys over girls in admissions to clinics and hospitals not only for psychiatric disorders (Andrews and Cappon report a sex ratio of 1.8:1 in their clinic) but also for physical disorders. But with the possible exception of Hinton and Bender, the above studies support Wing's (1966) contention that the excess of males with psychosis is greater than that occurring in most other psychiatric and physical disorders except perhaps conduct disorder, aphasia, and minimal brain dysfunction (Werry, 1968).

Age of Onset

Although the early papers on childhood psychosis describe it only in school-age children (e.g., Potter, 1933; Bradley & Bowen, 1941), increasing attention in the mental health field to children at younger age levels has demonstrated that psychosis can have its onset at any age from birth on (e.g., Fish, 1957; Kanner, 1943; Mahler, 1965; Reiser, 1963; Rutter & Lockyer, 1967), but for obvious reasons diagnosis is easier in older children. Bender (1956) stated that there were three peak periods of onset, namely, 0–2 years, 3–4½ years (the highest), and from 10–11½ years. Bender does not support this statement with any actuarial data. In their survey, Nicol and MacKay (1968) did find a peak incidence between 3–6 years although rates were then very low until puberty (13) when the highest rate was attained. Goldberg and Soper (1963) found that over 50% of their group developed symptoms before 3 years of age with very few thereafter. Rutter and Lockyer (1967) reported that in 54% of their sample of 63 children the onset of the psychosis was in early infancy and in all cases before 6 years. Many authors agree, however, that severity of the disorder is negatively correlated with age (e.g., Pollack, 1960; Wolff & Chess, 1964; Nicol & MacKay, 1968).

Physical and Biochemical Abnormalities (Other Than Neurological)

Bender (1947, 1956) suggested that growth and maturation tend to be either retarded or precocious, but offers no anthropometric data in support. Dutton (1964) and Simon and Gillies (1964) found minor abnormalities of growth and skeletal maturity as determined by anthropometric and radiological measures in a significant number of institutionalized psychotic boys most of whom were, however, severely retarded. Hinton (1963) found a group of 62 psychotic children seen in a clinic primarily for retarded children to be somewhat shorter than a normal control group and to have a high (24%) frequency of congenital anomalies. On the other hand, Goldfarb (1961) found the general physical characteristics of 24 psychotic children to be similar to that of a matched group of normal children and Reiser (1963) found the 240 children with psychosis of early childhood seen at the Putnam Center to be generally indistinguishable physically from normal children.

Böök, Nichtern, and Gruenberg (1963), in one of the very few studies of chromosomal structure in childhood psychosis (other than single case reports in which there is good reason to believe that the studies were done because of associated malformations leading to suspicion of chromosomal abnormality), found no striking or consistent abnormality in 10 psychotic children. In another study, Judd and Mandell (1968) examined the chromosomes of a group of 11 children who, using Rimland's checklist, met the most rigorous diagnosis of early infantile autism and found that there was no significant or consistent abnormality.

In a carefully controlled and documented study, Fowle (1968) examined the leukocytes of 26 psychotic children to see if the blood changes reputed to be found in adult schizophrenia were present. She found that, although there were consistent abnormalities such that she was able to predict whether the child was a normal, control, or psychotic (except in children 8 or above), these changes were identical to those occurring in children with virus infections or allergic conditions suggesting an immune response. Further, these changes were exaggerated by phenothiazine medication though 8 of the children were reported never to have had such treatment. Inasmuch as the changes were not *qualitatively*, only *developmentally*, abnormal, Fowle posited they might reflect in part a disorder of maturation as well as an immune response.

Tilton et al. (1966) listed 16 biochemical studies of psychotic children involving a variety of substances, including serum proteins and inorganic radicals, biogenic amines, and amino acids. With very few exceptions no abnormalities were found or, if present, were not peculiar to psychosis. Kety (1965), in an extensive review of the biochemical theories of schizophrenia, concluded that while there are several plausible theories, they have little experimental support to date. The same appears to be true of childhood psychosis.

Thus, nonneurological physical abnormalities are clearly not a necessary concomitant of childhood psychosis although they occur, particularly in growth and physical maturation, in a minority of psychotic children, especially those who are institutionalized and functionally retarded. Whether these abnormalities are any more common than in nonpsychotic children of comparable IQ remains to be established.

Neurological and Electroencephalographic Abnormalities

Bender (1947, 1956) has emphasized the frequency and the subtle nature of neurological abnormalities, particularly hypotonia, choreiform movements, whirling, and persistence of the tonic neck reflex, in childhood psychosis. Bender felt that major neurological abnormalities were infrequent and that unless a special neurological examination taking cognizance of these "soft" signs was performed, the psychotic child would be declared neurologically normal. Fish (1961) emphasized that the neurological disorder of childhood psychosis was not specific (being common in children with organic behavior disorders), but was instead a disorder of timing and integration of neurological maturation with retardation in some areas and precociousness in others. In both retrospective and prospective studies, she found that these deviations of development began in infancy and tended to be closely correlated with the degree of ultimate intellectual impairment. Goldfarb (1961) found that older psychotic children were differentiated from normal children by a variety of minor neurological abnormalities, notably hypotonia, whirling, disturbances of body schema, and abnormal righting and postural responses. Furthermore, these differences seemed to be largely confined to one subgroup of the schizophrenics, which he called organic. Similarly, Eaton and Menolascino (1966) and Hinton (1963) found a variety of minor abnormalities, principally clumsiness, hypotonia, or hypertonia in 40% and 56% respectively of their groups of psychotic children. Gittelman and Birch (1967) found neurological abnormalities (epilepsy, abnormal EEG, choreiform movements, pathological reflexes, myoclonic jerking) in 19% of 97 psychotic children with a further 13% possibly having dysfunctions.

A generally good, controlled study of Australian psychotic children (Gubbay, Lobascher, & Kingerlee, 1970; Lobascher, Kingerlee, & Gubbay, 1970), where diagnosis was based on the above nine points, found the psychotic children to have a much greater prevalence of abnormal birth histories and unequivocal evidence of neurological disorder (56%). The one criticism of this study is that all the psychotic children proved mentally defective and the control group was comprised of normal schoolchildren, instead of a group matched for IQ as was done by Rutter (1966). Similarly, Pollack, Miller, Berman, Bakwin, and Gittelman (1970) found 76 psychotic children to be much more frequently neurologically impaired (76%) than their sibs (17%) although the signs were nearly all "soft." The same criticism of the previous study, namely inappropriate control group, applies here too.

Other motor "abnormalities" frequently observed are stereotypies (Green, 1967; Hutt et al., 1965; Lebowitz et al., 1961; Lovaas, et al., 1965; Ritvo, Ornitz, & LaFranchi, 1968; Sorosky et al., 1968; Wolff & Chess, 1964). Stereotypies are discussed in detail in Chapter Four.

Rachman and Berger (1963) found that psychotic children differed from a comparable group of retarded children by their inability to stand still for a minute with eyes closed (Romberg Test) and by a greatly increased frequency of whirling. Major neurological conditions, principally epilepsy, were present in 12 out of 100 children with psychosis seen by Creak (1963). Rutter (1965a) found about 25% of his series of 63 psychotic children definitely to have a major neurological disease, principally epilepsy, and another 25% probably to have a neurological disease. Interestingly, in both these studies the epilepsy did not appear in many cases until some years after the initial diagnosis. Schain and Yannet (1960) found a history of seizures in 42% of 50 autistic children in a school for mental defectives where the diagnostic process was based solely on Kanner's criteria. On the other hand, Kanner and Eisenberg (Eisenberg, 1967) and the Putnam group (Reiser, 1963) found no neurological or EEG abnormalities in their large groups of autistic children.

EEG studies of psychotic children suggest that they have an excess (usually about 50%) of EEG abnormalities (Bender, 1947; Eaton & Menolascino, 1966; Fish & Shapiro, 1965; Goldman & Rosenberg, 1962; Gubbay et al., 1970; Hinton, 1963; Hutt et al., 1965; Kennard, 1965; Schain & Yannet, 1960; Taterka & Katz, 1955; White, DeMyer, & DeMyer, 1964), though a minority (Eisenberg, 1967; Reisner, 1963) do not find such abnormalities. Generally speaking these abnormalities are of the diffuse, slow dysrhythmic pattern often described as immature (Kennard, 1965) rather than clearly abnormal.

It appears, then, that studies, though not unanimous, generally find psychotic children to have an excess of minor neurological (especially motor) and electroencephalographic abnormalities when compared with normal and possibly neurotic children. However, the exact etiological and neuropathological significance of these abnormalities is quite uncertain and they are not confined to psychotic children, being common in normal children and those with mental retardation, behavior disorders, learning problems, and the so-called minimal brain-dysfunction syndrome (Kellaway, Crawley, & Maulsby, 1965; Freeman, 1967; Werry, 1968; White et al., 1964; see also Chapter Three). But there is some evidence, by no means unequivocal, that the abnormalities, particularly of the electroencephalogram, may be more severe in psychotic children (Fish & Shapiro, 1965; Kennard, 1965; Taterka & Katz, 1955).

Cognitive Functioning

Intelligence

Although childhood psychosis is apparently compatible with a normal level of intelligence (Andrews & Cappon, 1957; Bradley & Bowen, 1941; Goldberg & Soper, 1963; Goldfarb, 1961; Eisenberg & Kanner, 1956; Pollack, 1967; Potter, 1933; Rutter & Lockyer, 1967), these same studies and the ninth point of the British working party (a background of serious retardation) also show that childhood psychosis is frequently accompanied by general intellectual retardation, sometimes quite profound.

In a review of the literature, Pollack (1967) found 13 studies involving a total of 306 psychotic children in which IQ had been formally measured. One-third to one-half of the children diagnosed as psychotic had IQs below 70, two-thirds below 80, and less than one-quarter scored above 90, with preschool children generally having the lowest IQs.

Nicol and MacKay (1968) found that two-thirds of their sample of 126 psychotic children were functioning at a retarded level, though how this level was established is not stated.

Eaton and Menolascino (1966) found that of the *testable* children in their group of 32 psychotic children seen in a clinic for retarded children, 75% were retarded in varying degrees.

Goldfarb (1961) found the IQ distribution in his group of 24 severely psychotic children of school age to be bimodal with the organic subgroup having a mean IQ of 62 while in the nonorganic group it was 92. Goldberg and Soper (1963) found a similar bimodal IQ distribution, which they felt, on the basis of associated neurological signs, generally tended to confirm Goldfarb's findings. Lobascher et al. (1970) found all 25 of their group of psychotic children to be mentally defective, and Pollack et al. (1970) found 72% of their group of 76 to have IQs of less than 90 (mean IQ 70.5).

Gittelman and Birch (1967) found over 50% of 97 schizophrenic children to be retarded and this IQ to be related inversely to age at diagnosis and inversely to signs of neurological dysfunction and perinatal complications.

Follow-up studies (Fish et al., 1968; Gittelman & Birch, 1967; Eisenberg & Kanner, 1956; Pollack, 1967; Rutter, 1965a) further suggest that retardation present at the time of initial diagnosis tends to persist. Rutter found at a follow-up after five to ten years the retest reliability of the IQ to be $r = .80$. Gittelman and Birch (1967) found similar stability, and like Rutter, found the more retarded children to deteriorate if anything. Pollack (1960) has suggested, using data from Goldfarb's group and a comparative population of adult psychotics, that the younger the onset of psychosis, the greater the degree of intellectual impairment—a finding substantiated by Gittelman and Birch (1967) and Nicol and MacKay (1968). Bender's use of the term "pseudodefective" to describe the children in whom psychosis develops in the first two years of life clearly indicates her belief in this hypothesis.

Kanner (Eisenberg & Kanner, 1956; Kanner, 1943) and after him the British working party (Creak et al., 1961) have suggested that the retardation accompanying childhood psychosis is differentiated from general mental retardation by islets of normal or near-normal intellectual function revealed particularly on performance tests (such as the Seguin Form Board) or special abilities of the *idiot savant* kind. Rimland (1964) developed this argument at great lengths, but most of his evidence is of the anecdotal kind and there have been few formal studies of this hypothesis. Goldberg and Soper (1963) found that only 20% of their children exhibited such a phenomenon (though it might be argued that these children were not then really psychotic if these islets of normal intelligence were necessary to the diagnosis of psychosis). Rutter and Lockyer (1967) did find general support for this hypothesis in that in contrast to the clinic contrast group matched for IQ the psychotic children were generally superior on the subtests requiring manipulative or visuospatial skills or immediate memory while they were markedly inferior on any test involving the use or understanding of language. O'Connor and Hermelin (Hermelin, 1966) found likewise. However, Pollack (1967) cites a study by Cullies who found no difference between psychotic and mentally retarded children matched for IQ on a variety of verbal and performance tasks, and points out that "sparing" of certain abilities is not confined to psychotic children (indeed, it is often cited as diagnostic of brain damage) and that on the basis of long-term outcome, psychotic children who test retarded are, for all practical purposes, retarded. In an experimental study, Cowan, Hoddinott, and Wright (1965) found that IQ and negativism were inversely correlated, suggesting that the retardation in autistic children may be partly motivational in some cases.

Language

Impairment of language and speech function in psychotic children is one of the outstanding features of the disorder (e.g., Creak et al., 1961) and a frequent reason for referral. In a significant proportion, especially those where psychosis is of early onset, speech is absent—nearly half of Kanner's (Eisenberg & Kanner, 1956) and one-third of Gittelman and Birch's cases (1967) were still mute by the age of five and Kanner's remained so. The majority of Schain and Yannet's (1960) severely autistic children were mute. Clinical studies have suggested that when language is present or when it develops in previously mute psychotic children, it exhibits many abnormalities, some of fundamental language usage (pronominal reversal, extreme literalness, echolalia) (Eisenberg & Kanner, 1956; Rimland, 1964, pp. 14–15) and others of delivery (absence of inflection, mouthing of words, uneven coordination of speaking and breathing) (Rutter, 1965a). A number of experimental studies have analyzed the language and speech of psychotic children and the results of these generally confirm the clinical observations (Goldfarb, Braunstein, & Lorge, 1956; Wolff & Chess, 1964) though there are few studies to show whether these differences are characteristic of psychosis or of the commonly associated retardation (e.g., Weiland & Legg, 1964).

Mute psychotic children have not infrequently developed speech subsequently dependent apparently on their IQ (Rutter, 1965a) and the treatment they receive (e.g., Lovaas, Berberich, Perloff, & Schaeffer, 1966). In an experimental study using a memory task, Hermelin (1967) found autistic children to be significantly inferior to normal and retarded controls matched for vocabulary level in their ability to organize verbal material into meaningful clusters, though they actually had superior recall for words in general. Thus there is some evidence to suggest that a significant number of psychotic children have specific language disabilities (Rutter, 1965a).

Attention

Psychotic, especially autistic, children are commonly believed to be unresponsive to the environment. In the auditory area they frequently behave as if they were deaf—this is the reason many are first referred for medical attention, though as with other sensory modalities, auditory acuity is almost always normal (Goldfarb, 1961; Rimland, 1964, p. 9). In the visual area Wolff and Chess (1964) have shown that psychotic children have two kinds of abnormality as observed behaviorally, visual *avoidance* and *staring*, the former being more characteristic of the more severely psychotic children.

There have been a number of experimental studies examining attentional mechanisms. In a careful study of auditory responsiveness, Anthony (1958) found that in contrast to a neurotic control group from the same clinic, psychotic children generally showed either no response or rapid adaptation to a loud noise. In a series of studies Goldfarb (1964) demonstrated a selective inattention to the distance receptors of vision and hearing, especially when the latter involved language. Goldfarb (1961) further showed that this in-attention was not at the level of sensory acuity but rather appeared to be a secondary "screening out," perhaps resulting from an initial hypersensitivity to visual and auditory stimuli as suggested by Bergman and Escalona (1949) and Anthony (1958). On the other hand, in a meticulous laboratory study, Metz (1967) found that 10 autistic boys (mean age 8.4 years, Kanner's diagnostic criteria) tended to seek higher levels of auditory stimulation (verbal, musical, and scrambled) than a group of "successful" normal boys of similar age. Ten schizophrenic (i.e., late onset of psychosis) boys tended to be more variable than either group. Freedman, Deutsch, and Deutsch (1960) found that a group of schizophrenic children were significantly inferior to a normal control group in their reaction time to both auditory and visual stimuli. In a series of well-designed studies in which, unlike most other studies, mental age was carefully controlled, O'Connor and Hermelin (Hermelin, 1966; O'Connor & Hermelin, 1967) found that psychotic children generally behaved and responded to simple visual, auditory, tactile, and social cues similarly to subnormal children except when the cues were verbal. However, their responses to complex combinations of stimuli suggested their discrimination was impaired at this level. O'Connor and Hermelin found two possible causes of this inattention. First, psychotic children often responded to irrelevant dimensions and spent more time in nondirected staring or scanning and less time inspecting relevant material or, in short, were relatively speaking inattentive. This visual inattentiveness was also found in a free-field situation by Hutt et al. (1965). There is some evidence to suggest that stereotypies in psychotic children either primarily or secondarily screen out environmental stimuli and that psychotic children with and without stereotypies may constitute distinct groups as far as attention and responsiveness are concerned (see Chapter Four), which may explain some of the discrepancies on the studies just cited, as may motivational factors (Cowan et al., 1965).

Perception

Bender has frequently stressed the marked degree of perceptual and perceptual-motor disorder found in schizophrenic children, notably those relating to body image as seen on the Draw-A-Person Test and Bender-Gestalt Visual Motor Test (Bender & Helm, 1953). Using the same tests Taterka and Katz (1955) did demonstrate that psychotic children had a higher frequency of abnormalities, but these were also found in a group of children with primary and organic behavior disorders. Goldfarb (1961) also demonstrated an increased frequency of visual perceptual deficits in psychotic children. However, Safrin (1964) found that when mental age was controlled, psychotic and nonpsychotic children did not differ on tests of visual perception and visual motor function. Ornitz and Ritvo (1968) have summarized the evidence suggesting that there may be perceptual inconstancy in psychotic children from which they have elaborated an etiological theory (see below).

Thinking

A variety of other cognitive abnormalities has been demonstrated in childhood psychosis. Goldfarb (1961) found an increased frequency of impaired abstraction and categorization. Anthony (1958), using Piaget's developmental epistemological model, found psychotic children to have retarded intellectual development, notably a persistence of egocentricity as compared with neurotic children from the same clinic.

Quite certainly, psychotic children frequently exhibit profound abnormality of cognitive function so that many of them function in effect at the severely retarded level. Despite the contention of Creak (1963) and Pollack (1967) that the distinction between mental retardation and childhood psychosis is academic since they both are, from a functional point of view, very similar, there is some evidence to support Kanner's (1943) original contention that, especially in autism, this cognitive deficit involves the area of language to a disproportionately greater degree than in comparable retardates. This language deficit is associated with an inattentiveness to and an apparent lack of meaningfulness in verbal stimuli (receptive dysphasia). It may be that the inattentiveness is primarily because of shutting out stimuli or, secondary, because of a fundamental deficit of perception or associative learning. Though the abnormalities in the auditory system are more conspicuous because of the resultant language deficits, there appear to be similar but quantitatively smaller abnormalities in the visual system. Perceptual, perceptual motor, and integrative abnormalities also appear to be common. The increasingly sophisticated attempts, largely by means of operant conditioning, to remediate these fundamental cognitive deficits (Hewett, 1964, 1965; Lovaas, 1966; Lovaas, et al. 1966; Risley & Wolf, 1967) may hopefully shed some light on the widely held belief that psychotic children functioning at the retarded level have nevertheless normal or near normal intellectual potential (Creak et al., 1961). From a point of view of ultimate social adaptation, however, psychotic children who test at a retarded level presently appear to do somewhat worse than retarded children (Rutter, Greenfeld, & Lockyer, 1967).

Birth History

Pollack and Woerner (1966) summarized all the studies on abnormalities of pregnancy and delivery in which comparative data was used. There were five such studies: Hinton (1963), Knobloch and Pasamanick (unpublished data), Taft and Goldfarb (1964), Terris, Lapouse, and Monk (1964), and Vorster (1960), together involving over 600 children of whom over two-thirds had been diagnosed by Bender (Terris, Lapouse, and Monk, 1964). Two of the studies (by Vorster and by Taft & Goldfarb) excluded children with major CNS disease, while two others did not (Hinton, Knobloch, & Pasamanick). The sources of information varied (birth records or mother's histories) as did the source of control subjects (sibs, normal or neurotic coevals). Pollack and Woerner concluded that the five studies were practically unanimous in finding an excess of complications of pregnancy but no excess of prematurity (defined as low birth weight) associated with childhood psychosis. The evidence of an excess of a history of previous reproductive loss in the mother, postnatal illness, and birth complications was less clear but suggestive. Wing (1966, p. 28) states that in an epidemiological study Lotter found a significantly higher frequency of perinatal complications in the histories of autistic children as compared to their siblings. Lobascher et al. (1970) and Pollack et al. (1970) found an excess of complications in their groups of uncategorized psychotic children.

On the other hand, Kanner (Eisenberg, 1967), Schain and Yannet (1960), and Reiser (1963) reported no excess of complications of pregnancy and delivery in what is collectively a large group of children primarily with early infantile autism. Rimland (1964, pp. 112–117), reviewing the literature, suggested that there might be a relationship between retrolental fibroplasia and autism and, hence, that hyperoxia might be a possible causative factor. Glavin (1966), developing this idea more intensively, suggested that early infantile autism, like retrolental fibroplasia, might be caused by a rapid change in oxygen concentration rather than hyperoxia. However, the majority of papers cited by Rimland and Glavin consist of single case reports. Since rapid changes in oxygen level are most commonly, though by no means necessarily, associated with prematurity, the failure by the five studies cited by Pollack and Woerner (1966) to find an increase in the prematurity rate is difficult to reconcile with this hypothesis, though it is true that three of the studies are concerned primarily with the psychoses of later childhood instead of early infantile autism. Bender (1955), without offering any statistical data, states that the complications of delivery are important in the etiology of childhood psychosis, but she sees their role as only that of a precipitant. Fish et al. (1968) found complications of pregnancy and delivery to be common in the histories of psychotic children (a frequency rate of about 50%) but not more common than in a group of mentally retarded and behaviorally disturbed children. Gittelman and Birch (1967), using overly liberal criteria, found 34.9% of mothers to have had complications of pregnancy and delivery, a figure not strikingly different from the 31.9% reported by Rogers, Lillienfeld, and Pasamanick (1955) in the normal population.

Thus, although the evidence is by no means unanimous, the better studies suggest an excess of complications of pregnancy and delivery (excluding prematurity) in the histories of psychotic children as compared to normal and neurotic controls, though probably not to controls matched for IQ. While findings may support the thesis that psychosis is a part of Pasamanick's continuum of reproductive casualty (Pasamanick & Knobloch, 1955), such conclusions must be regarded somewhat cautiously in view of the still unresolved compatibility of concomitant major CNS disease with the diagnosis of psychosis and the possibility of selective recall by mothers of abnormal children. Also, such complications are common in the histories of normal children (Rogers et al., 1955) and their exact relationship to brain damage in the fetus is hence unclear (see Chapter Three).

Birth Order

Rimland (1964, p. 6), observing that over 50% of Kanner's cases were the first or only child, stated that the disease was primarily one of firstborn males. Reiser (1963) did not find this to be so in the 240 cases seen at the Putnam Center, but no precise statistics are cited. Bender (1955) found 39 of 90 psychotic children under the age of six (44%) to be firstborn. Creak (1963) found the frequency of first or only children to be also approximately 50%. Wolff and Chess (1964) found 50% of their sample of 14 were firstborn and the remainder last born. None was a middle child.

Wing (1966, pp. 25–27), summarizing English figures—mostly unpublished—involving 372 children, found that while there was no overall association with birth order there was a clear one between primacy of birth order in two-child families and later birth order in multiple sibships. Wing points out that these findings are open to both psychological (limiting the family after the birth of a defective child) and to biological findings (greater vulnerability of the first and later born). Rutter and Lockyer (1967) did not find any difference in ordinal position between 63 psychotics and matched clinic controls, but did find differences in sibship patterns somewhat similar to Wing's (excess of firstborn children in two-child families).

Socioeconomic Status

Kanner was first to suggest that autistic children came from higher socioeconomic backgrounds, a point greatly emphasized by Rimland (1964) as a differentiating criterion from other forms of childhood psychosis. Bender (1955), Creak and Ini (1960), Pittfield and Oppenheim (1964) and Wing (citing two unpublished studies) confirm the excess of higher socioeconomic backgrounds not only for autism but for all forms of psychosis. On the other hand, Wolff and Chess (1964) found parents from all socioeconomic groups, but the number of psychotic children was small (11). Rutter and Lockyer (1967) found a marked excess of higher socioeconomic backgrounds (55% versus 32%) in psychotic children as compared with matched clinic controls. In a study of 76 psychotic children, McDermott, Harrison, Schrager, Lindy, and Killins (1967) found that the social class of the children was consistent with the distribution in the general population, but the *symptomatology* differed with severe autism being much commoner in the professional and executive class, whereas thought disturbances were associated with both the skilled labor and professional-executive classes. Also noted was a tendency for the professional-executive parents to bring their children in at younger ages. Unfortunately, the significance of these findings is diluted by the large number of borderline psychotic (53) children in the group.

In a formal test of Rimland's corollary statement that parents of autistic children are uniformly of very high intellectual level, Levine and Olson (1968) administered a vocabulary test of intelligence to the parents of three children diagnosed as autistic on the basis of Rimland's checklist. Although all the parents had average or above intelligence, none was greatly so and none had completed college.

While there appears to be an excess of psychotic children, especially those with autism, from higher socioeconomic backgrounds this has yet to be demonstrated not to be a sampling artifact.

Personosocial Functioning of Parents and Families of Psychotic Children

Opinions on the frequency of pathological attitudes and disorders in the parents and families of psychotic children vary greatly. Some (Bender 1947, 1956; Bettelheim, 1956, 1967; Esman, Kahn, & Nyman, 1959; Kanner in Eisenberg & Kanner, 1956; Mahler, 1965; Rank, 1949; and Szurek, 1956) feel that childhood psychosis is very frequently (and in some cases always, e.g., Reiser, 1963; Szurek, 1956) accompanied by significant psychopathology in one or both parents. Kanner (Eisenberg & Kanner, 1956) felt that parents of autistic children were of the refrigerator type, namely highly intelligent obsessive people incapable of warmth. Mahler (1965), Rank (1949), and Reiser (1963) expressed a point of view that is essentially similar to that enunciated earlier by Kanner, namely, that the mothers of psychotic children are incapable of giving their child a warm sustaining relationship because of their own severe disturbance (psychosis, depression, and immaturity). Szurek (1956) feels that the parental psychopathology consists primarily of severe internalized unconscious conflicts within each parent, which result in marital friction and the utilization of the child by the parent for the solution of his own conflict. Szurek considers there is no particular specificity about the nature of these parental conflicts and Esman et al. (1958) hold a similar position. These views appear to have been derived largely from clinical interviews of varying duration, some psychoanalytic, some not. On the other hand, Klebanoff (1959) found that the mothers of psychotic children were intermediate between the mothers of disturbed brain-damaged children and mothers of normal children in the number of unhealthy parent-child attitudes they exhibited. Pitt-field and Oppenheim (1964) found little difference in parental attitudes between mothers of normal, mongol, and psychotic children, as did Anthony (1958) between mothers of psychotic and mothers of neurotic children from the same clinic. Creak and Ini (1960) found the mothers and fathers of 102 psychotic children to be a heterogeneous group with respect to emotional warmth, in fact, slightly under half were described as "outgoing." It is conspicuous that all these studies with relative negative findings have used attitudinal scales of varying levels of sophistication rather than clinical interviews. Rutter and Lockyer (1967), using an objective but somewhat remote index of parental adjustment, found that in contrast to a matched clinic control group, the proportion of psychotic children living in unbroken homes was normal. Ogdon, Bass, Thomas, and Lordi (1968), in a well-designed study, found the parents of autistic children to have significantly more psychopathology along several dimensions of the Rorschach (though not of Kanner's perfectionistic kind) than a matched group of parents of normal children.

Goldfarb (1961), using a structured interview in the child's home, found the family adequacy scores for the nonorganic schizophrenic subgroup to be significantly inferior, whereas those of the organic subgroup did not differ from normal children. The particular feature exhibited by the nonorganic child's family was what Goldfarb described as "parental perplexity." Similar (bimodal) results are reported from psychiatric interviews with parents of children with primary psychosis and with psychosis secondary to brain syndrome by Eaton and Menolascino (1966). Anthony (1958) found that the mothers of children who had been autistic since birth (primary) appeared to be more self-righteous than the mothers whose children had become psychotic after a relatively normal period (secondary) who appeared more perplexed. Ratings of emotional warmth by two independent observers showed that most of the cold mothers had primary autistic children, whereas most of the overprotective mothers had secondary autistic children.

The distribution of frank psychosis in the families of psychotic children has been found to be increased by Bender (1955), Fish et al. (1968), and Kallmann and Roth (1956), though in the latter case the majority of schizophrenics were preadolescent. However, Creak and Ini (1960), Kanner (Eisenberg & Kanner, 1956), Rutter (1965a), Rutter and Lockyer (1967), and Schain and Yannet (1960) did not find any increased frequency of psychosis.

Thus, there is considerable disagreement about the frequency and type of psychopathology in the families of psychotic children though, generally speaking, studies that find increased frequency are methodologically poor, using unstructured clinical interviews without control groups or "hard" data. When control groups are used, parents of psychotic children are found to be either no different from the parents of normal children or, if different, no more so than the mothers of disturbed or physically disabled nonpsychotic children. While it is tempting to give more credence to these controlled studies, the differences may be a result of the mode of measurement (clinical interview versus attitudinal scales), and it is a moot point as to which is the more valid technique. Thus, it seems best to conclude that the frequency of disorder in the parents of psychotic children is presently unestablished. Furthermore, the relationship in time of any parental disturbance to the onset of the child's psychosis is equally unestablished and some (Anthony, 1958; Bender, 1956; Klebanoff, 1959) argue that the parental disorder is largely reactive to having a psychotic child. The work of Goldfarb (1961) and others suggests that the frequency of parental disorder may vary according to the particular subclass of psychosis (see also Eaton & Menolascino, 1966; Rimland, 1964, pp. 74–75). It is also apparent that opinions on the frequency of parental and family disorder covary more with the investigator's predilection for a particular etiological theory than they do with the state of knowledge. Klebanoff's (1959) suggestion that centers which stress the psychogenesis of childhood psychosis should study intensively the parents of organically disordered children would seem to have much merit, though centers which favor the organic hypothesis might do the converse. However, all investigations could benefit from proper attention to the methodology of evaluating parent-child interaction (see Chapter Two).

Etiology

Etiological theories of childhood psychosis may be grouped according to the nature (psychological or organic) of the posited *primary* etiological agent. A recent, lucid and more detailed review of these theories can be found in Rutter (1970). Also useful particularly in conjunction with the former is Ward's overview (1970) since it gives more detailed coverage of psychogenic theories.

Organic Theories

In this view, children with psychosis or with particular subtypes thereof have an abnormally functioning CNS. The etiological agent may be considered genetic (Bender, 1955; Kallmann & Roth, 1956; Vaillant, 1963) or resulting from brain damage occurring mostly during the pre- and perinatal periods (Gittelman & Birch, 1967; Goldfarb, 1961; Pollack & Woerner, 1966; Pollack, 1967; Rutter, 1965a). Support cited for the brain damage hypothesis is the increased frequency of pre- and perinatal insults, neurological EEG abnormalities often observed in psychotic children. These supporting findings have been discussed in detail above and it will be recalled that their presence is not unanimously recognized and their exact neuropathological significance is uncertain. The genetic hypothesis draws most of its support from one study, that by Kallmann and Roth (1956), who concluded after an examination of the frequency of psychosis in the twins, parents, and siblings of 102 patients who became psychotic before the age of 15, that there was good evidence for a pattern of inheritance of the disorder similar to adult schizophrenia. The great majority of Kallmann and Roth's cases, however, became psychotic during later childhood, a group which comprises only the minority of psychotic children and which is thought to be different, resembling adult psychotics more closely.

Vaillant (1963), summarizing the twin studies of early infantile autism, found concordance in 7 of 10 sets of twins with 2 of the homozygous and the only fraternal set being discordant. However, Judd and Mandell (1968), in an extensive search of the literature, claimed that in only one case in which zygosity has been adequately established had there been discordance in homozygous twins and in that case there was reason to believe that the child had a chronic brain syndrome because of perinatal anoxia. Few of the studies of the families of psychotic children have shown an increased frequency of psychosis in relatives (see section on families of psychotic children), and there is some reason to suppose that in those which do (Bender, 1955; Fish et al., 1968) this may be no higher than in parents of all kinds of disturbed children.

Perceptions of the basic lesion or pathogenesis vary. Bender (1947, 1955, 1956) sees psychosis as a widespread encephalopathy developing during fetal life resulting in a variety of primary neurological abnormalities (vasovegetative, tone, mobility, and perceptual abnormalities) and of psychological symptoms secondary to the anxiety provoked by the child's impaired adaptational ability. Goldfarb (1961, 1964) has a similar view though he sees the deficits as more restricted, involving ego functions of perception, central integration, and motor execution. This results in a faulty interaction by the child with his environment and a failure in the feedback necessary to adapt his ongoing behavior to the environment. Unlike Bender, however, Goldfarb believes that this basic deficit may not necessarily be due to brain damage, but in some is due to the failure of the familial environment to provide clear cues, while in others a combination of organic and familial factors are at fault. Gittelman and Birch (1967) see the brain lesions as involving both input and response systems to a severe degree.

Rimland (1964) posits that there is a lesion in the reticular activating system (RAS) in autism occurring in the pre- or perinatal period, particularly as a result of prematurity, though the precise location of the lesion within the CNS is not crucial to the theory. He sees the fundamental dysfunction in autism as the inability "to relate new stimuli to remembered experiences" (p. 70). The failure of the autistic child to develop human relationships is a direct result of his inability to associate the relief of distress and biological tensions with his mother.

Schain and Yannet (1960) have a basically similar concept except that on the basis of an autopsy of an autistic child with seizures they postulate the lesion to be in the hippocampal affective circuit.

Hutt et al. (1965), from EEG studies, also posit a lesion in the RAS, but unlike Rimland, they see the dysfunction as chronic internal hyperarousal which shuts out incoming environmental stimuli so that the autistic child is relatively refractory to his environment.

Ornitz and Ritvo (1968) also offer a neurophysiological theory derived from Pavlovian theory and from recent studies on the neurophysiology of sleep. They argue that the basic dysfunction in childhood psychosis is perceptual inconstancy which, like Bender and Goldfarb, they see as preventing the child's differentiation of self from environment and from responding accurately to incoming stimuli. This basic dysfunction is a consequence of a neurophysiological disorder of a lack of balance between states of excitation and inhibition, which results in the disruptive breaking through into waking life of the phasic excitation and phasic inhibition seen in REM sleep. However, the supporting evidence they cite for this theory is mostly inferential and basically weak.

Rutter (1965a, 1968), though considering psychosis to be of heterogeneous (organic) etiology, feels that the central dysfunction in most cases is damage to the speech area of the brain, leading to receptive aphasia. This, in combination with other defects of perception, interferes with the child's interaction with his environment leading to the clinical syndrome. This theory has many affinities with those of Goldfarb and Rimland, except that the imperception of language is more emphasized. However, Rutter is careful to underline that aphasia cannot be the only dysfunction since congenitally aphasic children are not autistic.

Psychogenic Theories

In these, the etiology is perceived as primarily due to the way the environment, and most importantly the parents, interact with the child especially during infancy and early childhood. Though most of the proponents of the psychogenic point of view now admit the role of organic etiological factors such as a constitutional ego deficit in utilizing need fulfilling objects (Mahler, 1965), with the possible exception of Anthony (1958), they remain for all practical purposes psychogenically oriented, certainly in their writings and in their attitude to parents (see Kysar, 1968).

Psychoanalytic theories have been summarized by Alanen (1960). Freud saw psychosis as primarily a regression to the level of primary narcissism because of a constitutional fixation of libido at that level, but Alanen feels that the psychosis is an ego disorder, the ego having failed to develop adequately. He outlines four phases at which this ego development may become arrested. In the autistic child there is a failure to establish normal symbiosis which has been emphasized by Mahler (1965) and the Putnam group (Reiser, 1963). The primary cause may lie in the child's inability to utilize this relationship though emphasis is usually given to the inability of the mother to provide a normal loving relationship. In symbiotic psychosis there is a failure to resolve normal symbiosis between mother and child due most usually to an overprotective mother. In older children the problem is one of identification with abnormal parents, particularly those who are psychotic or behave psychotically toward the child (the transmission of irrationality). In later childhood and adolescence the abnormalities are largely those of role taking and identity formation as a result of profound disturbances in the family, both in its intrafamilial and larger environmental interactions.

Two psychoanalytic investigators who do not fit easily into this framework are Szurek (Boatman & Szurek, 1960; Szurek, 1956), who places great emphasis on the early and continuous distortion of the child's personality development by the anxiety induced from anxious parents who are in conflict within themselves and between each other, and Bettelheim (1956, 1967) who sees the autistic child's perception of the world as a dangerous place (akin to a Nazi concentration camp) in which he is completely at the mercy of cruel, unpredictable savage adults. For Bettelheim the pathogenic element lies in what he calls the "extreme situation" in which the child has been grossly rejected, brutalized or terrorized, mostly but not necessarily, by the parents. This seems to approximate to the early idea of psychic trauma. Bettelheim has been sharply criticized by Wing (1968) for his complete disregard for scientific objectivity in formulating his ideas, a criticism which, however, could be applied with equal cogency to most theorists, but particularly the psychoanalysts. In one of the most elegant and testable psychoanalytic theories, Anthony (1958) drew a distinction between primary and secondary autism. The former is a persistence of what is called in psychoanalytic theory, normal autism or the primary objectless state of the neonate. This persistence is postulated to result from the existence in the child of a constitutionally determined "thick" stimulus barrier that insulates the child from a normal interaction with his environment and hence prevents the development of object relations. In secondary autism, on the other hand, the child develops normally at first but because of the opposite kind of constitutional deficiency, namely a "thin" stimulus barrier, the child is hypersensitive (see Bergman & Escalona, 1949) and is driven into autism as a secondary protection against stimulus overload. In the case of the primary autistic child, a highly stimulating mother may be able to overcome the child's autism, while in the secondary case what is needed is a mother who will protect the child from overstimulation.

Kanner (Eisenberg & Kanner, 1956; Kanner, 1943, 1958, p. 743–758), like Mahler, considers early and prolonged emotional deprivation by "refrigerator-type" parents in a vulnerable child to be fundamental to the development of autism, although the precise pathogenesis is not clearly articulated but appears to have as much in common with Ferster's (1961) theory as with the psychoanalytic.

Behaviorist theories are among the most recent and, unlike other theories, grew out of animal experimentation instead of clinical observations of psychotic children. As a result, they highlight externally observable behavior by the child and his parents rather than inferences about feelings or motives. Nevertheless, the basic pathogenic mechanisms have much in common with some of those propounded by psychoanalysts. Ferster (1961) conceptualized the clinical symptomatology of the autistic child as essentially an impoverished repertoire of behaviors restricted in frequency and in complexity because of the failure of parents to reinforce or attend to the child's early adult-directed behaviors. Ferster posited that the kinds of parental behavior that would result in this would be unresponsiveness resulting from depression, physical illness, preoccupation with other activities, and active dislike of the child. He also noted that the few behaviors that the autistic child has, apart from self-stimulatory ones, are aversive or unpleasant for others and usually lead to prompt gratification of the child's wishes. Thus the basic pathogenic mechanism is an extinction through nonreinforcement of most normal social behaviors requiring any extensive parent-child interaction and the selective reinforcement of self-stimulatory behaviors and what Ferster calls "atavistic" behaviors, which have the capacity through their extreme disagreeableness to bring prompt environmental gratification.

Unlike most theorists, Ferster made certain testable predictions, though it is difficult to say how many have been post hoc due to a knowledge of the literature on psychotic children. The first prerequisite was that the general principles of operant conditioning would have to be valid for autistic children, which Ferster (1961) was able to demonstrate experimentally without difficulty, as were several other investigators (e.g., Hingtgen & Coulter, 1967; Lovaas, Schaeffer, & Simmons, 1965; Risley & Wolf, 1967). Ferster also predicted that because of the mitigating effect of siblings, relatives, and neighbors, autism would be rare and would occur much more commonly in the firstborn child and in socially isolated parents, all of which are fairly consonant with Kanner's observation of early infantile autism. The great virtue of Ferster's theory is its simplicity, its explicitness, and its emphasis on observable behavior in both parent and child, all of which make it one of the most testable and treatment-relevant theories.

Summary of Etiology

There is a great deal of evidence to suggest that psychotic children have a variety of perceptual and cognitive abnormalities that interfere significantly with their ability to interact in a meaningful way with their environment and that hence impede their acquisition of basic language, cognitive, and social skills. The etiology of these abnormalities is presently unknown, but the consensus of opinion appears to be moving increasingly toward the acceptance of some organic etiology or more probably etiologies with nonorganic environmental factors playing a variable role.

All theories of etiology and pathogenesis, whether organic or psychogenic, would benefit from formal testing. Many currently popular theories would no doubt fail to survive the rigor of prediction which is the essence of science. Since it is impossible to choose an etiological theory now solely on supporting evidence, criteria of post hoc explanatory value, heuristic qualities, testability, and applicability to treatment must be used as a basis by which to evaluate theories. Unfortunately, with the exception of Rutter's (1968) and Ferster's (1961), present theories seem to be strongest on the least important of these qualities, namely, post hoc explanation, and weakest on explicating treatment procedures and fostering significant research.

Treatment

Mode and intensity of treatment tend to reflect the investigator's ideas of etiology and pathogenesis. Thus, those who consider psychological variables of primary importance tend to favor intensive individual and family psychotherapy, whereas those who are organically oriented generally adopt a more pessimistic point of view using physical treatments and leaving the greater part of the child's management to others as in an environmental manipulations or reeducative procedures.

Psychotherapies

Tilton et al. (1966), in their annotated bibliography on childhood psychosis, list over 30 articles on the use of psychotherapy with psychotic children published between 1955 and 1964. With few exceptions these articles are purely descriptive and centered on a detailed discussion of a single or very small number of cases. Psychotherapeutic techniques differ to the extent to which they are centered on the child, the parent(s), or the whole family. Group therapy with psychotic children seems to be an infrequent treatment method.

Bettelheim (1956, 1967) is the strongest proponent of primarily child-centered individual therapy given in a residential setting where the child may be more effectively isolated from his parents. The goal is to provide the child with a need-satisfying person (all day long, every day of the year) who must act to reduce all environmental pressures on the child. In action this seems tantamount to extreme permissiveness and indulgence. In this way the psychotic child can overcome his fear of the environment and his arrested psychosexual development may proceed from its primitive level. Bettelheim differs somewhat from the traditional psychotherapeutic model in that he sees therapy continuing throughout the 24 hour period and primarily invested in child-care workers instead of in mental health professionals. Mahler (Mahler, 1965; Mahler, Furer, & Settlage, 1959), though also seeing the psychotic child's problem centered primarily in deficient need-satisfying relationship with his mother, sees the key to treatment in trying to reconstruct the early mother-child symbiosis with the mother a necessary part of this process. In her psychotherapy, which seems to follow the more traditional format of professional therapist and discrete sessions, the therapist assists this process of reconstitution through the use of psychoanalytic theory that enables an understanding of the child's behavior and hence facilitates the therapist's reactions to the child's unconscious needs. The traditional psychoanalytic concept of encouraging the patient to regress and work through actually (e.g., soiling) or symbolically (e.g., playing with clay) missed or unsatisfactory phases of psychosexual development appear to be as characteristic of Mahler's therapy as they are of Bettelheim's. However, although Mahler cautions against pushing the psychotic child too hard in therapy, she seems to favor the setting of more limits than Bettelheim and also stresses the necessity for the therapist to have at times an active instigating or educational role. The attitude of the therapist toward the mother appears to be essentially didactic, teaching her to meet the special dependent and educational needs of the psychotic child, though Mahler does stress the need for simultaneous treatment of the mother in some cases.

Szurek (1956) uses a classical psychoanalytic framework and sees the therapist's role as lending whatever assistance he can to ego, superego, or id, whichever needs it most at that particular moment in therapy. He also is among those who put greatest stress on the simultaneous treatment of parents, which is consonant with his idea of the child's incorporating the parental conflicts. Reiser (1963) considers that intensive psychoanalytically oriented psychotherapy two to three times a week for several years for both child and parents is necessary. More lengthy discussions of psychotherapeutic techniques with psychotic children are to be found in Caplan (1955), Ekstein, Bryant and Friedman (1958), Hammer and Kaplan (1967), LaVietes (1967), and Mahler et al. (1959).

Accurate evaluation of the effectiveness of psychotherapy in childhood psychosis is impossible since there are no published systematic studies using untreated or differently treated control groups diagnosed by the same investigator(s) and receiving the same additional treatments such as milieu therapy, occupational therapy, and remedial education. An unpublished study done in Vancouver (Ney, personal communication) showed 50 1-hour sessions of psychoanalytically oriented play therapy to be inferior to a similar number of operant conditioning sessions. Ney's study, though well-designed and controlled, suffers from the weakness that his therapists were relatively untrained subprofessionals.

Thus, one is left with the unsatisfactory state of attempting to evaluate the results of psychotherapy with psychotic children against some estimate of the untreated recovery rate, such as the recovery rate used by Levitt (1957, 1963) in the most comprehensive review of the effectiveness of psychotherapy with children. Unfortunately, in the first review Levitt specifically excluded psychotic children. In the second he cited three uncontrolled studies on psychotic children (Bender & Gurevitz, 1955; Kane & Chambers, 1961; Kaufman, Frank, Friend, Heins, & Weiss, 1962) showing improvement rates of 100%, 75%, and 75%, as compared with 72.5% in the untreated control group comprised of nonpsychotic dropouts from treatment waiting lists (hardly, unfortunately, a suitable comparative group since its prognosis is probably much better). Bettelheim (1967) recently reported a cure rate of 17 out of 40 (42%) and an improvement rate of 15 (38%) to give a total cure and improvement rate of 80%. Wing (1968), however, points to the total absence of objective criteria, either of diagnosis or improvement so that Bettelheim's figures are of dubious value.

Eisenberg (1957), in his scholarly review of the long-term course of childhood psychosis, states that one-quarter showed marked improvement (good social adjustment in adolescence) without treatment, while another third have a fluctuating course but manage to keep out of institutions. He suggests that a spontaneous improvement rate of about 60% can be expected if all degrees, however slight, are admitted. This is obviously a very unsatisfying inference, particularly since the diagnosis of childhood psychosis appears to have become rather more elastic than that used by Kanner and Eisenberg in their study with consequent probable improved spontaneous remission rates. In one of the better (insofar as indices of social function are concerned), though uncontrolled studies of long-term outcome after intensive individual psychotherapy, Brown (1963) found that of 129 children 54% appeared to be making some kind of adjustment in society though few were symptom-free. It should also be noted that the children in Brown's and the three studies cited by Levitt (1963) did not use psychotherapy as the sole treatment and that the criteria of improvement are extremely variable.

Until properly controlled studies such as those by Ney are instituted, the role of individual psychotherapy in the treatment of child psychosis must be regarded as of uncertain value.

Behavior Therapy

This is a relatively new technique. Of three recent reviews (Leff, 1968; Gelfand & Hartmann, 1968; Werry & Wollersheim, 1967), one (Leff) devoted specifically to childhood psychosis shows that the technique has already had a not inconsiderable application in childhood psychosis and enough to excite prejudicial judgments both pro (e.g., Rimland, 1965) and con (e.g., Bettelheim, 1967). The details of behavior therapy are discussed in Chapter Seven. In contrast to studies on the use of psychotherapy in the treatment of childhood psychosis, those on behavior therapy make the techniques and goals of treatment explicit, concentrate on items of observable behavior, require the therapist to be active and maintain control of therapy, reward good behavior and ignore or punish bad behavior *immediately* after its occurrence and, though these are by no means necessary correlates of behavior therapy, generally use controls (usually within subject) and generate objective assessment data. However, like studies on psychotherapy, the majority of reported instances of the use of behavior therapy concern only single or very small numbers of children.

Ferster (1961) first demonstrated that the principles of learning derived from animal experiments which underpin behavior therapy were, as with normal children, equally valid for autistic children. DeMyer and Ferster (1962) describe the use of an operant conditioning approach to the development of social behaviors in eight psychotic children. Target social behaviors such as responses to an adult, use of the toys, and verbalizations were built up in successive steps (or shaped) by rewarding the elements as they appeared with praise, cuddling, singing, rocking, etc. Therapy was carried out by child-care staff. Six children responded well to this treatment and two did not. DeMyer and Ferster were particularly impressed by the prospects behavior therapy offered for the utilization of relatively unskilled therapists. Wolf et al., (1964), by using aides and parents as therapists, were able to deal successfully with a psychotic child's refusal to wear glasses and other negativistic behaviors, and were also able to develop some language. Generally speaking, their approach was to reward desired behaviors with food and to punish bad behaviors by placing the child in isolation. At follow-up two years later behavioral improvement was found to have been maintained and a second course of treatment was given this time to develop behaviors appropriate for school. The same authors (Risley & Wolf, 1967) have described in detail with data and illustrations the techniques of establishing functional speech in several echolalic psychotic children using operant conditioning techniques.

Davison (1964, 1965), Hingtgen, Sanders, and DeMyer (1965), Hingtgen, Coulter, and Churchill (1967), Hudson and DeMyer (1968), Martin, England, Kaprowy, Kilgour, and Pilek (1968), and McConnel (1967), and Metz (1965) have described ways of improving the social skills and interaction of psychotic children using operant conditioning techniques generally similar to those described in detail by Risley and Wolf. Hewett (1964, 1965) established basic verbal reading and social skills in a similar manner in a 13-year-old autistic child. In a series of elegant and carefully documented studies Lovaas (Lovaas, Freitas, Nelson, & Whalen, 1967; Lovaas et al., 1965a, 1965b, 1966) successfully developed verbal, academic, and social behaviors simultaneously, extinguishing a variety of self-destructive and disruptive behaviors in a group of severely autistic children, several of whom were mute and older than Eisenberg's (1967) critical age of 5 years. Techniques used by Lovaas are generally similar to those described by Risley and Wolf (1967) with the exception that he (Lovaas et al., 1965b) used in addition painful electric shock both in the treatment of severely self-mutilating behavior and, more interestingly, as a means of developing human relationship in the autistic child by pairing the termination of the shock with physical contact from an adult. Also of interest is the demonstration by Lovaas (Lovaas et al., 1965a) and Baroff and Tate (1968) that self-destructive behavior appears to be externally instead of internally motivated as judged by its augmentation with attention. Baroff and Tate also successfully stopped self-mutilation in an autistic boy with painful electric shock. Hingtgen et al. (1967), Lovaas (Lovaas et al., 1967), and Risley and Wolf (1967) have drawn attention to the necessity of first developing imitation—a behavior frequently lacking in autistic children—as a prerequisite to the developing of many subsequent skills including verbal behavior.

In an unpublished controlled treatment study, Ney, Palvesky and Markeley subdivided each of the target behaviors (self-awareness, emotional relationships, imitation of adult behavior, and communication) into 25 steps and used attention and candy as reinforcers in the stepwise shaping of these target behaviors. The group was comprised of 20 psychotic boys aged 5–13 years, subdivided into two groups matched according to age, signs of organicity, length of hospitalization, amount of speech and adaptive behavior. Each subgroup was treated with 50 1-hour individual sessions of operant conditioning or psychoanalytically oriented play therapy with a crossover of treatments at midpoint. Progress was measured by psychological tests of development and intellectual function given before treatment and at the end of each phase. Generally speaking, the results showed operant conditioning to be superior to play therapy, which produced little change.

Though behavior therapy is still in its early states, it has already shown promise as a treatment of childhood psychosis, at least in its ability to teach basic social skills and to eliminate distressing clinical symptoms such as tantrums, self-destructive behavior, social withdrawal, mutism, and echolalia (Leff, 1968). Its explicitness and simplicity make it readily carried out by largely unskilled personnel, notably child-care aides and parents (Davison, 1964, 1965; DeMyer & Ferster, 1962; Hudson & DeMyer, 1968; Wolf et al., 1964). Its empirical conceptualization more readily permits investigation of its efficacy and also of its therapeutic components. However, behavior therapy shares with individual psychotherapy two important shortcomings, the amount of time that must be invested in a child (Lovaas, 1966; Fischer & Glanville, 1970) (this point is disputed by Leff, 1968) and its inability to make the psychotic child not readily distinguishable from a normal child (Leff, 1968). (Brown, 1963 noted this to be a similar failing of individual psychotherapy.) Nevertheless, for the reasons outlined above, behavior therapy appears to be one of the more promising developments in the treatment of psychosis, a conclusion consistent with that reached by other reviewers (Gelfand & Hartmann, 1968; Leff, 1968; Werry & Wollersheim, 1967).

Occupational, Milieu, and Educational Therapy

These treatment techniques are generally employed as part of a total treatment program of the psychotic child. However, there is little or no information relating to their specific components or effectiveness except in one excellent study by Wenar, Ruttenberg, Dratman, and Wolf (1967). Using the behavior rating instrument developed by Ruttenberg et al. (1966) as a dependent variable measure they compared 8 autistic children in a custodial program, 15 in an activity-educational milieu therapy program in a state hospital, and 9 in a psychoanalytically oriented day-care unit emphasizing emotional relationships. The day-care unit, which had the highest staff ratio (and hence success cannot be ascribed necessarily to the underpinning theory), proved more successful in producing changes in relationship, mastery, and psychosexual development after 1 year, but none of the children made progress in communication and vocalization. This, if anything, might be taken as a vindication of the problem-oriented approach of the behaviorists.

In an uncontrolled study, valuable chiefly for the explicitness of its therapeutic technology, Fischer and Glanville (1970) describe a programmed classroom-behavior shaping and educational method of teaching autistic children. However, Fischer and Glanville predict that it will take the majority of austistic children 10 years to complete the course which is basically a preschool program, after which 6 years of normal elementary school education would be required to obtain a minimal educational qualification.

Lovaas et al. (1966) and Risley and Wolf (1967) argue that the most compelling initial need of the psychotic child is to give him basic language skills and focusing thereon appears to have been reasonably successful. Wenar et al. (1967) focused on emotional relationships and also seem to have been successful. Thus, the question of evaluating methods of therapy becomes inextricably intertwined with defining goals of therapy. Until some agreement in this respect can be reached, meaningful comparisons between differing therapeutic modalities seem unlikely.

Physical Treatments

Metrazol and electric shock treatment have been used almost exclusively by Bender (1953) who claimed that they stimulate maturation and patterning as judged by EEG, anthropometric, and other data. At long-term follow-up, Bender found that a shock-treated group had a higher rate of fair-to-good adjustment (25%) than a group comprised largely of severe cases and those with uncooperative parents (4%). In assessing the validity of this difference it should be noted that the untreated group is hardly comparable, that 89% of the treated group were still schizophrenic at follow-up and that the spontaneous remission rate in childhood psychosis appears to be about 25% (Eisenberg, 1957).

Though it is possible, as suggested by Bender, that shock treatment may improve individual symptoms such as anxiety, there appears to be little evidence that it is able to influence significantly the long-term outcome.

Drug Treatment

Despite the undoubted frequency with which psychotropic medication is used in psychotic children there are few studies of their use exclusively with this group and fewer still in which adequate methodology permits an accurate interpretation of the findings (see general reviews by Eveloff, 1966; Grant, 1962. See also Chapter Eight of this volume.). Grant cites five studies of differing quality, suggesting chlorpromazine is of value, particularly in the hyperactive, agitated psychotic child. In a double-blind, cross over study of 28 schizophrenic children, Fish (1960) found amphetamine to be of no value, while diphenhydramine and several phenothiazines were effective. In general, diphenhydramine was more effective in younger retarded, not so severely disturbed psychotic children, trifluoperazine in most, but particularly the hypoactive psychotic child and chlorpromazine in the hyperactive child with psychosis. In a subsequent double-blind study (Fish & Shapiro, 1965) in which improvements were assessed by weekly global severity ratings of apparent satisfactory reliability (see above), the same author found chlorpromazine to be the most generally useful drug, especially in the more classically autistic children (Fish's types I and II). Diphenhydramine was helpful in the same type of psychotic child, but its action was weaker than chlorpromazine. Other kinds of psychotic children such as the pseudoneurotic and pseudopsychopathic responded almost as well to placebo as they did to other drugs. The improvement occurring with medication was limited and the basic grave impairment of function remained.

In a novel and heuristic way, Ferster and DeMyer (1961) studied the effect of another phenothiazine, prochlorperazine, in two dosage levels (.5 and 1 mg./kg.), compared with placebo in a two-choice match-to-sample visual discrimination task. They found that the drug significantly increased the number of responses, but any effect of the higher dosage level cannot be ascertained since it was confounded with order, reinforcement, and scheduling effects.

Freedman, Deutsch, and Deutsch (1960) examined the effects of hydroxyzine, a minor tranquilizer, on the reaction time to visual and auditory stimuli in 14 schizophrenic children aged 7 to 13 years. Each subject was tested twice, predrug and after two weeks of a total daily dosage of 60 mg. of hydroxyzine. It was found that reaction time to both kinds of stimuli did move closer to normal values after the drug administration, but they remained significantly inferior to those of a normal control group. However, this could have been merely a practice effect, since the normal control group was tested only once and no placebo control was used in the psychotic group. Incidental behavior observations suggested that the subjects' behavior in the test situation was improved, most noticeably a reduction in fear and general behavior disturbance, but this too could have been simply a habituation to the test situation. Rawitt (1959), in a double-blind crossover study in 40 boys of mixed diagnoses, aged 10 to 16 years, found that meprobamate even in fairly high dosage did not appear to be particularly helpful for those with diagnosis of psychosis, a finding essentially similar to that of others (see Grant, 1962).

Freedman, Ebin, and Wilson (1962) gave 100 mg. of LSD on a single occasion to 12 mute or near-mute psychotic children aged 6 to 12 years. The effect of the drug was judged by psychiatric observation throughout the time of effect (about 5 hours). The changes produced by the drug were facial flushing, posturing, ataxia, desire for physical contact, psychomotor excitation, possible hallucination, increased remoteness, and decreased eye contact. There was no change in verbal behavior except a general increment in preexisting vocalization patterns consonant with the general psychomotor excitation. Though the drug was given on one occasion only, Freedman et al. concluded on the basis of their observations that LSD was unlikely to be a useful tool in the treatment of childhood psychosis. In a methodologically very poor study, Bender (Bender, Goldschmidt, & Sankar, 1962; Bender, Cobrinik, Faretra, & Sankar, 1966) gave LSD and another psychotomimetic (UML) in doses of 150 mg. and 12 mg. respectively to hospitalized psychotic children from 1 to 18 months. From notations made by the psychiatrists and other ward personnel and some psychological tests it was concluded that the children, particularly younger autistic patients, showed significant improvement with reduction of anxiety, greater responsiveness, and improved social maturity.

Rolo, Krinsky, Abrahamson, and Goldfarb (1965) felt that Bender's results merited further investigation but only with much more exacting observation of behavioral changes. They therefore took movie films on repeated occasions in a set play situation before, during, and after the administration of 100 mg. of LSD given daily for one month. The several judges who examined the films were unable reliably to tell whether the child was receiving drugs or not. Simmons et al. (1966) studied the effects of 50 mg. of LSD in a pair of identical male autistic twins aged five years by means of several standard test situations (child in isolation, with a passive adult, and playing simple games with an adult). A variety of reliably observable behaviors such as vocalizations, stereotypies, smiles, physical contact with the adult, eye-to-face contact with the examiner, laughter, and smiling increased with medication, while self-stimulatory behavior decreased and a greater tendency for the subject to stay close to the adult was observed. This study is probably the most outstanding one in the pharmacotherapy of childhood psychosis for the care and rigor with which the behavioral effects of the drug have been measured, and it is hoped that it will serve as a model for other investigators, certainly as far as the short-term effects are concerned.

In another study Silberstein, Mandell, Dalack, and Cooper (1968) set a clearly defined and measurable goal, namely avoiding institutionalization trouble with police and dismissal from school. They then examined the relative efficacy of 2 treatment procedures in 48 psychotic children and adolescents of mean age 10 years, range 4 to 17 years, who had been recommended for hospitalization by two psychiatrists acting independently. The children were divided into 4 approximately equal matched (including for symptomatology) groups and given 4 different treatment conditions: trifluoperazine, placebo, parental counseling-placebo and parental counseling-trifluoperazine. Only two patients were treatment failures, so it was concluded that defining the treatment goal for the staff was more powerful than the treatment methods. This study may be crude and simplistic, but it does illustrate how meaningful evaluation can occur in the context of a clinical program.

In summary, there has been surprisingly little systematic investigation of the role of drugs in the management of childhood psychosis. The major tranquilizers, particularly the phenothiazine group of drugs, although they seem to have some utility in mitigating certain distressing behavioral symptoms, especially those of psychomotor excitation such as hyperactivity, they do not affect the basic psychotic process itself. LSD appears to be worthy of further investigation. No other drugs, except perhaps diphenhydramine (in younger psychotic children), appear to be of established value. Because of the paucity of good studies, the use of drugs with psychotic children should be regarded as experimental though there would seem to be little merit in adopting an entirely negative attitude such as that of Reiser (1963) who feels it may interfere with psychotherapy. As pointed out by Sprague and Werry (1971) in another context, there is a particular need to study the effect of drugs on the individual behavioral and cognitive abnormalities in childhood psychosis and the utility of medication not as an isolated treatment, but as a means of facilitating improved function, which can then be shaped and consolidated by other treatment approaches particularly those based on social learning principles.

Prognosis (See also Chapter Ten)

Ward (1963) reviewed follow-up studies on schizophrenic children and found very serious defects in most, particularly inadequate diagnostic criteria and the lack of thoroughness in follow-up assessment which tended to be described in vague, global terms such as recovered, greatly improved, etc. Other obfuscating variables characteristic of follow-up studies are the neglect of the importance of the age of onset, varying length of time of follow-up, and the fact that most children have had some kind of treatment, often of radically different kinds. All of these factors diminish greatly the significance of the studies to be reported below.

In an informal follow-up of Potter's (1933) 14 cases of childhood schizophrenia, Bennett and Klein (1966) located all except 2. Only one of the 14 had been discharged from a hospital. Of the remainder, 2 had died in an institution, 2 were retarded, 7 were typical deteriorated schizophrenics, and 2 seemed about the same as at admission. Bennett and Klein were impressed by the similarity between this group and institutionalized adult-onset schizophrenics which, of course, might be more a sign of the acculturating power of the mental hospital than of the similarity between childhood psychosis and schizophrenia.

Eisenberg (1967) summarized the literature until 1940 and found a recovery rate of approximately 7% in 132 cases reported by 7 authors. From a present-day perspective most of these children can be considered to have been untreated. Bender (1953), in her follow-up of almost 200 children, most of whom had received shock treatment, found 90% to be schizophrenic, though 25% were making a fair-to-good social adjustment as judged by their capacity to keep out of state institutions. Eisenberg (Eisenberg, 1957), in the follow-up of 63 autistic children seen by Kanner, found that 17 or about 25% appeared to be able to achieve minimal social adjustment as judged by their capacity to go to school and remain in the community. As with Bender's group, even those making a minimal adjustment showed residual signs of their psychosis, most notably social insensitivity described as a lack of savoir faire. Eisenberg found that the most important prognostic index was whether the child had learned to speak by the age of five years. Of those who did, half made some sort of scholastic and social adjustment, but for those who were still mute at five, only one out of a total of 20 subsequently developed language and made some adjustment.

Andrews and Cappon (1957) reassessed 21 autistic children of all ages and all degrees of severity after a relatively short period (1 to 2 years) using anecdotal reports. They found that 16 (80%) had shown at least some improvement, though 14 (70%) still had a significant residual autistic defect. Generally speaking, the degree of improvement seemed consistent with that predicted at the time of initial assessment based primarily on the degree of autism. Jackson (1958) found that of three psychotic children seen initially between the ages of 4 and 6 years, all had developed some language to a varying degree when seen at adolescence. Two originally diagnosed as having symbiotic psychosis appeared to have achieved marginal social adjustment as judged by work or by performance at school. All children had received intensive psychotherapy.

In a series of generally careful but uncontrolled studies from the Putnam Center, (Brown, 1960, 1963; Reiser & Brown, 1964) described the outcome of a large group (136) of children with psychoses of infancy and early childhood, almost all of whom had received intensive psychotherapeutic treatment. Age at follow-up ranged from 9 to 22 years, with the majority being under the age of 16. Approximately one-third were attending regular classes, another third special classes or special schools, and the remaining third were either in institutions or homebound. The level of academic skill was comparable to their educational placement. When overall psychological adjustment was rated by psychiatric evaluation or, when this was not available, by parental and school reports, it was found that practically none could be classified as normal and about half passed as no more disturbed than neurotic or schizoid. Considering the reluctance of psychiatrists to adjudge people normal, the significance of this latter finding is obscure and more credence should perhaps be paid to the educational placement so that at least one-third appear to be making reasonable adjustment. So few of the children had not been treated that its influence on prognosis could not be properly assessed. Handicaps additional to psychosis such as an overtly psychotic parent, neurological, EEG and physical abnormalities present at the time of diagnosis generally reflected a poor outcome. In a more detailed study on the prognostic value of a wide variety of historical, demographic, treatment, and clinical-symptomatological variables, Brown (1960) studied the worst and best quartiles in long-term status. Using two independent raters, she found that the two groups could be differentiated only by the severity of the clinical symptomatology, particularly a greater degree of withdrawal, the absence of speech after the age of 3, and few siblings. No treatment variables appeared influential, but because of the small number of children not treated this was difficult to evaluate. Thus, the outcome in this intensively treated group appears to be rather similar to that in Eisenberg's untreated group and substantiates the value of the presence or absence of speech as a prognostic variable.

Kane and Chambers (1961) found that after varying periods of time 75% of a group of 40 psychotic children mostly from intact families were described as improved in questionnaires sent to their parents, including 35% who were described as remarkably improved. Of the 4 children who were nonverbal at the time of diagnosis, all had developed language. All of the children had received comprehensive treatment in an inpatient setting. Kaufman et al. (1962) found that in a group of 40 psychotic children, 75% experienced considerable diminution or remission of symptoms during a 4- to 5-year period of intensive treatment (day and inpatient care and psychotherapy). Diagnostic criteria and means of evaluating change are not stated. Comparing the most and least improved quartiles on a variety of variables, Kaufman et al. found that clinical and demographic variables and length of treatment did not appear to influence outcome, whereas therapist variables (amount of emotional investment, constancy and ability to synchronize the total therapy) and one parental variable, willingness to support improvement in the child, did augur a good outcome. Creak (1963), using social adjustment criteria, found that of 100 cases of childhood psychosis seen by her 17% were attending regular schools, 40%, special schools, and 43% were permanently institutionalized as severely mentally retarded. Creak felt that the most important prognostic criterion was the possibility of the child establishing some kind of relationship. Of the children, 9% had developed clear evidence of major CNS disease (epilepsy, encephalopathy).

Annell (1963) reviewed the German literature on the prognosis of childhood schizophrenia and found it consistent in regarding schizophrenia developing before the age of 10 to have an extremely unfavorable prognosis. No details of these German language studies were given by which to assess their merit and it is also likely that the diagnostic criteria differ (probably on the conservative and hence more severely disturbed side) than those used in North America. Annell studied the prognosis and indices of prognosis in 115 psychotic children seen in her clinic at Upsala, 5 to 15 years previously, in whom the symptoms of psychosis had developed before the age of 10 years. The age of subjects at follow-up ranged from 15 to 23 years. The group was divided into two broad categories, the schizophrenic syndromes and other psychoses, most of which appear to have been organic and hence not germane to the present discussion. Annell's diagnostic criteria were rather vague, being "by a subjective estimate" of presence and degree of psychotic symptoms not further defined, but her definition of psychosis appeared to be primarily one of severity of disturbance. Treatment given to the children appeared to have been largely insulin therapy and psychotropic drugs. Follow-up status was determined in the majority by psychiatric examination or report. In the remainder, assessment was by interviewing family members, teachers, or employers. Of the 62 children with a diagnosis of the schizophrenic syndrome, approximately 50% were schizophrenic at follow-up, 25% schizoid, and 25% healthy. About 50% were working or at school while the remainder were in institutions or homebound (mostly the schizophrenic). An IQ of less than 80, the absence of any precipitating factor, the presence of autism and stereotypies, and a history of severe mental disturbance in the family were significantly correlated with the diagnosis of schizophrenia at follow-up. On the other hand, a diagnosis of encephalitis or other somatic illness precipitating the psychosis were negatively correlated. The value of Annell's carefully analyzed study is diminished by the fact that the statistical methods have been applied only to the data after its collection instead of beginning with the reliability of the diagnostic and assessment measures.

In the most thorough and best controlled study, Rutter (Rutter, 1965a, 1966; Rutter et al., 1967; Rutter & Lockyer, 1967) examined 63 children who had been previously diagnosed at the Maudsley Hospital as psychotic and whose case histories on reexamination were considered by Rutter to make the diagnosis of childhood psychosis unequivocal. He then compared their follow-up status with that of a nonpsychotic behaviorally disturbed group from the same clinic matched for sex, age, IQ, and date of first referral. The average age at the time of diagnosis was 6 years and at follow-up 15½ years. None of the children showed paranoid ideation, hallucinations or delusions which, together with the absence of psychosis in their parents and siblings at the time of diagnosis, led Rutter to the conclusion that Kanner's distinction between childhood psychosis and schizophrenia was indeed valid (Eisenberg & Kanner, 1956; Rimland, 1964). In general, children of average intelligence at the time of diagnosis had made progress, whereas those who were more retarded, particularly with an IQ below 50, had deteriorated, probably because of institutionalization, a fate that had befallen the majority in this category. There was a surprisingly high correlation between the IQ at the time of diagnosis and at follow-up (.80) even for the nonspeaking children. Rutter concluded that the IQ at the age of 5 years, even in mute psychotic children, was a very good predictor of their status 10 years later and superior to Eisenberg's (1967) criterion of language status at 5 years. (In fact, half of the mute children with IQ's above 50 subsequently developed speech).

When the most stringent criteria were applied, about 25% of the children were found to have unquestionable abnormalities of the CNS, mostly epilepsy which, in the majority of cases, had developed only during follow-up generally at adolescence. Of the children who had or who had subsequently developed language, almost all had abnormalities of speech, notably echolalia or abnormal speech patterns. Although there was improvement in over 50% of the children in many of the symptoms (with the notable exceptions of language retardation and various self-stimulatory behaviors), in overall social adjustment only 14% were functioning well while 25% were making a marginal adjustment with evidence of clear abnormality. These figures were significantly worse than the control group, particularly with respect to employment. However, the number institutionalized (44%) was not different from the control group. The best outcome occurred in children who had attended schools where they had received an unusual amount of individual attention both academic and social as contrasted with children of similar IQ who had not. Though grossly abnormal EEG records and other organic signs indicated a poor prognosis, Rutter felt that this was simply due to their association with a low IQ and the clearest prognostic indicator was IQ, particularly when less than 55.

Fish and her co-workers at Bellevue (Fish et al., 1968), using diagnostic procedures discussed above, set out formally to test observations from earlier work that in younger psychotic children prognosis was related to severity of impairment of development, particularly that involving language. Thirty-two children of mean age 3.2 years were grouped on the basis of language development. At follow-up 2 to 6 years later when the mean age of the children was 7 years, this initial grouping was found to be predictive of their language development and all children whose initial speech development had been 33% or less than the expected level for their age still exhibited gross degrees of language impairment. Only three children of the total were found to be functioning above the defective level though 20% of the children were in regular classes. Fish et al. concluded that the most accurate prognostic index in the young psychotic child is the degree of developmental impairment, particularly involving language. This would seem to be consistent with the views of Eisenberg (1957) and Rutter (1965a). Also valuable was the response of the child to placebo, a good response auguring a better outcome. Of no prognostic values was a history suggestive of organicity or a family history of psychosis both of which were common and independent of the state of language development at diagnosis. Fish et al. also concluded that it is possible in a single psychiatric examination of the kind she uses to make accurate predictions not only about long-term prognosis, but also about short-term response to treatment procedures.

Gittelman and Birch (1967) found that of 43 children seen 2 to 10 years previously (mean 6 years), about 50% had shown improvement according to somewhat vague criteria. This improvement was found to be significantly related to IQ at diagnosis (> 90) and to being first seen before 5. Over one-half of the children were in psychiatric hospitals (15) or other residential care (6) or at home not attending school (4), and all except 5 of the remainder were in some kind of special educational placement. One of the interesting findings of this study was that the children with lower IQ's tended to be rediagnosed as mentally retarded, which Gittleman and Birch (1967) interpreted as reflecting the focal symptom.

Szurek (personal communication) reported a 54% improvement rate in a large group of children with uncomplicated psychosis seen at the Langley Porter Institute. About half of the total group had received treatment as outlined above, but the relationship of improvement to treatment and also the exact criteria by which improvement was judged was not stated. Similarly, Levobici, Diatkine, Lavondes, Debray, and Shentoub (1967) reported a 50% good social adjustment at long-term follow-up (10 to 20 years) in a group of 23 children. Autism and early onset were unfavorable prognostic indices, but further details on diagnosis or treatment were not available in the English abstract.

Follow-up studies of childhood psychoses leave much to be desired. Methods of establishing diagnosis and subsequent status are seldom stated and their reliabilities are rarely ascertained. Further complications are added by the variations in age of onset of psychosis, length of time intervening between diagnosis and follow-up, and kinds and amount of treatment. Ward (1963) has also criticized the prevalent tendency to describe status in terms of social functioning instead of in psychotic symptomatology, though it is possible to argue that the social functioning is the more pertinent criterion from a clinical point of view. All this makes it very difficult to attempt to draw conclusions about the outcome of childhood psychosis but nevertheless some will be attempted. Though, as pointed out by Eisenberg (1967), the prognosis of childhood psychosis appears to have improved over the past 30 years, a significant proportion of psychotic children, probably in excess of 50%, will still exhibit serious impairment of social adjustment in adolescence or young adulthood. Although there is less conflict about outcome as judged by social functioning, there is considerable disagreement about the follow-up psychiatric diagnosis with some finding a high proportion of adult schizophrenia and others finding the majority to be virtually indistinguishable from the severely mentally retarded. The single most important prognostic index appears to be the child's IQ, whether judged by tests of intelligence, language, or development. In contrast to British studies, the majority of American studies do not find that a significant number of psychotic children later develop organic CNS conditions such as epilepsy. At the present it is not possible to evaluate the effects of various kinds of treatment on long-term outcome. Certain intensively treated groups appear to have an improvement rate greater than the 60% considered by Eisenberg (1957) compatible with spontaneous improvement, but these are also the groups in which diagnosis appears to be most elastic. Long-term studies that begin with adequate and reliable diagnosis and that attempt to control some of the crucial variables are needed before definitive statements about prognosis and the effect of treatment on it can be made with any assurance. In the meantime, it would seem that predictions about the outlook for any individual psychotic child with or without treatment would appear to be unwarranted except perhaps in predicting ultimate IQ and its social consequences.

Conclusions

The central issues in childhood psychosis devolve onto four main areas:

1. Is there a condition (or conditions) of childhood psychosis and if so how can it be delineated?

Clinical consensus rather than careful demonstration suggests that the notion of a discrete disorder is useful in determining clinical action and advice. However, the rules for making the diagnosis are vague and responsible for many of the contradictory findings. It is, however, probable that there is a central core of cases that all clinicians could agree to be psychotic if they could agree on delimiting criteria such as coexistent neurological disease. Beyond this common core (chiefly a dimension of severity), clinicians vary greatly on the elasticity with which they make the diagnosis. Until some of the concepts, rules, and practices of empirical approaches to classification as outlined in Chapter One are applied to the study of behaviors thought to be involved in psychosis, no great advances in defining what exactly comprises childhood psychosis can be expected.

2. What is the etiology?

Studies of etiology will not have much significance until the problem of classification is solved. Currently, concepts of etiology generally fall into two classes: organic and psychogenic. The evidence for the organic in the form of abnormal birth histories, minor associated neurological and physical abnormalities, preponderance of males, and severe concomitant cognitive abnormalities is strong, but the evidence is largely circumstantial and not incompatible with the psychogenic view. It might be described as credible but not complete. On the other hand, evidence for the psychogenic view derives from almost uniformly poor and inadequate investigation. The evidence that the condition is not homogeneous but that there are certain subgroups (including those in which psychogenic factors may play some, though not necessarily a primary, role) is strong. How these etiological factors, whether organic or psychogenic, produce the fundamental defect of an inability meaningfully to interpret environmental events—notably those of linguistic or social connotation—is obscure, but most easily explained by organic theories on the basis of lesions of the interpretative cortex.

The relationship to adult schizophrenia is unclear, but suggestion is strong that psychosis observable at or shortly after birth is unrelated, whereas that occurring after five years of age is related.

3. What is the treatment?

Evidence that any treatment has a dramatic or durable effect is lacking. Behavioral techniques are among the few that have attempted to match clinical effort and theorizing with outcome and process evaluations, but the changes so far have been limited in scope to specific behaviors or symptoms. Small changes involve the same considerable investment of time and effort as do the unproven psychotherapeutic and milieu techniques.

4. What is the outcome?

Despite enormous efforts at treatment the outcome for most psychotic children is poor with less than one third capable of any kind of independent life. The best single predictor of final adaptive level is intellectual functioning at the time of diagnosis. Although many psychotic children may appear to have "islets of intelligence," most are and will remain at least functionally mentally retarded with the added handicap of severe behavioral disturbance.

Directions for Future Research

After the above, it is not difficult to point out the desiderata of a good study. It should achieve as many of the following as possible:

1. Use testable theory (whether organic or psychogenic).
2. Define operationally the behavioral, social, or biological parameters of subjects it calls psychotic.
3. Define outcome and process variables in measurable terms.
4. Use normally accepted ways of controlling for error and for determining the specificity of any independent variable condition to psychosis.
5. Address itself to important and researchable issues in diagnosis, etiology, treatment, and cost/benefit analysis of programs.

References

Andrews, E., & Cappon, D. Autism and schizophrenia in a child guidance clinic. *Canadian Psychiatric Association Journal,* 1957, **2**, 1–25.

Annell, A. The prognosis of psychotic syndromes in children. *Acta Psychiatrica Scandinavica,* 1963, **39**, 235–241.

Anthony, J. An experimental approach to the psychopathology of childhood: Autism. *British Journal of Medical Psychology,* 1958, **31**, 211–225.

Anthony, J., & Scott, P. Manic-depressive psychosis in childhood. *Journal of Child Psychology and Psychiatry,* 1960, **1**, 53–72.

Baroff, S., & Tate, B. The use of aversive stimulation in the treatment of chronic self-injurious behavior. *Journal of the American Academy of Child Psychiatry,* 1968, **7**, 454–470.

Bender, L. Schizophrenia in childhood. *The Nervous Child,* 1942, **1**, 138–140.

Bender, L. Childhood schizophrenia: Clinical study of one hundred schizophrenic children. *American Journal of Orthopsychiatry,* 1947, **17**, 40–55.

Bender, L. Childhood schizophrenia. *Psychiatric Quarterly,* 1953, **27**, 663–681.

Bender, L. Twenty years of clinical research on schizophrenic children with special reference to those under six years of age. In G. Caplan (Ed.), *Emotional Problems of Early Childhood.* New York: Basic Books, 1955. Pp. 503–515.

Bender, L. Schizophrenia in childhood: Its recognition, description and treatment. *American Journal of Orthopsychiatry,* 1956, **26**, 499–506.

Bender, L., Cobrinik, L., Faretra, G., & Sankar, D. The treatment of childhood schizophrenia with LSD and VML. In M. Rinkel (Ed.), *Biological Treatment of Mental Illness.* New York: L. C. Page, 1966.

Bender, L., Goldschmidt, L., & Sankar, D. Treatment of autistic schizophrenic children with LSD-25 and UML 491. *Recent Advances in Biological Psychiatry,* 1962, **4**, 170–177.

Bender, L., & Gurevitz, S. Results of psychotherapy with young schizophrenic children. *American Journal of Orthopsychiatry,* 1955, **33**, 162–170.

Bender, L., & Helm, W. A qualitative test of theory and diagnostic indicators of childhood schizophrenia. *Archives of Neurology and Psychiatry,* 1953, **70**, 413.

Bennett, S., & Klein, H. Childhood schizophrenia: Thirty years later. *American Journal of Psychiatry,* 1966, **122**, 1121–1124.

Bergman, P., & Escolona, S. Unusual sensitivities in very young children. In *Psychoanalytic Study of Child*. Vol. 3–4. New York: International Universities Press, 1949. Pp. 333–352.

Bettelheim, B. Schizophrenia as a reaction to extreme situations. *American Journal of Orthopsychiatry*, 1956, **26**, 507–518.

Bettelheim, B. *The Empty Fortress*. New York: Free Press, 1967.

Boatman, M., & Szurek, S. The etiology of schizophrenia: A clinical study of childhood schizophrenia. In D. Jackson (Ed.), *The Etiology of Schizophrenia*. New York: Basic Books, 1960.

Böök, J. A., Nichtern, S., & Gruenberg, E. Cytogenetical investigations in childhood schizophrenia. *Acta Psychiatrica Scandinavica*, 1963, **39**, 309–323.

Bradley, C. Neurology and psychiatry in childhood. In R. McIntosh and C. Hare (Eds.), *Proceedings of the Association for Research in Nervous and Mental Diseases*. Baltimore: Williams and Wilkins, 1954.

Bradley, C., & Bowen, M. Behavior characteristics of schizophrenic children. *Psychiatric Quarterly*, 1941, **15**, 298–315.

Brown, J. Prognosis from presenting symptoms of preschool children with atypical development. *American Journal of Orthopsychiatry*, 1960, **30**, 382–390.

Brown, J. Follow-up of children with atypical development (infantile psychosis). *American Journal of Orthopsychiatry*, 1963, **33**, 855–861.

Caplan, G. (Ed.) *Emotional Problems of Early Childhood*. New York: Basic Books, 1955.

Cowan, P., Hoddinott, B., & Wright, B. Compliance and resistance in the conditioning of autistic children: An exploratory study. *Child Development*, 1965, **36**, 913–923.

Creak, M. Childhood psychosis: A review of 100 cases. *British Journal of Psychiatry*, 1963, **109**, 84–89.

Creak, M., Cameron, K., Cowie, V., Ini, S., MacKeith, R., Mitchell, G., O'Gorman, G., Orford, F., Rogers, W., Shapiro, A., Stone, F., Stroh, G., & Yudkin, S. Schizophrenic syndrome in childhood. *British Medical Journal*, 1961, **2**,

Creak, M., & Ini, S. Families of psychotic children. *Journal of Child Psychology and Psychiatry*, 1960, **1**, 156–175.

Davison, G. A social learning therapy programme with an autistic child. *Behaviour Research and Therapy*, 1964, **2**, 149–159.

Davison, G. The training of undergraduates as social reinforcers for autistic children. In L. Ullmann and L. Krasner (Eds.), *Case Studies in Behavior Modification*. New York: Holt, Rinehart and Winston, 1965. Pp. 146–148.

DeMyer, M., & Ferster, C. Teaching new social behavior to schizophrenic children. *Journal of the American Academy of Child Psychiatry*, 1962, **1**, 443–461.

Dutton, G. The growth pattern of psychotic boys. *British Journal of Psychiatry*, 1964, **110**, 101–103.

Eaton, L., & Menolascino, F. Psychotic reactions of childhood. Experiences of a mental retardation pilot project. *Journal of Nervous and Mental Disorders*, 1966, **143**, 55–67.

Eisenberg, L. The course of childhood schizophrenia. *Archives of Neurology and Psychiatry*, 1957, **78**, 69–83.

Eisenberg, L. The classification of the psychotic disorders in childhood. In L. Eron (Ed.), *Classification of Behavior Disorders*. Chicago: Aldine, 1966. Pp. 89–111.

Eisenberg, L. Psychotic disorders I. Clinical features. In A. Freedman, H. Kaplan, and H. Kaplan (Eds.), *Comprehensive Textbook of Psychiatry*. Baltimore: Williams and Wilkins, 1967. Pp. 1433–1438.

Eisenberg, L., & Kanner, L. Childhood schizophrenia. *American Journal of Orthopsychiatry*, 1956, **26**, 556–564.

Ekstein, R., Bryant, K., & Friedman, S. Childhood schizophrenia and allied conditions. In L. Bellak and P. Benedict (Eds.), *Schizophrenia: A Review of the Syndrome*. New York: Logos Press, 1958. Pp. 555–693.

Esman, A., Kahn, M., & Nyman, L. The family of the schizophrenic child. *American Journal of Orthopsychiatry*, 1959, **29**, 455–459.

Eveloff, H. Psychopharmacologic agents in child psychiatry. *Archives of General Psychiatry*, 1966, **14**, 472–481.

Ferster, C. Positive reinforcement and behavioral deficits of autistic children. *Child Development*, 1961, **32**, 437–456.

Ferster, C., & DeMyer, M. Increased performances of an autistic child with prochlorperazine administration. *Journal of Experimental Analysis of Behavior*, 1961, **4**, 84.

Fish, B. The detection of schizophrenia in infancy. *Journal of Nervous and Mental Diseases*, 1957, **125**, 1–24.

Fish, B. Drug therapy in child psychiatry: Pharmacological aspects. *Comprehensive Psychiatry*, 1960, **1**, 212–227.

Fish, B. The study of motor development in infancy and its relationship to psychological functioning. *American Journal of Psychiatry*, 1961, **117**, 1113–1118.

Fish, B., & Shapiro, T. A typology of children's psychiatric disorders: I. Its application to a controlled evaluation of treatment. *Journal of the American Academy of Child Psychiatry*, 1965, **4**, 426.

Fish, B., Shapiro, T., & Campbell, M. Long-term prognosis and the response of schizophrenic children to drug therapy: A controlled study of trifluoperazine. *American Journal of Psychiatry*, 1966, **123**, 32–39.

Fish, B., Shapiro, T., Campbell, M., & Wile, R. A classification of schizophrenic children under five years. *American Journal of Psychiatry*, 1968, **124**, 1415–1423.

Fish, B., Shapiro, T., Halpern, F., & Wile, R. The prediction of schizophrenia in infancy III: Ten-year follow-up report of neurological and psychological development. *American Journal of Psychiatry*, 1965, **121**, 768–775.

Fischer, I., & Glanville, B. Programmed teaching of autistic children. *Archives of General Psychiatry*, 1970, **23**, 90–94.

Fowle, A. Atypical leukocyte pattern of schizophrenic children. *Archives of General Psychiatry*, 1968, **18**, 666–679.

Freedman, A., Deutsch, M., & Deutsch, C. Effects of hydroxyzine hydrochloride on the reaction of the performance of schizophrenic children. *Archives of General Psychiatry*, 1960, **3**, 153–159.

Freedman, A., Ebin, E., & Wilson, E. Autistic schizophrenic children. *Archives of General Psychiatry*, 1962, **6**, 203–213.

Freeman, R. Special education and the electroencephalogram: Marriage of convenience. *Journal of Special Education*, 1967, **2**, 61–73.

Gelfand, D., & Hartmann, D. Behavior therapy with children: a review and evaluation of research methodology. *Psychological Bulletin*, 1968, **69**, 204–215.

Gittelman, M., & Birch, G. Childhood schizophrenia: Intellect, neurologic status, perinatal risk, prognosis and family pathology. *Archives of General Psychiatry*, 1967, **17**, 16–25.

Glavin, J. Rapid oxygen change as possible etiology of RLF and autism. *Archives of General Psychiatry*, 1966, **15**, 301–309.

Goldberg, B., & Soper, J. Childhood psychosis or mental retardation: A diagnostic dilemma. *Canadian Medical Association Journal*, 1963, **89**, 1015–1019.

Goldfarb, W. *Childhood schizophrenia*. Cambridge, Mass.: Harvard University Press, 1961.

Goldfarb, W. An investigation of childhood schizophrenia. *Archives of General Psychiatry*, 1964, **11**, 621–634.

Goldfarb, W., Braunstein, P., & Lorge, S. A study of speech patterns in a group of schizophrenic children. *American Journal of Orthopsychiatry*, 1956, **26**, 544–555.

Goldman, D., & Rosenberg, B. Electroencephalographic observations in psychotic children. *Comprehensive Psychiatry*, 1962, **3**, 93–112.

Grant, Q. Psychopharmacology in child emotional and mental disorders. *Pediatrics*, 1962, **61**, 626–637.

Green, A. Self-mutilation in schizophrenic children. *Archives of General Psychiatry*, 1967, **17**, 234–244.

Group for the Advancement of Psychiatry. *Psychopathological Disorders in Childhood: Theoretical Considerations and a Proposed Classification*. New York: Group for Advancement of Psychiatry, 1966, 251–258.

Gubbay, S. S., Lobascher, M., & Kingerlee, P. A neurological appraisal of autistic children: Results of a Western Australian survey. *Developmental Medicine and Child Neurology*, 1970, **12**, 422–429.

Hammer, M., & Kaplan, A. *The Practice of Psychotherapy with Children*. Homewood, Ill.: Dorsey Press, 1967.

Haworth, M., & Menolascino, F. Video-tape observations of disturbed young children. *Journal of Clinical Psychology*, 1967, **23**, 135–140.

Hermelin, B. Educational and psychological research. In J. K. Wing (Ed.), *Early Childhood Autism*. Oxford: Pergamon Press, 1966. Pp. 159–175.

Hermelin, B. Coding and immediate recall in autistic children. *Proceedings of the Royal Society of Medicine*, 1967, **60**, 563–564.

Hewett, F. Teaching reading to an autistic boy through operant conditioning. *The Reading Teacher*, 1964, **17**, 613–618.

Hewett, F. Teaching speech to an autistic child through operant conditioning. *American Journal of Orthopsychiatry*, 1965, **35**, 927–935.

Hingtgen, J., & Coulter, S. Auditory control of operant behavior in mute autistic children. *Perceptual and Motor Skills*, 1967, **25**, 561–565.

Hingtgen, J., Coulter, S., & Churchill, D. Intensive reinforcement of imitative behavior in mute autistic children. *Archives of General Psychiatry*, 1967, **17**, 36–43.

Hingtgen, J., Sanders, B., & DeMyer, M. Shaping cooperative responses in early childhood schizophrenia. In L. Ullmann and L. Krasner (Eds.), *Case Studies in Behaviour Modification.* New York: Holt, Rinehart and Winston, 1965.

Hinton, G. Childhood psychosis or mental retardation: A diagnostic dilemma. II. Paediatric and neurological aspects. *Canadian Medical Association Journal,* 1963, **89**, 1020–1024.

Hudson, E., & DeMyer, M. Food as a reinforcer in educational therapy of autistic children. *Behaviour Research and Therapy*, 1968, **6**, 37–43.

Hunt, B. Schizophrenia in childhood. *Pediatric Clinics of North America*, 1958, **5**, 493–512.

Hutt, S., Hutt, C., Lee, D., & Ounsted, C. A behavioral and electroencephalographic study of autistic children. *Journal of Psychiatric Research*, 1965, **3**, 181–197.

Jakoda, H., & Goldfarb, W. Use of standard observation for psychological evaluation of non-speaking children. *American Journal of Orthopsychiatry*, 1957, **27**, 745–754.

Jackson, L. Non-speaking children: Seven years later. *British Journal of Medical Psychology*, 1958, **31**, 92–103.

Judd, L., & Mandell, A. Chromosome studies in early infantile autism. *Archives of General Psychiatry*, 1968, **18**, 450–456.

Kallmann, F., & Roth, B. Genetic aspects of preadolescent schizophrenia. *American Journal of Psychiatry*, 1956, **112**, 599–606.

Kane, R., & Chambers, G. Improvement—real or apparent? *American Journal of Psychiatry*, 1961, **117**, 1023–1027.

Kanner, L. Autistic disturbances of affective contact. *Nervous Child,* 1943, **2**, 217–250.

Kanner, L. General concept of schizophrenia at different ages. In R. McIntosh and C. Hare (Eds.), *Proceedings of the Association for Research in Nervous and Mental Diseases. Neurology and Psychiatry in Childhood.* Baltimore: Williams and Wilkins, 1954.

Kanner, L. *Child Psychiatry.* Springfield, Ill.: Charles C Thomas, 1958.

Kaufman, L., Frank, T., Friend, J., Heins, L., & Weiss, R. Success and failure in the treatment of childhood schizophrenia. *American Journal of Psychiatry,* 1962, **118**, 909–1015.

Kellaway, P., Crawley, J., & Maulsby, R. Electroencephalogram in psychiatric disorders of childhood. In W. Wilson (Ed.), *Applications of Electroencephalography in Psychiatry.* Durham, N.C.: Duke University Press, 1965.

Kennard, M. Application of EEG to psychiatry. In W. Wilson (Ed.), *Applications of Electroencephalography in Psychiatry.* Durham, N.C.: Duke University Press, 1965.

Kety, S. Biochemical theories of schizophrenia. *International Journal of Psychiatry,* 1965, **1**, 409–446.

Klebanoff, L. Parental attitudes of mothers of schizophrenic, brain-injured and retarded, and normal children. *American Journal of Orthopsychiatry,* 1959, **29,** 445–454.

Kysar, J. E. The two camps in child psychiatry: A report from a psychiatrist-father of an autistic and retarded child. *American Journal of Psychiatry,* 1958, **125,** 103–109.

La Vietes, R. Psychotic disorders II—Treatment. In D. Freedman and H. Kaplan (Eds.), *Comprehensive Textbook of Psychiatry.* Baltimore: Williams and Wilkins, 1967. Pp. 1438–1442.

Lebowitz, N., Colbert, E., & Palmer, J. Schizophrenia in children. *American Journal of Diseases of Children,* 1961, **102,** 25–27.

Leff, R. Behavior modification and the psychosis of childhood. *Psychological Bulletin,* 1968, **69,** 396–409.

Levine, M., & Olson, R. Intelligence of parents of autistic children. *Journal of Abnormal and Social Psychology,* 1968, **73,** 215–217.

Levitt, E. The results of psychotherapy with children: An evaluation. *Journal of Consulting Psychology,* 1957, **21,** 189–196.

Levitt, E. Psychotherapy with children: A further evaluation. *Behaviour Research and Therapy,* 1963, **1,** 45–51.

Levobici, S., Diatkine, R., Lavondes, V., Debray, R., & Shentoub, V. Eléments d'une recherche concernant l'avenir éloigné des psychoses de l'enfant. *Revue de Neuropsychiatrie infantile,* 1967, **15,** 13–18.

Lovaas, O. A program for establishment of speech in psychotic children. In J. Wing (Ed.), *Early Childhood Autism.* Oxford: Pergamon, 1966. Pp. 115–144.

Lovaas, O., Berberich, J., Perloff, B., & Schaeffer, B. Acquisition of imitative speech by schizophrenic children. *Science,* 1966, **151,** 705–707.

Lovaas, O., Freitag, G., Gold, V., & Kassorla, I. Experimental studies in childhood schizophrenia: Analysis of self-destructive behavior. *Journal of Experimental Child Psychology,* 1965a, **2,** 67–84.

Lovaas, O., Freitas, L., Nelson, K., & Whalen, C. The establishment of imitation and its use for the development of complex behavior in schizophrenic children. *Behaviour Research and Therapy,* 1967, **5,** 171–181.

Lovaas, O., Schaeffer, B., & Simmons, J. Building social behavior in autistic children by use of electric shock. *Journal of Experimental Research on Personality,* 1965b, **1,** 99–109.

Mahler, M. On child psychosis in schizophrenia: Autistic and symbiotic infantile psychosis. In *Psychoanalytic Study of the Child.* Vol. 7. New York: International University Press, 1952.

Mahler, M. On early infantile psychosis. The symbiotic and autistic syndromes. *Journal of the American Academy of Psychiatry,* 1965, **4,** 554–568.

Mahler, M., Furer, M., & Settlage, C. Severe emotional disturbances in childhood: Psychosis. In S. Arieti (Ed.), *American Handbook of Psychiatry.* New York: Basic Books, 1959. Pp. 816–839.

Martin, G., England, G., Kaprowy, E., Kilgour, K., & Pilek, V. Operant conditioning of kindergarten—class behavior in autistic children. *Behaviour Research and Therapy,* 1968, **6,** 281–294.

McDermott, J., Harrison, S., Schrager, J., Lindy, J., & Killins, E. Social class and mental illness in children: The question of childhood psychosis. *American Journal of Orthopsychiatry*, 1967, **37**, 548–557.

Menolascino, F. Psychosis of childhood: Experiences of a mental retardation pilot project. *American Journal of Mental Deficiency*, 1965, **70**, 83–92.

Metz, J. Conditioning generalized imitation in autistic children. *Journal of Experimental Child Psychology*, 1965, **2**, 389–399.

Metz, J. Stimulation level preferences of autistic children. *Journal of Abnormal Psychology*, 1967, **72**, 529–535.

Ney, P., Palvesky, A., & Markeley, J. The relative effectiveness of operant conditioning and play therapy in schizophrenic children. Unpublished paper.

Nicol, H., & MacKay, J. Psychoses in children in British Columbia. Paper presented at 1968 meeting of Canadian Psychiatric Association, Regina, Saskatchewan.

O'Connor, N. The experimental study of psychotic children. *Proceedings of the Royal Society of Medicine*, 1967, **60**, 560–563.

O'Connor, N., & Hermelin, B. The selective visual attention of psychotic children. *Journal of Child Psychology and Psychiatry*, 1967, **8**, 167–179.

Ogdon, D., Bass, C., Thomas, E., & Lordi, W. Parents of autistic children. *American Journal of Orthopsychiatry*, 1968, **38**, 653–658.

Ornitz, E., & Ritvo, E. Neuropsychological mechanisms underlying perceptual inconstancy in autistic and schizophrenic children. *Archives of General Psychiatry*, 1968, **19**, 22–27.

Pasamanick, B., & Knobloch, H. Brain damage and reproductive casualty. *American Journal of Orthopsychiatry*, 1960, **30**, 298–305.

Pittfield, M., & Oppenheim, A. Child-rearing attitudes of mothers of psychotic children. *Journal of Child Psychology and Psychiatry*, 1965, **5**, 51–57.

Polan, C., & Spencer, B. Check-list of symptoms of autism in early life. *West Virginia Medical Journal*, 1959, **55**, 198–204.

Pollack, M. Comparison of childhood, adolescent and adult schizophrenia. *Archives of General Psychiatry*, 1960, **2**, 652–660.

Pollack, M. Mental subnormality and "childhood schizophrenia." In J. Zubin (Ed.), *Psychopathology of Mental Development*. New York: Grune and Stratton, 1967.

Pollack, M., Miller, R., Berman, P., Bakwin, R., & Gittelman, M. A developmental, pediatric, neurological and psychiatric comparison of psychotic children and their sibs. *American Journal of Orthopsychiatry*, 1970, **40**, 329–330.

Pollack, M. & Woerner, M. Pre- and perinatal complications and "childhood schizophrenia": A comparison of five controlled studies. *Journal of Child Psychology and Psychiatry*, 1966, **7**, 235–242.

Potter, H. Schizophrenia in children. *American Journal of Psychiatry*, 1933, **12**, 1253–1268.

Rachman, S., & Berger, M. Whirling and postural control in schizophrenic children. *Journal of Child Psychology and Psychiatry*, 1963, **4**, 137–155.

Rank, B. Adaptation of psychoanalytic technique for the treatment of young children with atypical development. *American Journal of Orthopsychiatry*, 1949, **19**, 130–139.

Rawitt, K. The usefulness and effectiveness of Equanil in children. *American Journal of Psychiatry*, 1959, **115**, 1120–1121.

Reiser, D. Psychosis of infancy and early childhood. *New England Journal of Medicine*, 1963, **269**, 790–798 and 844–850.

Reiser, D., & Brown, J. Patterns of later development in children with infantile psychosis. *Journal of the American Academy of Child Psychiatry*, 1964, 3, 650–667.

Rimland, B. *Infantile Autism*. New York: Appleton-Century-Crofts, 1964.

Rimland, B. Breakthrough in the treatment of mentally ill children. Paper presented at meeting of Society for Autistic Children, New York and Washington, D.C., 1965.

Risley, T., & Wolf, M. Establishing functional speech in echolalic children. *Behaviour Research and Therapy*, 1967, **5**, 73–88.

Ritvo, E., Ornitz, E., & LaFranchi, S. Frequency of repetitive behavior in early infantile autism and its variants. *Archives of General Psychiatry*, 1968, **19**, 341–347.

Rogers, M., Lilienfeld, A., & Pasamanick, B. Pre- and para-natal factors in the development of childhood behavior disorders. *Acta Neurologica et Psychiatrica Scandinavica*, 1955. Supp. 102.

Rolo, A., Krinsky, L., Abramson, H., & Goldfarb, L. Preliminary method study of LSD with children. *International Journal of Neuropsychiatry*, 1965, **1**, 552–555.

Ruttenberg, B., Dratman, M., Fraknoi, J., & Wenar, C. An instrument for evaluating autistic children. *Journal of the American Academy of Child Psychiatry*, 1966, **5**, 453–478.

Rutter, M. The influence of organic and emotional factors in the origins, nature and outcome of child psychosis. *Developmental Medicine and Child Neurology*, 1965a, **7**, 518–528.

Rutter, M. Book review of *Infantile Autism* by B. Rimland. *Journal of Child Psychology and Psychiatry*, 1965b, **6**, 132–133.

Rutter, M. Behavior and cognitive characteristics. In J. Wing (Ed.), *Early Childhood Autism*. Oxford: Pergamon Press, 1966. Pp. 51–81.

Rutter, M. Concepts of autism—a review of research. *Journal of Child Psychology and Psychiatry*, 1968, **9**, 1–25.

Rutter, M., & Lockyer, L. A five to fifteen year follow-up study of infantile psychosis I. Description of sample. *British Journal of Psychiatry*, 1967, **113**, 1169–1182.

Rutter, M., Greenfeld, D., & Lockyer, L. Five to fifteen year follow-up study of infantile psychosis II. Social behavioural outcome. *British Journal of Psychiatry*, 1967, **113**, 1183–1199.

Safrin, R. Differences in visual perception and in visual motor functioning between psychotic and non-psychotic children. *Journal of Consulting Psychology*, 1964, **28**, 41–45.

Schain, R., & Yannet, H. Infantile autism. *Pediatrics*, 1960, **57**, 560–567.

Silberstein, R., Mandell, W., Dalack, J., & Cooper, A. Avoiding institutionalization of psychotic children. *Archives of General Psychiatry*, 1968, **19**, 17–21.

Simmons, J., Leiken, S., Lovaas, O., Schaeffer, B., & Perloff, B. Modification of autistic behavior with LSD-25. *American Journal of Psychiatry,* 1966, **122**, 1201–1211.

Simon, G., & Gillies, S. Some physical characteristics of a group of psychotic children. *British Journal of Psychiatry,* 1964, **110**, 104–107.

Sorosky, A., Ornitz, E., Brown, M., & Ritvo, E. Systematic observations of autistic behavior. *Archives of General Psychiatry,* 1968, **18**, 439–448.

Sprague, R., & Werry, J. Methodology of psychopharmacological studies with the retarded in N. Ellis (Ed.), *International review of research in mental retardation,* Vol. 5, New York: Academic Press, 1971. Pp. 147–219.

Szaz, T. The myth of mental illness. *American Psychologist,* 1960, **15**, 113–118.

Szurek, S. Psychotic episodes and psychotic maldevelopment. *American Journal of Orthopsychiatry,* 1956, **26**, 519–543.

Taft, L., & Goldfarb, W. Prenatal and perinatal factors in childhood schizophrenia. *Developmental Medicine and Child Neurology,* 1964, **6**, 32–43.

Taterka, J., & Katz, J. Study of correlations between electroencephalographic and psychological patterns in emotionally disturbed children. *Psychosomatic Medicine,* 1955, **17**, 62–72.

Terris, M., Lapouse, R., & Monk, M. The relation of prematurity and previous fetal loss to childhood schizophrenia. *American Journal of Psychiatry,* 1964, **121**, 476–481.

Tilton, J., & Ottinger, D. Comparison of the toy play behavior of autistic, retarded and normal children. *Psychological Report,* 1964, **15**, 967–975.

Tilton, J., DeMyer, M., & Loew, L. *Annotated Bibliography on Childhood Schizophrenia 1955–1964.* New York: Grune and Stratton, 1966.

Ullmann, L., & Krasner, L. What is behavior modification? In L. Ullmann and L. Krasner (Eds.), *Case Studies in Behavior Modification.* New York: Holt, Rinehart and Winston, 1965. Pp. 1–15.

Vaillant, G. Twins discordant for early infantile autism. *Archives of General Psychiatry,* 1963, **9**, 163–167.

Vorster, P. An investigation into the part played by organic factors in childhood schizophrenia. *Journal of Mental Science,* 1960, **106**, 494–522.

Ward, A. Early infantile autism—diagnosis, etiology and treatment. *Psychological Bulletin,* 1970, **73**, 350–362.

Ward, T. The course of childhood schizophrenia. *Diseases of the Nervous System,* 1963, **24**, 211–220.

Weiland, I., & Legg, D. Formal speech characteristics as a diagnostic aid in childhood psychosis. *American Journal of Orthopsychiatry,* 1964, **34**, 91–94.

Wenar, C., Ruttenberg, B., Dratman, M., & Wolf, E. Changing autistic behavior: The effectiveness of three milieus. *Archives of General Psychiatry,* 1967, **17**, 26–34.

Werry, J. Studies on the hyperactive child IV: An empirical analysis of the minimal brain dysfunction syndrome. *Archives of General Psychiatry,* 1968, **19**, 9–16.

Werry, J., & Wollersheim, J. Behavior therapy with children: A broad overview. *Journal of the American Academy of Child Psychiatry,* 1967, **6**, 346–370.

White, P., DeMyer, W., & DeMyer, M. EEG abnormalities in early childhood schizophrenia. *American Journal of Psychiatry,* 1964, **120**, 950–958.

Wing, J. Diagnosis, epidemiology and etiology. In J. Wing (Ed.), *Early Childhood Autism*. Oxford: Pergamon, 1966. Pp. 3–50.

Wing, J. Review of B. Bettelheim, The empty fortress. *British Journal of Psychiatry*, 1968, **114**, 788–791.

Wolf, M., Risley, T., & Mees, H. Applications of operant conditioning procedures to the behavior problems of an autistic child. *Behaviour Research and Therapy*, 1964, **1**, 305–312.

Wolff, S., & Chess, S. A behavioral study of schizophrenic children. *Acta Psychiatrica Scandinavica*, 1964, **40**, 438–466.

Chapter Six

The Assessment of Psychopathology in Children

K. Daniel O'Leary[1]

> To be interested in diagnosis marked one as a person who did not see the light. Nosological classification was a sterile waste of time, for every case was an individual, and yet all development followed the same basic dynamic pattern. . . . What was necessary—for all—was simply to bring into consciousness all those thoughts and impulses that had been repressed into the unconscious (p. 91).

This statement by R. L. Jenkins (1964) depicts the attitude toward diagnosis in child psychiatry during the 1930s when Jenkins was in training. Critiques of the diagnostic enterprise as normally practiced continue to be made by many authors (Kanfer, 1967; Greenspoon & Gersten, 1967; Patterson, 1967). The criticisms have been so compelling that some simply ignore diagnosis as a major concern. Despite the repeated criticisms of diagnosis and the lack of validation for classification schemes (Zigler & Phillips, 1961; see also Chapter One), many psychologists spend the major portion of their time making diagnostic evaluations (Meehl, 1959). This persistent use of diagnosis

---

[1] The author is indebted to Susan G. O'Leary for editorial assistance during the preparation of this manuscript.

in the face of insufficient validation puzzles some of the clinician's colleagues. In writing about projectives, Kelly (1954) stated, "The curious state of affairs wherein the most widely (and confidently) used techniques are those for which there is little or no evidence of predictive validity is indeed a phenomena appropriate for study by social psychologists" (p. 288). One might then ask why the clinical psychologist's diagnostic behaviors have not extinguished.

Prior to the 1960s there were very few therapeutic techniques with children that were validated by research, and Eysenck's (1952a) and Levitt's (1963) critiques of psychotherapy probably convinced many clinicians that their therapeutic endeavors were of little value. In contrast to therapy, diagnostic schemes at least had the semblance of something scientific. Therapists who gave parents diagnostic summaries about their children that were filled with clinical cliches were probably seen as highly competent clinicians and thus they persisted with their time-honored, yet often invalid, procedures. As Ulrich, Stachnick, & Stainton (1963) demonstrated, almost all college students who took personality tests and then received *identical* personality interpretations indicated that the interpretations were either good or excellent. Aside from the ability to do research, diagnostic skill is the major factor that differentiates the clinical psychologist from other members of the mental health team. Furthermore, in the majority of state and federal institutions, diagnoses are required by law. Thus, there are a number of reasons why the diagnostic behaviors of clinical psychologists have been maintained. This seemingly fruitless activity—at least from the researcher's vantage point— does indeed often have positively reinforcing consequences for the diagnostician that are independent of psychologists' abilities to treat the child.

The clinician probably does not employ the above rationale in his use of diagnostic techniques; diagnosis is seen as a valuable enterprise for other reasons. Kessler (1966) noted in her book on child psychopathology that diagnosis originally meant "thorough understanding" and many psychologists today act as if a diagnosis does imply knowledge about the etiology and treatment of a child. The penchant for diagnostic labeling stems partly from the medical model where disordered behavior is viewed as a symptom of some underlying cause and where labeling points to a body of research information concerning treatment. However, several investigators (Cattell, 1957; Eysenck, 1952b) have asserted that a diagnostic system can be valuable even if its classes are only minimally related to etiology and treatment. Eysenck has repeatedly emphasized that diagnosis is a basic scientific enterprise similar to taxonomy which is characteristic of all science. Although classification necessarily results in loss of uniqueness, the possible gain such as facilitation of data communication could compensate for the loss. As was pointed out in Chapter One, classification allows one to relate variables to the similarity resulting from class membership. As Zigler and Phillips (1961) noted, "Class membership conveys information ranging from the descriptive similarity of two phenomena to a knowledge of the common operative processes underlying the phenomena" (p. 608).

Despite the arguments that may be logically advanced in defense of the taxonomic value of classification, especially for purposes of advancing research, differential diagnosis is not clinically useful until it relates to treatment or etiology. I shall examine the extent to which three major approaches to the diagnosis of children's behavior problems provide valid information regarding etiology and—more importantly—treatment. It should be emphasized that this chapter will concern itself largely with behavior problems often considered social in nature such as problems in peer, parent, and teacher relations. Intellectual assessment and diagnosis of brain damage (see Chapter Three) will not be considered. The three approaches to assessment that will be discussed are projective, dimensional, and target analyses.

Projective Techniques

The development of projective tests as a clinical tool is largely a result of conceptualizing projection as a defense. Defensive projection, or the externalization of impulses unacceptable to the ego, is held to occur because conscious recognition of these impulses is painful to the ego. Freud referred to projection as a defense mechanism that operates unconsciously so that emotionally unacceptable impulses are unconsciously rejected and attributed to others. Thus projective tests were originally utilized in a clinical manner to reflect the individual's unacceptable, unconscious impulses.

Frank (1948), a pioneer in projective techniques, promoted the view that projective tests tap the inner world of an individual and reveal feelings and desires of which the individual is not aware. Murray also felt that projectives evoke responses of one's private world and commented as follows:

> If the pictures are presented as a test of imagination, the subject's interest, together with his need for approval, can be so involved in the task that he forgets his sensitive self and the necessity of defending it against the probing of an examiner, and before he knows it he has said about an invented character that apply to himself, things which he would have been reluctant to answer to a direct question. As a rule the subject leaves the test happily unaware that he has presented the psychologist with what amounts to an X-ray picture of his inner self (p. 550).[2]

---

[2] Murray's statement was taken from Zubin, Eron, and Schumer (1965, p. 550). The

Certainly not all projective theorists (Zubin, Eron, & Schumer, 1965) are in agreement with Murray, but it is widely believed that a projective test can reveal information that cannot be obtained by other methods (Halpern, 1953; Lindzey, 1952).

The use of projective tests with children and their application in psychotherapy was expounded by Halpern (1953). She felt that the Rorschach could provide one with information concerning prognosis and the procedures to be used in psychotherapy. Furthermore, Halpern felt that with the Rorschach one could determine whether symptoms were transitory or chronic. Halpern noted:

> . . . the test results will indicate whether or not the child has the ability to make an emotional contact with others, as well as the level at which such a contact will be made and the ends to which it will be employed. The child who gives no color answers or perhaps only one color answer will be difficult to reach because he has turned away from the environment and is minimally responsive to emotional pressure from the outside (p. 263).

Since there is a decided pragmatic emphasis in this chapter and since lengthy discussions of methodological problems such as stimulus ambiguity and reliability of projectives can be found in other sources (Murstein, 1963; Zubin, Eron, & Schumer, 1965), this evaluation of projectives will be made primarily on the basis of their clinical utility. The issues of awareness and sign versus global projective assessment will be discussed, since the practitioner's defense of the continued usage of projectives often revolves around these issues. Finally, the future of projective testing as it relates to assessment and treatment will be considered.

Predictive Validity: Rorschach

Research regarding the usefulness of the Rorschach in differential diagnosis is rather limited[3] and often contradictory. Despite the conflicting results, a few studies that have been cross-validated indicate that one may be able to predict emotional disturbances in children from the Rorschach. Ames' publication with her associates of *Child Rorschach Responses* in 1952 presented

---

author's discussion of projectives was influenced by the excellent books on projective techniques by Murstein (1963) and Zubin, Eron, and Schumer (1965).

[3] See Zubin, Eron, and Schumer (1965) for review of differential diagnosis pp. 203–209.

normative Rorschach data on children from two to ten years old. In this publication, Ames listed "danger signs" that could be considered pathological in children. Elkins (1958) investigated the usefulness of Ames' danger signs by comparing Rorschach records of 40 disturbed children with records of a control group matched for age, sex, and IQ. The disturbed children had been referred to a child guidance clinic; the nondisturbed children were described as "well-adjusted" by their teachers. Contrary to expectations, nondisturbed children had significantly more "danger signs" than the disturbed children.

Ames (1959) questioned the severity of disturbance present in the children used in the Elkins (1958) study, and thus she reassessed the diagnostic usefulness of the Ames' danger signs by comparing Rorschach records of boys who were "clearly disturbed" with a normal control group matched for age, sex, intelligence, and socioeconomic status. In order to insure behavioral differences in the criterion groups, 50 severely disturbed boys were selected from 500 clinical cases. Ames compared the Rorschach records of the disturbed and normal children on the presence of a modified list of the 16 danger signs proposed earlier (1952). Seven of the 16 danger signs occurred more frequently in the protocols of the disturbed group. However, the practical significance of the danger signs is limited by Ames' use of greatly differing groups where decisions with regard to presence or absence of emotional disturbance might have been made without any test. If 15 minutes of discussion with a "clearly disturbed" child or his significant others would allow a clinician to differentiate him from his normal counterpart, routine administration and scoring of the Rorschach are clearly a waste of time for such decisions. Despite the cross-validation of the "danger signs," Ames deemphasized their value in favor of other diagnostic indicators that have not been validated with children. She (1959) concluded:

> An examiner's total impression of a Rorschach response will in most cases reveal much more than any checking of list of signs, no matter how adequate that list may be. Thus, emotional disturbance in a child subject is revealed by such things as going over and over the same blot area, by consistent dissatisfaction with responses, by extreme unevenness of responses, by presence of various kinds of shock responses (as described by Phillips and Smith) (p. 297).

Cobrinik and Popper (1961) investigated the relationship between the Rorschach manifestations of thought disturbance and other test indicators of disturbance. In addition, they were interested in the extent of thought disturbance at different age levels. The subjects were 48 boys between the ages of 7 and 13 years in residential treatment at a state hospital. All children had reportedly been diagnosed schizophrenic according to criteria used by Bender (1956) (see Chapter Five). The analysis of thought disturbance was based on perceptual distortions (F-) and deviation in the elaboration (E-) of the child's perceptions. Of the 48 children, 23 diagnosed as schizophrenic gave *no* evidence of thought disturbance, but of those children indicating disturbance, a large proportion demonstrated numerous instances. There was a sharp decline in the manifestation of thought disturbance after 11 years of age, and this result confirmed earlier work of Beck (1954) who found a decline in thought disturbance as children reach early adolescence.

Draguns, Haley, and Phillips (1967) presented a useful, detailed review of Rorschach content as utilized both in the United States and abroad. Although they noted that H, human response, repeatedly emerged as a predictor of favorable response to treatment in schizophrenics, neurotics, and problem children, they also stated that all such predictive indicators should be considered tentative, "as there are research reports which failed to uncover the reflection of treatment effect in any of the Rorschach content scores" (p. 16). Draguns et al. (1967) concluded that none of the traditional content classifications of Rorschach responses corresponded to a diagnostic category, a defense mechanism, or a dynamic constellation.

Proponents of the Rorschach argue that it is unfair to assess validity of the Rorschach by correlating it with fallible criteria, such as a diagnostic grouping, and that Rorschach responses should be related to more reliable criteria if a true picture of the test's validity is to be obtained. Haley, Draguns, and Phillips (1697), who also reviewed nontraditional uses of content indicators with a number of reliable criteria, stated that there was some overlap between content measures and their behavioral referents that could not be attributed to chance, but that the overlap was far from approaching correspondence.

Despite Halpern's (1953) testimonial that the Rorschach protocol provides a child therapist with information concerning the severity, prognosis, and planning of therapy, the evidence certainly does not support such a broad claim. There does seem to be some correspondence between Rorschach indices and behavior, but research involving the complex mediating variables that influence such correspondence has only begun. Problems of base rates in the evaluation of children's Rorschach responses are rarely discussed. As Meehl and Rosen (1955) pointed out, in order for a psychological test to be efficient, the test must make possible a greater number of correct decisions than could be made on the basis of the base rate alone. At this point, the Rorschach appears to qualify as an instrument for research, but it has not met requirements which demonstrate its utility in the decision-making process of diagnosis or treatment.

Predictive Validity: TAT

Murstein (1963) reviewed some of the pertinent literature concerning the validity of the TAT. He reported one study (by Cox and Sargent) in which generally positive results were found regarding the differentiation of disturbed and nondisturbed children. A second study by Leith and Schafer compared TAT records of psychotic children with maladjusted, nonpsychotic children matched for age and IQ. This study yielded generally positive results, but the data were only partially analyzed, and no conclusive statement could be made. Despite some successful results in group differentiation, Murstein concluded that "application of the TAT as a medium for psychiatric diagnosis would seem to be an injudicious use of time . . . [since the evidence suggests that the TAT has] minimal statistical validity which is insufficiently precise for individual prediction" (p. 287, 296). In general, a test must be highly reliable and must have a small standard error of measurement before it can successfully predict in an individual case. The TAT does not meet this criterion with respect to predicting diagnostic categories.

There are a number of studies, however, indicating that at times TAT responses may predict behaviors such as aggression, which are more specifically defined than diagnostic categories. Mussen and Naylor (1954), utilizing a lower-class group of boys who had been referred to a Research Bureau because of disorderly conduct, found that fantasy aggression as assessed by the TAT did relate to aggressive behavior as rated by ward attendants. Kagan (1956) demonstrated a positive relationship between frequency of fighting themes on the TAT and teachers' ratings of fighting. James and Mosher (1967) found a positive relationship between sociometric ratings of aggression in adolescent boys' thematic aggression to low ambiguity cards, but not to high ambiguity cards.

Sternlight and Silverg (1965) investigated the relationship between overt aggression as rated by a psychiatrist and an attendant and fantasy aggression (TAT) in retarded children. The 60 moderately retarded (IQs of 50 to 69) children in this study were divided into two matched groups of 30 each. The aggressive group was described as "very acting out, hostile, and destructive," whereas the other group was considered docile and conforming. The groups were matched in terms of age, sex, ethnic origin, and length of stay in the institution. The amount of fantasy aggression was assessed by 11 TAT cards and scored according to the system of Mussen and Naylor (1954). No difference in fantasy aggression between the two groups were obtained.

Megargee and Cooke (1967) investigated the relationship between projective test measures of aggression (TAT and Holtzman Inkblot) and overt aggressive behavior of adolescent delinquents. TAT and Inkblot aggression were related to 11 criterion measures: 4 measures of antisocial behavior in the community, 3 measures of aggressive behavior as observed by others while the child was in custody, and 4 measures of aggressive habit patterns reported by the boy himself. Aggression as assessed by the TAT related to only 1 of the 11 criterion measures of aggression—school conduct. There were several significant relations between the Holtzman Inkblot scales and the criteria of overt aggression. They concluded:

> For the clinician who might wish to use these scales in the prediction of overt aggression in the individual case, the results are quite discouraging. The paucity of significant findings, the low order of those which were obtained, and the contradictory modes of relationship to the criteria all suggest that the task of behavioral prediction with these instruments is one to be approached with great caution (p. 58).

General Measurement Issues

As mentioned in the introduction to this chapter, clinical psychologists persist in their use of projectives despite research questioning their utility. A frequent defense made for the use of projectives often runs as follows: "True, you take each projective or sign index separately and the data looks poor. No clinician does that! He looks at the test and the client's protocol, he uses some kind of complex analysis about the way in which those indices interrelate, and he then arrives at some decision based upon his impression of *all* those indices." As should be clear now, the diagnostic validity of the Rorschach and TAT is minimal when single or sign indicators are used to predict a diagnostic or behavioral criterion. A slightly more complex use of the Rorschach signs or TAT indicators is to utilize a ratio of one index to another. For example, one ratio is M (responses containing human movement) over C (responses based on color). This ratio is called the experience balance and is said to reflect when one's perceptions are based on his inner life (when movement predominates over color).

These frequently used ratios of projective scores do not offer a fruitful alternative to single indicators since as Cronbach (1965) noted, these ratios are notoriously unreliable. More complex relations among indices might include linear regression models and configural analyses models. Research with the MMPI using these more complex models has been quite disappointing to those who would argue for such models using diagnostic tools. Goldberg (1965) assessed the predictive success of "expert" MMPI diagnosticians versus linear and configural models based on actuarial tables in predicting a psychotic-neurotic criterion. Linear composites of single scale scores outperformed the complex configural analyses based on the actuarial data and the global assessments of all diagnosticians. To expect a clinician to operate more effectively than a computer in utilizing Rorschach, TAT, or MMPI scores for prediction seems unreasonable. It is possible that linear composites of scores on a projective test could be constructed to efficiently predict behavior. However, such a procedure would have to be undertaken with caution. Those who argue for combining all of the information obtained in a Rorschach or TAT must realize that the success of two or more predictors is a function of the redundance or correlation among the predictor variables as well as the relationships of each to the criterion. Only where the correlations among the predictor variables are low can one expect to combine these predictor variables and arrive at a useful multiple prediction equation.

There is no clear demonstration that children reveal feelings on the TAT of which they are not aware. Even if the TAT or Rorschach reflects variables influencing the child's behavior which are not verbalized by the child, the utility of the test still depends on its incremental validity. That is, the test should reveal information not already in the social history or in other readily available information so that there is some increment in predictive efficiency. It is likely that one could discover the information revealed in a child's projective protocol from a discussion with the parent, guardian, or ward attendant or by direct observation. Furthermore, because of the present nature of projective methodology, hypotheses based on projective protocols must be validated by direct observation of the child or by parental report. In short, a projective "test" hardly seems a useful circumvention of direct observation or parental conferences.

Summary

Even when the behavioral criterion is specific, results concerning the relationship of responses on a projective protocol and overt behavior are conflicting. Although over 2000 articles have been written concerning projective tests, there is no simple answer to the question posed by Skolnick (1966): Is the relationship between fantasy and behavior direct, inverse, or nonexistent? McClelland (1966) noted that Skolnick spoke of *tests*, of *projective* expressions of motives, and the relation of *fantasy* to *behavior*. McClelland argued as follows:

> Actually, the TAT is not a test in the conventional sense; it is a sample of operant behavior, that is, thoughts. The term projective creates a kind of pseudoproblem by suggesting that we must study the relation between what a person's motives "really" are and what he "projects": a person "is" just as much what he says in response to a TAT card as he is to anything else he does. And since when is fantasy not behavior . . . Let us redefine the problem as a study of the relationship between thought and action (p. 479).

McClelland's reinterpretation in which fantasy is simply considered as one form of behavior (thought) that can be related to another type of behavior (action) brings much of projective work within the framework of experimental psychology. As McClelland said,

> What all this points to is that we must stop arguing about such global generalizations and get on with the business of defining *under what conditions* correlations between thought and action will be positive, negative, or nonexistent. This essentially reduces what has tended to be a special problem in the literature of psychology to the more general problem of understanding the conditions under which any two types of responses are related to each other (p. 480).

Despite the possible rapprochement envisioned by McClelland, at present, projective devices simply do not warrant the time required for their administration, scoring, and interpretation. The validity coefficients that do exist are so low that they have little or no value for individual treatment decisions. More importantly, the information that is sometimes obtained could often be acquired from simpler and less expensive methods. In light of the lack of any incremental validity of projective tests, psychologists who persist in their use should seriously reevaluate their moral obligations to their clients. The administration and interpretation of Rorschach protocols—when not executed within a research context—clearly seems a waste of time. If a physician continued to assess disorders with an instrument that could not differentiate abnormal from normal tendencies, we would be appalled. It is time psychologists took a sharp look at their own activities lest they find themselves guilty of the same malpractice as our mythical physician.

Dimensional Approaches

The dimensional approach to assessment has long been advocated by Eysenck (1961) whose concern has mainly been with adults. He argues that disorders can be viewed in terms of dimensions of behavior instead of in terms of mental disease entities. As we have seen in Chapter One, there is considerable evidence to suggest that the psychopathology of childhood can be viewed in just such terms.

At the same time, a number of problems related to the measurement of these patterns of deviant behavior remain. As was also noted in Chapter One, a persistent problem has been the extent to which different methods of measuring the same pattern produce similar results. That is, if a child is rated high on conduct disorder on a behavior checklist is he also rated high on this pattern from case history data or on the basis of personality questionnaire?

Stated differently, to what extent is there factor-matching across different data domains? Quay (1966) obtained factor scores of young delinquents from behavior ratings, questionnaires, and case history data and intercorrelated these scores across subjects. The resultant coefficients were cast into a multi-trait, multimethod matrix described by Campbell and Fiske (1959). Frequently the correlation between different factors measured in different domains was almost as high as the correlation between the same factors measured in different domains. For example, the correlation between inadequate-immature scores as measured by a behavior rating and neurotic-disturbed scores as measured by case history information (.01) was not different from the correlation between inadequate-immature scores as measured by a behavior rating and inadequate-immature scores as measured by case history information (−.01). There was some suggestion of cross-domain matching for psychopathy and neuroticism when information was obtained from behavior ratings or case histories, but the cross-domain relationships were quite low for these two dimensions (average $r = .11$).

Data of a similar nature has also been presented by Quay and Parsons (1970). They interrelated scores on rating history and questionnaire measures of the four patterns described in Chapter One. Again, very low correlations were obtained between measures of the same factor from different instruments. The absence of significant cross-domain matching makes it difficult to argue strongly for a dimensional approach to assessment until better agreement from different measurement techniques can be obtained.

Much controversy continues over the problem of factor-matching across data domains (Becker, 1960; Becker, 1961b; Cattell, 1961a; Cattell, 1961b; Peterson, 1965). Certainly the evidence fails to support any one-to-one matching or secure linkage of behavior rating factors and questionnaire factors (Becker, 1960; 1961a). As Peterson (1965) pointed out, if questionnaires and ratings are in fact measuring personality traits, the traits should manifest some constancy over methods, over situations, and to some extent over time. If conditions of minimal validity are to be met, the intercorrelations between various measures of a given trait ought to be higher than the intercorrelations between different measures (Campbell & Fiske, 1959). At the same time, if the situational contribution to behavior is taken seriously and predictions of a pattern of behavior in a number of situations are desired, there are advantages in low intercorrelations among the predictors—if the predictors all relate to the criterion.

Validity

Let us now examine the extent to which factorially derived measures have been related to useful external criteria concerning the etiology and treatment of different behavior problems. Jenkins (1966) reanalyzed the case history data collected by Hewitt and Jenkins (1946) and extracted five symptomatic clusters: shy-seclusive children, overanxious-neurotic children, hyperactive children, undomesticated children, and socialized delinquents. The coded data on these children also included information concerning family background. Jenkins (1966) related the symptomatic groups to their family backgrounds and found characteristic and different backgrounds for each group.

The two groups of inhibited children (shy-seclusive and overanxious) nearly always lived with both natural parents. The aggressive children in the other three groups (hyperactive, undomesticated, and socialized delinquent children) were less likely to be with both natural parents. Mothers of aggressive children were seen as openly hostile, whereas mothers of inhibited children were not. Aggressive children also felt rejected by their mothers. It was felt that this rejection may have been associated with a change of parental figures and maternal hostility may have stimulated hostile, rebellious, aggressive responses in the children. It was hypothesized that rejection by the parents led to an inadequate development of conscience and guilt feelings.

Jenkins found that the overanxious-neurotic children had more histories of long or repeated illnesses than the shy-seclusive children. Overanxious children's fathers had more education than the shy-seclusive children's fathers. Perhaps more importantly, nearly half of the overanxious-neurotic children had mothers who were ". . . described as neurotic because of extreme nervousness, compulsions or evident emotional complexes" (p. 454). Jenkins concluded: "The overanxious-neurotic child appears more frequently in more educated families (which are prone to set higher standards) and with neurotic mothers, who are themselves anxious, and the more discouraged shy-seclusive child more frequently has an ill, handicapped or inadequate mother" (p. 455).

Undomesticated children were characterized as negativistic, defiant of authority, vengeful, sullen, maliciously mischievous, and having temper outbursts. Their backgrounds often included ". . . an unstable mother unable to relate herself to responsibility, and either a pregnancy unwanted by the mother or maternal rejection occurring after birth but while the child is still in infancy . . . Lack of sufficient maternal love and acceptance in early life is a significant factor in this reaction" (p. 456). The socialized delinquent was characterized by a bad neighborhood and by neglect in a large uneducated family. In this group, paternal deficiencies were most predominant; in more than half the cases the father was dead, and in more than two-fifths of the cases the father was alcoholic.

The hyperactive group had appeared to be more age-limited than other syndromes and ". . . under favorable conditions children probably more often outgrow it spontaneously than is the case with other symptom groups" (p. 457).

Becker and Krug (1964) used a type of multivariate analyses described as a circumplex model to produce a set of constructs that were systematically related to each other in terms of a two-factor space. Factors derived from ratings made by kindergarten teachers and by each parent that showed systematic intercorrelations were approximately ordered in a circular fashion in terms of their closeness to each other. Some of the more interesting findings of Becker and Krug were that both children's personality and children's conduct problems were highly associated with father's hostility and physical punishment. Girls with hostile-punitive fathers were most withdrawn and distrusting in the father's presence and there was some tendency for this pattern of behavior to be exhibited in the school and in the presence of the mother. Girls with highly anxious, maladjusted mothers showed a pattern of introversion or withdrawal in school, while at home, particularly with the mother, these girls tended to show primarily hostile behavior. Hostility and child-rearing anxiety of mothers was associated with hostile, defiant, and distrusting behavior of boys as seen by teachers. It should be emphasized that Becker and Krug's results support theoretical conceptions that view behavior as shifting with situational pressures, rather than conceptions that assume fixed traits.

The validity of dimensional approaches can be evaluated not only with respect to their etiological contributions but also with respect to their ability to differentiate or screen one group of children from another. Successful differentiation of child clinic patients from siblings of child patients and nonclinic children was made by Speer (1971) using the Behavior Problem Checklist of Peterson and Quay (1967). He had parents of 173 child patients and the parents of 445 nonclinic children complete the Behavior Problem Checklist. Parent ratings differentiated such children on three of the four Behavior Problem Checklist factor scales, namely, Conduct Disorder, Personality Disorder, and Inadequacy-Immaturity. The clinic children were not significantly different from the nonclinic children on the Socialized Delinquency scale. In a longitudinal study, Pimm (1967) demonstrated the usefulness of a screening device for detection or "early selection" of emotional problems in first-grade children. Details of the results of reliability, normative data, and factor analysis conducted in the early development of this screening device were reported by Pimm and Rogers (1966) and Pimm, Quay, and Werry (1967). The screening device predicted those first-grade children who were likely to have adjustment problems in grade four. Children identified as "emotionally disturbed" differed from "normal" children in terms of frequency of referral to special services, academic retardation, number of strappings, and adjustment as rated by fourth-grade teachers.

Quay and Levinson (1967) have presented results concerning the prediction of institutional adjustment of delinquent boys. Scores were obtained from case history data behavior ratings and questionnaires to measure the dimensions of psychopathic, neurotic-disturbed, immature, and socialized delinquency. The finding of poor adjustment among high psychopathy scorers was almost uniform. The transfer rate of these boys was higher; they spent more time in segregation; they received poorer grades; and their stay was longer. In short, high scorers on psychopathy did not benefit from the institutional program as much as other boys.

In a follow-up effort Ingram, Gerard, Quay, and Levinson (1970) selected a group of psychopathic delinquents for an experimental treatment program. Results indicated some improvement in the institutional adjustment of the experimentals as compared to a group of controls.

Additional research about differences between groups selected on the basis of various measures has already been discussed in Chapters One and Two. Such studies lend validity to the various measures of the dimensions as well as providing data about the patterns of deviant behavior themselves.

In terms of criteria necessary for a dimensional classification scheme the internal criteria seem to have been demonstrated. That is, the dimensions are relatively independent and objective, and the dimensions are obtainable from more than one kind of data. There are demonstrable relationships of factors or dimensional scores with parental variables, important social behaviors, and some basic psychological processes. However, as Humphreys (1962) emphasized, it would seem appropriate to regard the results of the factor analysis as the basis for hypothesis formation instead of as a method of hypothesis testing. Although the basic patterns of deviant behavior have been related to concurrent behavior assessments and to etiology, the patterns have only as yet begun to provide information with regard to planning a treatment program or to predicting differential responsiveness to various remediation procedures (Young, 1965; Quay, 1969; Gerard, 1970).

In summary, factor analytic approaches to the assessment of childhood psychopathology have aided greatly in reducing a myriad of deviant behaviors to a small number of relatively reliable and consistent dimensions. For those concerned with arriving at a conceptual scheme that organizes deviant child behavior in a meaningful way, the multivariate approach should provide some closure. In addition, data from group studies is accumulating which relates dimensions of behavior to important etiological variables. As yet, however, for prediction and aid in treatment planning, the utility of the dimensional approach requires much additional research.

Target Assessment

An alternative approach to traditional diagnostic tests and predictive measures is to focus directly on target behaviors. Target assessment generally refers to the observation of a child's undesirable behaviors, but a complete assessment would include observations of the child's appropriate behaviors and important environmental variables. The term "target behavior" was used by Paul (1966) regarding the outcome research in psychotherapy. He discussed the selection of subjects in terms of "target behaviors" with the goal of treatment being to change these behaviors in a specific direction. Target assessment has evolved with and is generally based on the same assumptions as the behavior modification approach to treatment (see Chapter Seven). A search for an underlying cause of behavior based on unconscious factors and defensive efforts to ward off anxiety as discussed by Kessler (1966) is not undertaken. Rather, as Olson emphasized in 1934, cures can be achieved by treating the symptom itself. He noted that where ". . . the symptom is the result of the repetition of some phase of behavior that has satisfying consequences, there is a clear analogy to the laws of learning and . . . removal of the symptom through direct work on a learning basis is synonymous with cure" (p. 374). As will be discussed later, the slogan "If you eliminate the symptom, you have effected a cure" had led to some oversimplification in treatment and conceptualization of problems, but the direct focus on current problem behaviors has had many beneficial consequences.

One of the important features of target assessment is that it provides information that has direct implications for treatment. The distinction between assessment and treatment is often necessarily vague, and the two procedures are integrally related. The diagnostician's job is (1) to identify the target behaviors to be increased or decreased in frequency or changed in topography, (2) to identify the environmental factors that elicit, cue, or reinforce the target behaviors, and (3) to identify what environmental factors can be manipulated to alter the child's behavior (Ullmann & Krasner, 1965).

Selection of Target Behaviors

The selection of target behaviors usually begins by having the parent, teacher, or guardian present his concept of "the problem." Thus in large measure, "Maladaptive behavior is behavior that is considered inappropriate by those key people in a person's life who control reinforcers" (Ullmann & Krasner, 1965, p. 20). In some cases, it may be sufficient to deal only with the complaint as presented by the parent. However, there are many situations in which a therapist may decide it is more important to modify behaviors other than those suggested by the parent or other key persons.

Parents usually present a number of behaviors or problems they wish to have changed. In light of client skepticism concerning the efficacy of psychotherapeutic endeavors, it is probably wise for the therapist to focus initially on a behavior that is both important to the parents and relatively easy to change. A successful modification of this behavior would tend to increase the parent's confidence in the therapist's effectiveness. In a number of instances one aspect of therapy may involve teaching the parents to modify the child's behavior themselves. Selecting a behavior that is easy for the parents to modify will illustrate to the parents that they can change both their own and the child's behavior. The therapist must realize that the parents' behavior must be shaped and reinforced as well as the child's behavior.

Another consideration that should influence the selection of the target behavior is how the modification of one behavior effects changes in other behaviors. For example, a parent may bring an enuretic child, who has poor grades and few friends, to the clinic. The parent may view the child's lack of friends as the main problem. Depending on the age of the child, however, it is possible that enuresis would be the most useful target behavior to modify. A recent study by Baker (1969) suggests that successful treatment of enuresis alone may be accompanied by favorable changes in other problem behaviors. It is doubtful that an increase in the number of the child's friends would have eliminated the problem of enuresis.

Another example in which careful selection and modification of the target behavior can influence the development of other behaviors involves increasing the cooperative play of a shy child who has a very low frequency of speech. Since an increase in the child's level of speech can serve to maintain cooperative behavior, it would probably be judicious to focus on the child's verbal behavior initially. To attempt to increase cooperative play without first dealing with the lack of speech could prove to be a frustrating exercise.

A target assessment approach usually focuses on an undesirable behavior. However, in many cases even if one could eliminate the undesirable behaviors, treatment may be only partially successful if behaviors incompatible with the undesirable behavior are not developed. The elimination of one undesirable behavior is no guarantee that other undesirable behaviors will not occur. If the frequency of fighting is decreased in a child who has few cooperative play skills, it is likely that he will adopt other modes of interaction that are already in his repertoire, such as swearing (O'Leary, Thomas, & Becker, 1968). With such a child it may be necessary to teach appropriate play behaviors while simultaneously attempting to eliminate the undesirable behaviors. Great controversy has arisen over the symptom-substitution issue, which has implications for assessment and treatment. The issue of symptom substitution seems to be a pseudoproblem that should be cast in different language. The problem might better be viewed as behavior-substitution. Since man is always behaving—in one way or another—removing or suppressing one behavior demands perforce that another behavior occur. In short, there is always behavior substitution! Depending on the probability of responses to particular situations, we can obtain either desirable or undesirable behavior when one undesirable behavior is removed. Following treatment, if the behavior remaining or being newly displayed is desirable, the case is often called a cure. If an undesirable behavior remains or newly occurs, the phenomena is called symptom substitution. Most importantly, one needs to be attuned to the situations in which elimination of undesirable behaviors might lead to other undesirable behaviors (Cahoon, 1968).

The importance of considering more than the circumstances immediately preceding a problem behavior can critically influence the behaviors one decides to change. This point is clearly exemplified in the treatment of alcoholism. Many studies report frequent relapses where conditioned aversion techniques are applied to drinking per se (Blake, 1967). It is possible that a long-established drinking pattern may involve an extensive chain of behaviors of which drinking is the terminal result. There may be behaviors in this chain that would be more desirable to control than drinking itself. For example, a therapist may find that his client drinks only when depressed and that depression is usually preceded by a fight with his wife. Focusing on the client's marital problems may reduce his drinking more quickly than punishing the drinking itself. Such an approach could be interpreted as a search for an underlying cause, but it should be noted that the search for the initial behaviors in the chain can often be made on the basis of observable events alone. In a sense, all therapists—whether of a psychodynamic or behavior modification tradition—are searching for causes in that they are looking for the determinants of behavior (Bandura, 1968)! It is in the conception of the determinants, however, where real differences exist (e.g., in libidinal or intrapsychic conflicts or in chains of reinforcing and eliciting events; *focus* on current factors versus *focus* on early childhood factors).

With regard to behavior therapy, Eysenck and Rachman (1965) stated, "All treatment of neurotic disorders is concerned with habits existing *at present*; the historical development is largely irrelevant" (p. 12). The emphasis on behaviors in the existing situation and the current controlling factors is quite useful, but it should not exclude the use of relevant historical information. The following example illustrates the importance of historical information. The treatment of a mute child based on observation of the target behavior would probably begin with the shaping of very rudimentary vocalizations. Such would have been the case in a local hospital had it not been for an astute observation by a psychologist who noticed that a nonverbal girl diagnosed as schizophrenic, mental defective, and hard of hearing blushed every time he winked at her. Assuming that a complex verbal history usually accompanies the development of a sophisticated behavior like blushing, he escorted her to his office, and confronted her with the assertion that she could talk, whereupon she did.[4] A less astute observer might not have avoided a naive application of speech therapy unless the social history had noted the previous verbal repertoire of the girl. The use of developmental or historical information is also illustrated in the findings of Sidman, Hernstein, and Conrad (1957) who established avoidance behavior in monkeys and then delivered occasional free shocks independently of the monkeys' behavior. The result was an *increase* in response rate. The same stimulus was used both for establishing the avoidance response and for testing the effects of free shock, and such data have implications for treatment of children. If disruptive behavior is essentially a fear-motivated avoidance response, then punishment might lead to more disruption.

Types of Target Behavior Assessment

Once the target behavior has been selected, the therapist follows one of at least two possible courses of action. Both courses have the function of further describing the target behavior and the situation in which it occurs and of guiding the therapist toward the selection of a treatment. The two approaches to assessment can be described as functional and static (Ferster, 1965). In general, the distinctive difference between these two methods of diagnosis is the extent to which the factors controlling the target behavior are analyzed and manipulated. This distinction is evident in two approaches to dealing with the target behavior of a temper tantrum. A functional assessment of tantrum episodes might include describing the situations that precipitate the tantrum, the characteristics of the tantrum itself, and the reaction of the parents, peers, or teachers to the tantrum. Variables such as parental attention would then be manipulated to discover which of the variables was controlling the tantrum episodes. In a static approach to assessment only the characteristics of the tantrum would be analyzed after which modification of the tantrum would ensue with a less detailed analysis of the environmental variables that had been controlling the tantrums.

One of the major differences between the functional and static methods of target behavior assessment and traditional approaches to diagnosis concerns the situation in which the assessment is conducted. Diagnosis using pro-

---

[4] Personal communication, Bennett Roth, Kings Park State Hospital, Kings Park, N.Y.

jective techniques is generally conducted in a clinic office or playrom. The diagnosticians using a dimensional approach rely heavily on the observations provided by others, e.g., teachers and parents. In a target assessment approach the diagnostician focuses on direct observation of the child in the situation in which the problem behavior occurs wherever possible. Diagnosis *in situ* increases the probability that the important controlling variables in the child's environment will be considered in the development of a treatment procedure. In addition to parent and teacher reports, target assessments will often involve observing the parent-child or teacher-child interactions in the home or classroom.

A typical target assessment in a classroom setting would proceed by first carefully defining the behavior to be changed. The definition should be made as objective as possible so that another person could agree on the occurrence of the behavior. For example, the full definition of vocalization might be as follows: Any nonpermitted "audible" behavior emanating from the mouth. This category includes answering without being called on, moaning, yawning, belching, crying, shouting, and "operant" coughs. The category excludes vocalization in response to teacher's question, sneezing, and automatic coughing.

After delineating the definition of a target behavior, such as vocalization, its presence is noted in specific time units during specific lessons (O'Leary & O'Leary, in press). For example, one might watch a child continuously, but the presence or absence of vocalization would be noted every 15 seconds. The occurrence of vocalization may be noted by a teacher aide, a psychologist, or even by the teacher herself. However, if the teacher observes the behavior herself she probably will choose small time blocks to observe the child, e.g., for two-minute periods each hour. If two observers watch the child, the reliability of their observations is assessed by recording the frequency of agreements per time unit (e.g., 30 sec.) over the number of agreements plus disagreements. For example, let us assume that two observers watched a child for 10 30-second time intervals, and their observations were as follows where V refers to the presence of vocalization. The reliability of such observation would be the number of agreements divided by the number of agreements plus disagreements or 8/10 = 80%. (See Fig. I.)

| Observer 1 | V | – | V | V | V | – | – | V | – | V |
| Observer 2 | V | – | – | V | V | – | – | – | – | V |

Bijou and his colleagues have conducted a number of field-experimental studies that involve the functional assessment of children's behavior. The collection of data in a functional assessment as described by Bijou (1965) includes the following procedures: "(a) observing and recording changes in frequency of occurrence, or frequency and duration of occurrence of one class of behavior (for example, time spent on climbing equipment), (b) recording the stimulus consequences of behavior usually in terms of changes in the behavior of the teacher (for example, giving attention, praise, or support) and the behavior of other children (for example, running away, and (c) using samples extending over the full school day or the majority of school hours" (p. 63).

The results of one study by Bijou's associates involving excessive crawling in a three-year-old girl will be presented to exemplify how target behaviors can be assessed functionally (Harris, Johnston, Kelley, & Wolf, 1964). Observations of this child during the third week of school indicated that she spent more than 80% of her time in off-feet positions. Most importantly it was observed that crawling behavior frequently drew the attention of teachers. On-feet behaviors such as standing and walking, which occurred infrequently, seldom drew such notice. After the initial or base line observations had been taken, the teacher was told to attend to the child only when she was standing, walking, or running. Initially, it was necessary to attend to behaviors which approximated standing, such as pulling herself up almost to her feet to hang up her coat. Within a week after initiating the procedure of teacher attention to on-feet behavior or approximations thereof, the child acquired a "close-to-normal pattern of on-feet behavior." In order to see whether the change from crawling to on-feet behavior was related to the change in the teacher's behavior, the procedures were reversed; that is, the teacher once again attended to crawling and other off-feet behavior but not to any on-feet behavior. The authors stated that by the second day the child had reverted to her old pattern of play and locomotion. The observational records showed that the child was off her feet 80% of the class session. To assess whether on-feet behavior could be reestablished, the teachers again reversed their procedures and attended to the child only when she was on her feet. On-feet behavior rose immediately, and by the fourth day, the child spent about 62% of her time on her feet.

Another study that involved the functional assessment of behavior is instructive because of the difficulties encountered in discovering the variables that were controlling the children's behavior. Wahler, Winkel, Peterson, and Morrison (1965) studied parent-child interaction in a clinic playroom. Three boys ranging from four to six years and their mothers participated in this study. Observations of the children's deviant behavior and behavior incompatible with the deviant behavior were made. The mothers were asked to play with their children just as they might at home. In addition to records of the child's behavior, observations were made of the mother's reactions to the child's deviant behavior. As the authors note, data from two of the three cases indicated that the mother's social behavior may have been functioning as a powerful class of positive reinforcers for a child's deviant behavior as well as for his normal prosocial behavior. In both of these cases the response rates of the children's disruptive behaviors were reduced when their mother's contingent behavior was eliminated; similarly, the rates were increased when the mother's behavior was again made contingent. In short, the child's deviant behavior was functionally related to the mother's behavior. There was little change in the rate of deviant behavior in the third case when the child's mother was instructed to ignore deviant behavior and to respond enthusiastically to cooperative behavior. The experimenters were unable after five sessions to determine the source of control of the deviant behavior of the third child. It was thus decided to stop searching for the controlling stimulus events and to concentrate on the most practical means of eliminating the child's behavior. The mother was instructed to isolate the boy in an empty room immediately following any of the child's deviant behavior which consisted of "oppositional responses" or failing to comply with the mother's requests. The social isolation did function as a very effective punishment technique and reduced the frequency of the child's deviant behavior.

Careful functional analysis of children's behavior that relates the behavior to its eliciting or reinforcing stimuli cannot always be made, as in the case just described. In such cases it would seem reasonable to (1) rely on past research regarding treatment, (2) make a static assessment of the child's behavior, and (3) treat him accordingly. There may be many behaviors that clinicians will learn to treat successfully even though they cannot determine the controlling etiological or maintaining factors. It is quite obvious that certain medical problems such as cancer can be successfully treated although their specific etiologies are not known. A very useful alternative to functional assessment is to conduct a static analysis of the child's behavior by observing the form, intensity, frequency, and other qualitative or quantitative aspects of the behavior.

O'Leary and Becker (1967) used a static approach to assess the problem behaviors in a third-grade adjustment class. Based on the teacher's description of the children's inappropriate behaviors, observations of the following behaviors were made: pushing, answering without raising one's hand, chewing gum, eating, name calling, making disruptive noise, and talking. It was noted that the daily mean of deviant behavior ranged from 66 to 91 percent. A token reinforcement program was then instituted. The daily mean of deviant behavior during the token program ranged from 3 to 32 percent. The program was equally successful for all children observed, and anecodotal evidence suggested that the children's appropriate behavior generalized to other school situations.

The systematic control of variables in a functional approach to assessment has significantly increased our knowledge of the variables important in the control and treatment of problem children. The use of static assessment and consequent treatment has verified the applicability of many new techniques. A less frequently utilized form of target assessment is ecological assessment, which consists of direct recording of behavior as it occurs in the given habitat of the individual without any manipulation of variables. As Wright (1967) and Barker (1965) noted, the model of manipulation and control of environmental determinants of behavior strongly dominates the psychological approach to studying human behavior, whereas the sciences of physics and chemistry have relied heavily on information concerning the incidence in nature of the phenomena in question. Ullmann and Krasner (1965), although operating within the model of manipulation of environmental variables, emphasized the analysis of the subject's social situation as being the most important area of diagnosis. They continued by saying that as one makes such analyses one becomes ". . . vitally interested in the study of social class, institutions and groups as they influence the types of reinforcement, and behavior that might be available for manipulation" (p. 28).

In contrast to some traditional approaches that place major emphasis on important determinants of behavior within the individual, ecological assessment emphasizes the significance of social and environmental variables. The massive influence of the "flower generation" and the Hippie culture has convinced many parents of the powerful influence of peers, but experimental studies concerning peer influence have only begun to assume major importance (Patterson, Bricker, & Greene, 1964). Ecological assessment may provide useful information regarding the probability that a newly learned behavior will be maintained by the child's natural environment. Such an analysis in turn can suggest what types of therapeutic interventions may be successful.

Buehler, Patterson, and Furniss (1966) ecologically described how a peer group tends to reinforce delinquent responses and punish socially conforming responses. Using a framework of interpersonal communication that included both verbal and nonverbal behavior, Buehler et al. described all interactions of delinquent girls and staff members in a detention home. The behaviors were later coded with regard to the level of communication, in accordance with delinquent or socially approved norms, and the peer responses to the behavior. The results of this study indicated that attention to the delinquent behavior of an individual within a peer group setting was generally nonverbal. Attention on a nonverbal level took the form of interest, ignoring, sneering, etc. Buehler, Patterson, and Furniss (1966) found that regardless of the size of the institution, peer responses to delinquent behavior were largely "reinforcing," i.e., approximately 75% of the children's delinquent behavior was followed by approval from peers. On the other hand, behaviors indicating compliance with social norms were punished. For example, if a girl identified with the social norms of the institution by indicating that she was going to get a job and stay out of trouble, the peer group would punish her for such statements. Furthermore, the staff members of the detention homes tended to react indiscriminately to the delinquent behavior. It was hypothesized that the peer influence had much more importance than the reactions of the staff in maintaining and changing behavior.

An ecological assessment of patients' behavior in a mental hospital (Gelfand, Gelfand, & Dobson, 1967) indicated that patients' prosocial and psychotic behavior was inconsistently reinforced by patients, nurses, and nursing assistants. Although similar to the results of Buehler, Patterson, and Furniss (1966) in that patients reinforced inappropriate behavior, these results indicated that the patients responded to other patients' inappropriate behavior less frequently than did the nursing assistants and nurses. Gelfand et al. argued that nurses probably reinforced a considerable amount of psychotic behavior unintentionally, e.g., by treating the patient sympathetically to establish feeling of self-worth. They further stated that for patients' inappropriate behavior in the typical ward situation ". . . the best response would be to ignore the patient since even punitive responses can serve as positive reinforcers" (Allen & Harris, 1966) (p. 203). This advice may be well founded in some instances, but O'Leary, Becker, Evans, & Saudargas (1969) found that ignoring disruptive behavior and praising appropriate behavior of children in a classroom with some very disruptive boys resulted in pandemonium. A careful assessment of factors controlling disruptive behavior is necessary before one should advise a parent, teacher, or ward attendant to simply ignore disruptive behavior. Prerequisites for such advice include knowledge that the child has appropriate behavior in his repertoire to replace the disruptive behavior, knowledge that adult attention is reinforcing, and knowledge that peer attention to disruptive behavior of a reinforcing nature is minimal.

From the studies of Buehler et al. and Gelfand et al. it seems obvious that training of ward personnel would be very useful, but if differences between these studies are reliable, one would concentrate on the peers as a reinforcing culture when dealing with children, whereas emphasis on the reinforcing aspects of the nurses and nursing assistants might be most useful on adult psychiatric wards.

Assessment of the behavior of attendants, nursing assistants, parents, and teachers can often be done reliably under standard conditions in situ, but many clinicians simply cannot take the time for direct observation. In addition, even when time is no deterrent, the presence of an observer in a naturalistic setting may greatly influence the behavior in question. One of the most impressive devices to measure environmental influences was developed by R.

Wolf (1966). In an attempt to predict academic success, a summary of the conceptions that guided the development of his devices is in order.

1. Specific environments are postulated to influence development of specific characteristics. For example, there may be a specific environment for the development of independence.
2. Seek environmental variables that are hypothesized to *directly* influence the development of certain characteristics.
3. Sample a variety of environmental conditions hypothesized to be related to a characteristic and summarize these determinants via psychometric procedures.
4. Systematically relate measurements of environments to measurements of an individual.

In assessing the climate in the home for achievement motivation (one of 21 process characteristics used in measuring academic achievement), Wolf measured such variables as parental concern for academic achievement, social pressure in the home for academic achievement, the rewards accorded academic accomplishments, and parental knowledge of the educational progress of the child. In short, a major concern was what parents did, not what parents were in terms of status, economic well being, or some other demographic variable.

The correlation between the total rating of the intellectual environment and general intelligence was +.69; the correlation between I.Q. and achievement battery scores was +.76; and the correlation between the total environmental rating and the total achievement battery score was +.80. Even more impressive was the multiple correlation of +.87 between I.Q. and overall environmental rating for academic achievement with the total achievement battery score. Most importantly, Wolf demonstrated that the addition of a measure of environment greatly enhances the estimation of academic achievement. This chapter is largely concerned with assessment of social behaviors, not intellectual behavior, but the general approach outlined by Wolf could be adopted to measure environments for aggression, dependency, and other social behaviors. Such assessment devices could be extremely valuable in ecological assessments. They could alert the therapist to parental behaviors that require modification and they could be of great benefit to people who make placement decisions about children. Wolf obtained his data via interviews, and although interview data has often been notoriously poor, Wolf's focus on conditions likely to promote particular behaviors suggests that interview data can be useful. The psychometrician has long known that the closer one's predictor is to his criterion, the greater his prediction will be. It is time that the clinician pays greater attention to this fact and focuses on the problem as it occurs in a particular environment. Seven replications of the study by Wolf have now been conducted with virtually identical results.[5] His model serves as a prototype of an assessment method which might allow clinical psychologists to predict social behaviors such as aggression and dependence and to exceed the usual ceiling of a validity coefficient of .40 seen in the traditional personality and assessment literature. Most importantly, his approach combines a direct focus on target behavior while retaining some of the classic psychometric features of good predictive devices.

Interviewing: The Universal Method of Data Collection

Despite one's theoretical biases, the interview is a universal tool for obtaining information about a child and his environment. Regardless of the tests or assessment devices used, some form of interview occurs. However, the material one collects in an interview and the meaning assigned to that material vary greatly depending on one's theoretical bent.

Psychodynamically oriented clinicians [who typically use projective data] rely chiefly on their intuitive inferences about the symbolic and dynamic meanings of the client's verbal behavior. Trait-oriented psychometric assessments [dimensional approach] investigate either the accuracy of the client's statements as indices of his non-test behavior, or treat his verbalizations as signs of his relative position on a personality dimension or on a criterion variable. A social behavior analysis of language [a target approach] . . . [is designed] to decipher the content of what is being conveyed and to discover its behavioral referents and consequences (Mischel, 1968, p. 238).

Since there is greater rapprochement between the dimensional and target approach than between the projective approach and the former two approaches, and because the former approaches have greater clinical utility, a discussion follows concerning some interview procedures which might be used by someone who uses dimensional assessment devices, a target approach or the combination of the two.

Tests or checklists like those described in the dimensional section are frequently used in clinics as a basis for some discussion in the parent interview. The checklist or rating scale may be completed before the first inter-

---

[5] Personal communication, R. Wolf, 1969.

view along with a general family questionnaire which asks questions about occupation of parents, ages, and number of siblings, the child's current problem, a history concerning developmental landmarks such as walking and talking, and some factors that might contribute to the problem at present. The checklist can be used to compare the child in question to "normal" children and to other known clinic and hospital samples—giving the interviewer some rough idea of the severity of the problem. In addition, the checklist or rating scale can be used as a method of insuring that information will be obtained about a wide variety of problems that could not be readily obtained in a one- or two-hour interview. Finally, as evidenced in the section on dimensional assessment, a person's score on a certain dimension may provide etiological or predictive information about the child's problem.

As was mentioned earlier, the dimensional approach is not specific enough to give detailed information about the target behaviors or their controlling factors. Consequently, a detailed examination of the target behavior and its controlling variables is necessary. In addition to factors already mentioned in the target behavior section, one should attempt to answer the following questions during the assessment interview(s): What brought the clients here at this particular time? By whom were they referred? Do the parents agree on the problem? What do they believe caused the problem? What procedures have the parents used in the past to deal with the problem and how long have such procedures been tried? Is there consistency between parents in applying such procedures? How do the parents feel about the child, i.e., do they like him? If so, how do they show it? Do they dislike the child? Do they desire institutionalization? Do the parents feel great guilt about causing the child's problem? Do the parents take the child's side in most matters where there is a school dispute? Do they want the child's class or grade placement changed? How willing are the parents to change their behavior? How much conceptual change is necessary on the parents' part before any treatment should be initiated? What expectations do the parents have about what can be done for the child? Have there been any dramatic changes in the child's environment recently, e.g., death of family member, separation, divorce, birth of child? If so, what have been the child's reactions to such events? What are the child's assets? What does the child like to do? What would the child work for? Is medical or intellectual assessment needed? Do the parents require treatment about their own problems independent of their problems with the child? What types of direct observation are needed?

Answers to the above questions will obviously be biased but they provide valuable information. Most importantly, they give a therapist a certain feeling about the family and the parents' attitudes and behavior toward the child. In all instances where possible, try to have both parents present at the initial interview. Having the father there stresses the importance of the interview.

It helps bring about his cooperation in the treatment problem, it allows for some assessment about the truthfulness (or biases) of the mother's report, and most importantly, the fathers' involvement in a treatment program is positively correlated to reported behavior change of success in treatment (Gluck, Tanner, Sullivan, & Erickson, 1964).

Interviews with children—particularly young children—are often difficult and provide little information about the target problems. Nonetheless, some time should generally be spent with the child or with the child and his parent(s) together. Often the latter is necessary with preschool children simply because the child is afraid when left alone with a strange adult. Most importantly, the therapist can make some assessment of the child's physical appearance, his general interview demeanor, and his relations with his parents. However, one should be cautious in drawing conclusions based on the interview with the child. The child may be delightful in an interview yet be a hellion in school or at home.

Because children's behavior differs so greatly from one situation to another, where possible, parents or teachers should be asked to record the frequency of target behaviors in a daily log book. Such recording not only allows for optimal evaluation of treatment procedures, it often points out that certain problems are almost nonexistent whereas others may be particularly important. Such recording is so important that certain treatment procedures often should not proceed before the parents have kept good records of the behaviors in question. An expectation should be conveyed in the initial interview that recording is crucial to the treatment. Although interviewing and verbal reporting of events can be helpful, nothing substitutes for a good record of behavioral events and their antecedents and consequences when those factors are noted immediately!

Needed Assessment Techniques

The shift in focus of diagnosis and assessment from internal variables to external observable variables necessitates the development of new assessment devices. The observational technique used by Bijou and his associates, which focuses on the frequency of behavior in a specific time interval, has provided a very useful assessment approach. In addition, variables such as the intensity or loudness of a child's behavior seem to be influenced by therapeutic manipulations in a classroom (Thomas, Becker, & Armstrong, 1968; O'Leary, Becker, Evans, & Saudargas, 1969), but measures of behavioral intensity are almost nonexistent within the child literature in behavior modification to date. It is quite conceivable that some of the richness and variety in behavior as depicted by Wright's ecological description (1967) will be adopted as the measuring techniques become more sophisticated. One of the instructions to the observers described by Wright is as follows.

Give the "how" of everything the subject does. It is assumed that everything a child does is done *somehow*. No child ever just walked, for example. The first time the subject walked he did so slowly, haltingly, awkwardly, unsteadily. . . . Common speech and literature confront us with countless differing ways in which persons walk, smile, sit . . . and we know that the differences from one way to the next are often behaviorally crucial (p. 51).

Wright presented evidence showing that some variables in his child records such as affect and mood could be reliably observed and analyzed. The literary quality of Wright's specimen records is appealing to some and his procedures represent an initial step in providing psychologists with a rich fund of data. However, such data has not been incorporated within any child diagnostic schema as yet. The retrieval of information from the ongoing moment-to-moment behavior of a child as depicted by Wright is an extremely arduous task. The specimen record does not include built-in provisions for qualification. There is a heavy dependence on observers and little reliance on instrumentation. Nonetheless, an observational or diagnostic scheme that combines frequency of various responses and some of the variables mentioned by Wright such as intensity and mood might be a fruitful approach.

Kanfer and Saslow (1965) provide a very useful summary of general categories of information that one should obtain in planning a course of therapy with adults. Their suggestion of analyzing a client's social behavior as it relates to normative patterns of behavior should be emphasized. In dealing with a child it is useful to know what percentage of children are enuretic at certain ages, what percentage of children fight at various ages, length of utterances of children, and percentage of various deviant behaviors in a classroom. In addition, it would be useful to know what percentage of time a teacher or ward attendant has to respond to an average child in order to maintain his behavior. The practicing clinician might well find Peterson's (1968) elaborations of the (1) observation, (2) interview, and (3) experiment useful in executing a target assessment approach.

Historically, assessment and diagnostic procedures have focused largely on the attitudes, feelings, and behaviors of the *child* that require change. The work by Bijou and his associates concerning a functional analysis of a child's behavior combines an assessment of *both* the child's behavior and the variables controlling the behavior. The ecological assessments of R. Wolf, and Patterson and his associates focus largely on the stimulus factors that might control a child's behavior. At this point, however, if one wishes to assess the effectiveness of stimulus to see whether it will be a positive reinforcer, a negative reinforcer, or a neutral stimulus, one has to make the following test: One observes an operant response which has some stable strength for a child. Then conditions are arranged so that the stimulus to be evaluated such as praise is consistently presented to the child as a consequence of that response. If the response increases in strength as a function of the praise, the praise may be classified as a positive reinforcer (Bijou & Baer, 1961). Obviously, there are some common stimuli that ordinarily serve as positive reinforcers such as the verbal statements "That's good," and "You're doing a fine job." Nonetheless, we cannot assume that such statements will serve a reinforcing function for all children. There are several recent attempts to assess a wide variety of reinforcing stimuli of adults by pencil and paper tests (Geer, 1965; Cautela & Kastenbaum, 1967). In addition, there is evidence concerning the effectiveness of various factors related to an adult's social reinforcing power such as sex (Hill & Stevenson, 1965), institutionalization (Stevenson & Fahel, 1961), and deprivation and satiation (Gerwitz, 1967), and there is research assessing the "incentive" value of various objects such as balloons and bubble gum by the paired comparisons method (Witryol & Fisher, 1960). However, assessment of the so-called "reinforcing" stimuli for children and later testing of the reinforcing effect of these stimuli has not been done systematically.

Even though there would probably be an imperfect correlation between what a child says he likes and what in fact proves reinforcing, a description of probable positive and negative reinforcers for a child could aid in a therapeutic plan. There is also a need for techniques that can reliably assess internal emotional responses. One may wish to integrate both classical and operant conditioning procedures with children (Lazarus, Davison, & Polefka, 1965), but at present the assessment of levels of anxiety in children must be made largely on the basis of clinical hunches. Present knowledge of the relationships between overt and covert behavior in children is minimal. Telemetry devices may help to provide such information, but assessments of child behavior in field-experimental or clinical settings may be fraught with a great deal of variability extraneous to the dependent measure in question. However, one example of ingenious use of diagnostic instrumentation is provided by Lang and Melamed (1969) who successfully used psychophysiologic recording in the treatment of a nine-month-old infant with persistent vomiting.

There is evidence that the verbal behavior of children can be manipulated in a way that dramatically influences their motor behavior (Luria, 1963; O'Leary, 1968), but the extent to which children's verbal behavior influences their motor behavior under nonmanipulated conditions remains uncertain. Clinical observations would seem to indicate that a child's verbal self-descriptions such as "I'm dumb" or "I'm clumsy" would affect his behavior in important ways. Obviously verbal and motor behavior can be related in various temporal orders, but with children it may be a great deal easier to change a child's own verbal self-descriptions by changing his motor behavior than vice versa. This view does certainly not discount the possibility that verbal or cognitive change could be a useful adjunct or corollary procedure in effecting motor changes. Nonetheless, as many effective teachers know, it is easier to reduce a child's statements "I'm dumb" by shaping up academic behavior than to continually tell him he is not dumb. In short, the old adage, "it is easier to get a person to behave his way into thinking properly than to think his way into behaving properly" is especially pertinent to the treament of children.

Target assessment is one attempt to resolve dissatisfactions with projective, clinical and psychometric techniques; however, currently this approach to children's disorders may appear to provide little more than a detailed enumeration of specific behavior problems. To those who are searching for a conceptual scheme which will order a vast amount of data, such an emuneration may not be pleasing. At present it would seem most fruitful to make detailed specifications of problem behaviors and as many of the associated important etiological and treatment variables as possible. Though a catalog of target behaviors is not conceptually neutral, such a catalog can be utilized by any theoretical framework. Nonetheless, as one begins to recognize the full import of the situational specificity of behavior and the crucial role of environmental determinants in the regulation of behavior, one will also see that present, broad, clinically derived conceptual schemes used in the diagnostic and treatment decisions may be practically useless. Children quickly learn to discriminate times and places in which they are reinforced and punished, and only with precise treatment specification of stimulus determinants of behavior across times and situations can one hope to obtain generalizations of appropriate behavior. Furthermore, if the catalog of target behaviors includes most of the problem behaviors presented to a clinician, the individual clinicians who are not satisfied with such an enumeration can build their own conceptual schema to interrelate the vast diversity of behaviors. However, they should not force others to adopt such schemes unless they can demonstrate their utility.

The clinical psychologist working in almost any state institution might despair at the suggestion of changing his diagnostic focus from dispositional states and trait approaches to target behaviors. However, it is my impression that if such psychologists continue to use devices such as the TAT, Rorschach, and questionnaires unrelated to etiology and treatment, they will soon find their roles usurped by social workers and action-oriented social psychiatrists who are tired of attending rather fruitless case conferences which discuss internal dynamics of a child. The service-oriented clinical psychologist has a psychoeducational task, and there are now methods available to teach many new behaviors (see Chapter Seven). If one has to place a child into a diagnostic classification system—as often is required by law in state institutions—he can use the target assessment approach to give him information for such categorization. Admittedly, the classification schemes used in most state institutions are based on different assumptions than the target assessment approach, but laws and state diagnostic schemes change slowly, and consequently I recommend that a psychologist gain minimal information necessary to utilize the existing classification system and then get on with the business of treatment or a more detailed analysis of the eliciting and maintaining factors as quickly as possible.

Conclusion

At this point one might ask whether there should be any integration among the three assessment approaches. From a diagnostic standpoint the projectives have not fulfilled their expectations, and any large-scale attempt at integrating projective methodology with other assessment procedures seems unlikely. As Zubin, Eron, and Schumer (1965) pointed out in their epilogue,

> . . . as the criteria for evaluating projective techniques begin to be spelled out, it becomes more and more apparent that projective techniques are not very efficient and that there are more direct techniques for eliciting the kind of material claimed to be unique to them. Prediction of total or global behavior is virtually impossible, it might be noted, but there is some success in predicting rigidly and narrowly defined "specific" behavior under certain types of experimental conditions. But projectives arose as the need for predicting "nonlaboratory" behavior became greater—for example, prognosis in therapy. It is with respect to the latter type of prediction that the failures of projective techniques have been most glaring (p. 609).

Nonetheless, as Zubin et al. emphasized, clinicians will give up tools such as the Rorschach and TAT only when they are provided with better tools. Attempts to champion against their use have been made repeatedly, but with little avail. Whether dimensional and target approaches to assessment will take their place among projectives as a major diagnostic tool by practicing clinicians remains to be seen. It should be emphasized, however, that some of the assumptions of projective methodology and dimensional or target assessment often differ radically.

The integration suggested by McClelland (1966) offers a possible rapprochement between projective methodology and other assessment approaches, and could do much to stimulate useful research that would bring projective methodology in close contact with general experimental psychology. McClelland proposed that a response to a projective "test" could be regarded as an operant behavior and treated like other operants. Within such a framework one could then relate responses on projective tests to other operant behaviors such as aggression or cooperative behavior as assessed by a target approach. Despite this possible rapprochement, at present projective "tests" qualify only as research instruments whose validity remains to be demonstrated, and those psychologists who persist in their routine use should seriously reevaluate their own behavior.

The dimensional approach to assessment has produced results that indicate that four patterns describe a large portion of variance in case histories, behavioral ratings, and questionnaire data of deviant children. The dimensions are reliable and sufficiently precise for group prediction; and the major dimensions of neuroticism and psychopathy have been related to conditionability of particular responses or treatment outcome. In addition, the dimensional approach does provide one with a conceptual scheme that aids in the integration of a wide variety of data and in the communication of this data. However, while swearing, stealing, and lying are all included in the conduct problem domain, a particular treatment may influence only one of these behaviors in a particular child. A change score on a conduct disorder scale or a general rating does not indicate which of the behaviors was modified by one's treatment procedures. Consequently, a target approach that focuses on the repeated observation of specific behaviors would seem a necessity in conduction research where one wishes to conclude that particular behaviors were modified by a particular treatment.

Traditional assessment procedures simply have not provided adequate tools for individual prediction and they fail to provide for the uniqueness of individual children with disruptive behaviors that occur with great frequency and intensity under certain situations but not under other situations.

To specify the significant behaviors and the stimulus conditions in which the behaviors occur for each child, as is done in a target approach, may seem like an arduous task. However, in the future, psychologists may be able to classify children according to specific common target behaviors and responsiveness to treatment programs, and thus provide a much more useful and precise classification scheme than exists now. Psychology's reliance on medicine for both diagnostic and treatment models has led clinicians to expect that they can devise tests which can quickly provide them with crucial information for treatment. However, when one assesses the sugar metabolism of a child, one can be reasonably certain that the major determinants of the metabolic rate will not change drastically when the child returns home on the day after his sugar metabolism test. On the other hand, the major determinants of a young child's behavior in the clinic may be drastically different from those variables that control his behavior at home. Barrett's (1965) advice to assess behavior over repeated occassions in specified situations is very well founded. If the problem behavior occurs at home, the specified situation would be the home not the clinic. On the other hand, if the problem behavior occurs at school, the assessment should be done at school.

At the outset of this chapter it was mentioned that in recent years anyone interested in diagnosis was viewed as one who did not see the light. Today a person who proceeds to treat a child with little regard for the variables that maintain a child's behavior and no regard for the development of the behavior should be marked as one who does not see the light. In fact, as "therapy" becomes more specified and can be carried out by parents, teachers, and attendants, diagnosis may again become a major and prestigeful role of the clinical psychologist. As Greenspoon and Gersten (1967) mentioned,

> . . . the therapeutic community has tended to bring all people, non-medical as well as medical, who have frequent contact with the patient, into the psychotherapy picture. Thus the psychologist is confronted with the problem of providing information that can be used to deal with the patient to personnel who may not have the requisite knowledge of dynamic psychology (p. 849).

Unlike a good deal of information obtained from traditional psychological tests, a target assessment approach that utilizes functional analysis, static assessment, and ecological assessment can provide information which is specific and which could be easily understood and applied by the wide range of personnel involved in today's mental health programs.

References

Allen, K. E., & Harris, F. R. Elimination of a child's excessive scratching by training the mother in reinforcement procedures. *Behavior Research and Therapy,* 1966, **4**, 79–84.

Ames, L. B. Further check on the diagnostic validity of the Ames danger signals. *Journal of Projective Techniques,* 1959, **23**, 291–298.

Ames, L. B., Learned, J., Metraux, R. W., & Walker, R. N. *Child Rorschach responses: developmental trends from two to ten years.* New York: Hoeber-Harper, 1952.

Baker, B. L. Symptom treatment and symptom substitution. *Journal of Abnormal Psychology,* 1969, **74**, 42–49.

Bandura, A. Modeling approaches to the modification of phobic disorders. Paper presented to Ciba Foundation Symposium, London, 1968.

Barker, R. G. Explorations in ecological psychology. *American Psychologist,* 1965, **20**, 1–14.

Barrett, B. H. Acquisition of operant differentiation and discrimination in institutionalized retarded children. *American Journal of Orthopsychiatry,* 1965, **35**, 862–885.

Beck, S. J. *The six schizophrenias: Reaction patterns in children and adults.* New York: American Orthopsychiatric Assn., 1954.

Becker, W. C. The matching of behavior rating and questionnaire personality factors. *Psychological Bulletin,* 1960, **57**, 201–212.

Becker, W. C. Comments on Cattell's paper on "perturbations" in personality structure research. *Psychological Bulletin,* 1961a, **58**, 175.

Becker, W. C. A comparison of the factor structure and other properties of the 16PF and the Guilford-Martin inventories. *Educational and Psychological Measurement,* 1961b, **21**, 393–404.

Becker, W. C., & Krug, R. A circumplex model for social behavior in children. *Child Development,* 1964, **35**, 371–396.

Bender, L. Schizophrenia in childhood: Its recognition, description, and treatment. *American Journal of Orthopsychiatry,* 1956, **26**, 499–506.

Bijou, S. W. Experimental studies of child behavior, normal and deviant. In L.

Krasner & L. P. Ullmann (Eds.), *Research in behavior modification.* New York: Holt, Rinehart, & Winston, 1965. Pp. 56–81.

Bijou, S. W., & Baer, D. M. *Child Development.* Vol. 1. *A systematic and empirical theory:* New York: Appleton-Century-Crofts, 1961.

Blake, B. G. A follow-up of study of alcoholics treated by behavior therapy. *Behavior Research and Therapy,* 1967, **5,** 89–94.

Buehler, R. E., Patterson, G. R., & Furniss, J. M. The reinforcement of behavior in institutional settings. *Behavior Research and Therapy,* 1966, **4,** 157–167.

Cahoon, D. D. Symptom substitution and the behavior therapies. *Psychological Bulletin,* 1968, **69,** 149–156.

Campbell, D. T., & Fiske, D. W. Convergent and discriminant validation by the multitrait-multimethod matrix. *Psychological Bulletin,* 1959, **56,** 81–105.

Cattell, R. B. *Personality and motivation structure and measurement.* New York: World Book, 1957.

Cattell, R. B. Cattell replies to Becker's "comments." *Psychological Bulletin,* 1961a, **58,** 176.

Cattell, R. B. Theory of situational, instrument, second order, and refraction factors in personality structure research. *Psychological Bulletin,* 1961b, **58,** 160–174.

Cautela, J. R., & Kastenbaum, R. A reinforcement survey schedule for use in therapy, training, and research. *Psychological Reports,* 1967, **20,** 1115–1130.

Cobrinik, L., & Popper, L. Development aspects of thought disturbance in schizophrenic children: A Rorschach study. *American Journal of Orthopsychiatry,* 1961, **31,** 170–179.

Cronbach, L. J. Statistical methods applied to Rorschach scores: A review. In B. Murstein (Ed.), *Handbook of Projective Techniques.* New York: Basic Books, 1965. Pp. 355–394.

Draguns, J. G., Haley, E. M., & Phillips, L. Studies of Rorschach content: A review of the research literature. Part 1: Traditional content categories. *Journal of Projective Techniques and Personality Assessment,* 1967, **31,** 3–32.

Elkins, E. The diagnostic validity of the Ames "Danger Signals." *Journal of Consulting Psychology,* 1958, **22,** 281–287.

Eysenck, H. J. The effects of psychotherapy. *Journal of Consulting Psychology,* 1952a, **16,** 319–324.

Eysenck, H. J. *The scientific study of personality.* London: Routledge, Kegan Paul, 1952b.

Eysenck, H. J. *Handbook of abnormal psychology.* New York: Basic Books, 1961.

Eysenck, H. J. *Experiments in behavior therapy.* New York: Macmillan, 1964.

Eysenck, H. J., & Rachman, S. *The causes and cures of neuroses.* San Digeo: Knapp, 1965.

Ferster, C. B. Classification of behavioral pathology. In L. Krasner & L. P. Ullmann (Eds.), *Research in behavior modification.* New York: Holt, Rinehart, & Winston, 1965. Pp. 56–81.

Frank, L. K. *Projective methods.* Springfield, Ill.: Charles C. Thomas, 1948.

Geer, J. H. The development of a scale to measure fear. *Behavior Research and Therapy,* 1965, **3,** 45–54.

Gelfand, D. M., Gelfand, S., & Dobson, W. R. Unprogrammed reinforcement of patients' behavior in a mental hospital. *Behaviour Research and Therapy*, 1967, **5**, 201–208.

Gerard, R. E. *Differential treatment: A way to begin*. Washington, D.C.: Bureau of Prisons, U.S. Department of Justice.

Gewirtz, J. L. Deprivation and satiation of social stimuli as determinants of their reinforcing efficacy. In Hill, J. P. (Ed.), *Minnesota Symposium on Child Psychology*, Minneapolis, Minnesota: University of Minnesota Press, 1967, pp. 3–56.

Gluck, M. R., Tanner, M. M., Sullivan, D. F., & Erickson, P. Follow-up evaluation of 55 Child Guidance Cases. *Behavior Research and Therapy*, 1964, **2**, 131–134.

Goldberg, L. R. Diagnosticians vs. diagnostic signs: The diagnosis of psychosis vs. neurosis from the MMPI. *Psychological Monographs*, 1965, **79**, Whole No. 602.

Greenspoon, J., & Gersten, O. D. A new look at psychological testing: Psychological testing from the standpoint of a behaviorist. *American Psychologist*, 1967, **22**, 848–853.

Haley, E. M., Draguns, J. G., & Phillips, L. Studies of Rorschach content: A review of research literature. Part 2: Non-traditional uses of content indicators. *Journal of Projective Techniques and Personality Assessment*, 1967, **31**, 3–38.

Halpern, F. *A clinical approach to children's Rorschachs*. New York: Grune & Stratton, 1953.

Harris, F. R., Johnston, M. K., Kelley, C. S., & Wolf, M. M. Effect of positive social reinforcement on regressed crawling of a nursery school child. *Journal of Educational Psychology*, 1964, **55**, 35–41.

Hewitt, L. E., & Jenkins, R. L. *Fundamental patterns of maladjustment, the dynamics of their origin*. Springfield: State of Illinois, 1946.

Hill, K. T., & Stevenson, H. W. The effect of social reinforcement vs. nonreinforcement on sex of E on the performance of adolescent girls. *Journal of Personality*, 1965, **33**, 30–36.

Humphreys, L. G. The organization of human abilities. *American Psychologist*, 1962, **17**, 475–483.

Ingram, G. L., Gerard, R. E., Quay, H. C., & Levinson, R. B. An experimental program for the psychopathic delinquent: Looking in the correctional waste basket. *Journal of Research in Crime and Delinquency*, 1970, (Jan.) 24–30.

James, P., & Mosher, D. L. Thematic aggression, hostility-guilt, and aggression behavior. *Journal of Projective Techniques and Personality Assessment*, 1967, **31**, 61–67.

Jenkins, R. L. *Diagnoses, dynamics, and treatment in child psychiatry*. Psychiatric Research Report, No. 18, October 1964.

Jenkins, R. L. Psychiatric syndromes in children and their relation to family background. *American Journal of Orthopsychiatry*, 1966, **36**, 450–457.

Kagan, J. The measurement of overt aggression from fantasy. *Journal of Abnormal and Social Psychology*, 1956, **52**, 390–393.

Kanfer, F. H. Directions in behavior modification research or where the insufficiencies are. Paper presented at the Second Annual Institute of Man's Adjustment in a

Complex Environment: The Behavior Therapies. Veteran's Administration Hospital, Brecksville, Ohio, May 1967.

Kanfer, F. H., & Saslow, G. Behavioral analysis: An alternative to diagnostic classification. *Archives of General Psychiatry*, 1965, **12**, 529–538.

Kelly, E. L. Theory and techniques of assessment. *Annual Review of Psychology*, 1954, **5**, 281–310.

Kessler, J. W. *Psychopathology of childhood*. Englewood Cliffs, New Jersey: Prentice-Hall, 1966.

Lang, P. J., and Melamed, B. G. Case report: Avoidance conditioning of an infant with chronic ruminative vomiting. *Journal of Abnormal Psychology*, 1969, **74**, 1–8.

Lazarus, A. A., Davison, G. C., Polefka, D. A. Classical and operant conditioning factors in the treatment of a school phobic child. *Journal of Abnormal Psychology*, 1965, **70**, 225–229.

Levitt, E. E. Psychotherapy with children: A further evaluation. *Behavior Research and Therapy*, 1963, **1**, 45–51.

Lindzey, G. Thematic Apperception Test: Interpretive assumptions and related empirical evidence. *Psychological Bulletin*, 1952, **49**, 1–25.

Luria, A. R. Psychological studies of mental deficiency in the Soviet Union. In N. R. Ellis (Ed.), *Handbook of Mental Deficiency*, New York: McGraw-Hill, 1963. Pp. 353–387.

McClelland, D. C. Longitudinal trends in the relation of thought to action. *Journal of Consulting Psychology*, 1966, **30**, 479–483.

Meehl, P. E. Some ruminations on the validation of clinical procedures. *Canadian Journal of Psychology*, 1959, **13**, 102–128.

Meehl, P. E., & Rosen, A. Antecedent probability and the efficiency of psychometric signs, patterns, or cutting scores. *Psychological Bulletin*, 1955, **52**, 194–216.

Megargee, E. I., & Cooke, P. E. The relation of TAT and Inkblot aggressive content scales with each other and with criterion of overt aggressiveness in juvenile delinquents. *Journal of Projective Techniques and Personality Assessment*, 1967, **31**, 48–60.

Mischel, W. *Personality and assessment*. New York: Wiley, 1968.

Murstein, B. I. *Theory and research in projective techniques*. New York: Wiley, 1963.

Mussen, P. L., & Naylor, H. K. The relation between overt aggression and fantasy aggression. *Journal of Abnormal and Social Psychology*, 1954, **49**, 235–240.

O'Leary, K. D. The effects of self-instruction on immoral behavior. *Journal of Experimental Child Psychology*, 1968, **6**, 297–301.

O'Leary, K. D., & O'Leary, S. G. *Classroom management: The successful use of behavior modification*. New York: Pergamon Press, in press.

O'Leary, K. D., & Becker, W. C. Behavior modification of an adjustment class: A token reinforcement program. *Exceptional Children*, 1967, **33**, 637–642.

O'Leary, K. D., Thomas, D. R., & Becker, W. C. The effects of isolation, discussion of rules, and other procedures on aggressive behavior of a kindergarten boy. Unpublished manuscript, University of Illinois, 1968.

O'Leary, K. D., Becker, W. C., Evans, M., & Saudargas, R. Token reinforcement in a public school: A replication and systematic analysis. *Journal of Applied Behavior Analysis*, 1969, **2**, 3–14.

Olson, W. C. Diagnosis and treatment of behavior disorders of children. National Society for the Study of Education. *Thirty Fourth Yearbook*, 1934. Pp. 363–397.

Patterson, G. R. Prediction of victimization from an instrumental conditioning procedure. *Journal of Consulting Psychology*, 1967, **31**, 147–152.

Patterson, G. R., Bricker, W., & Greene, M. Peer group reactions as a determinant of aggressive behavior in nursery school children. Paper presented to APA, September 1964.

Paul, G. L. *Insight vs. desensitization in psychotherapy*. Stanford: Stanford University Press, 1966.

Peterson, D. R. Scope and generality of verbally defined personality factors. *Psychological Review*, 1965, **72**, 48–59.

Peterson, D. R. *The clinical study of social behavior*. New York: Appleton-Century-Crofts, 1968.

Pimm, J. B. Early detection of emotional disturbance in a public school setting: A three year follow-up. Paper presented at the annual meeting of the Canadian Psychological Association, Ottawa, June 1967.

Pimm, J. B., & Rogers, J. A behavior checklist approach. Paper presented to the annual meeting of the Ontario Psychological Association, January 1966.

Pimm, J. B., Quay, H. C., & Werry, J. S. Dimensions of problem behavior in first grade children. *Psychology in the Schools*, 1967, **4**, 155–157.

Quay, H. C. Personality patterns in preadolescent delinquent boys. *Educational and Psychological Measurement*, 1966, **26**, 99–110.

Quay, H. C. Dimensions of problem behavior and educational programming. In P. S. Graubard, (Ed.), *Children against schools*. Chicago: Follett, 1969.

Quay, H. C., & Levinson, R. B. The prediction of institutional adjustment of delinquent boys: Preliminary results. Unpublished manuscript. University of Illinois, Urbana, 1967.

Quay, H. C., & Parsons, L. B. The differential behavioral classification of the juvenile offender. Washington, D.C.: Bureau of Prisons, U.S. Department of Justice, 1970.

Quay, H. C., & Peterson, D. R. Manual for the Behavior Problem Checklist. Mimeo., 1967.

Sidman, M., Herrnstein, R. J., & Conrad, D. G. Maintenance of avoidance behavior by unavoidable shock. *Journal of Comparative and Physiological Psychology*, 1957, **50**, 553–557.

Skolnick, A. Motivational imagery and behavior over twenty years. *Journal of Consulting Psychology*, 1966, **30**, 463–478.

Speer, D. C. The behavior problem checklist (Peterson-Quay): Baseline data from parents of child guidance and nonclinic children. *Journal of Consulting and Clinical Psychology*, 1971, **36**, 221–228.

Sternlight, M., & Silverg, E. F. The relationship between fantasy aggression and overt hostility in mental retardates. *American Journal of Mental Deficiency*, 1965, **70**, 486–488.

Stevenson, H. W., & Fahel, L. S. The effect of social reinforcement of institutionalized and noninstitutionalized normal and feebleminded children. *Journal of Personality*, 1961, **29**, 136–147.

Thomas, D. R., Becker, W. C., & Armstrong, M. Prediction and elimination of disruptive classroom behavior by systematically varying teacher's behavior. *Journal of Applied Behavior Analysis*, 1968, **1**, 35–46.

Ullmann, L. P., & Krasner, L. *Case studies in behavior modification.* New York: Holt, Rinehart, & Winston, 1965.

Ulrich, R. E., Stachnick, T. J., & Stainton, S. R. Student acceptance of generalized personality interpretations. *Psychological Reports*, 1963, **13**, 831–834.

Wahler, R. G., Winkel, G. H., Peterson, R. F., & Morrison, D. C. Mothers as behavior therapists for their own children. *Behavior Research and Therapy*, 1965, **3**, 113–134.

Witryol, S. L., & Fisher, W. F. Scaling children's incentives by the method of paired comparisons. *Psychological Reports*, 1960, **7**, 471–474.

Wolf, R. The measurement of environments. In A. Anastasi, (Ed.), *Testing problems in perspective*, Washington: American Council on Education, 1966.

Wright, H. F. *Recording and analyzing child behavior.* New York: Harper & Row, 1967.

Young, G. C. Personality factors and the treatment of enuresis. *Behavior Research and Therapy*, 1965, **3**, 103–105.

Zigler, E., & Phillips, L. Psychiatric diagnosis: A critique. *Journal of Abnormal and Social Psychology*, 1961, **63**, 607–618.

Zubin, J., Eron, L. D., & Schumer, F. *An experimental approach to projective techniques.* New York: Wiley, 1965.

Chapter Seven

Behavior Therapy
Alan O. Ross

Basic Assumptions

Behavior therapy is based on the assumption that principles of learning can be applied to the treatment of psychological disorders that find their manifestation in behavior and it can thus be defined as the correction of psychological disorders through the systematic and explicit application of principles of learning.

Psychological disorders can be said to fall into two major categories: Deficient behavior and maladaptive behavior. In cases of behavior deficits, the individual has failed to learn adaptive responses in his environment. The responses missing from his repertoire may be verbal, as in speech deficiency; intellectual, as in mental deficiency; social, as in the child lacking skills in peer relations; or muscular, as in children who have failed to acquire control over eliminative functions or in those who lack such skills as dressing, feeding, or riding a tricycle. Behavior deficits may also entail failures to attend to or discriminate relevant stimuli, as may be the case, for example, in a child who "won't listen." Lastly, behavior deficiencies include instances where social and other secondary reinforcers have not acquired reinforcing properties.

In cases of maladaptive behavior, the individual has responses available in his repertoire but he emits these responses under inappropriate circumstances. Responses may be adaptive at one developmental stage but not at another, or they may be adaptive in one setting, but in another. Since the environment defines what is adaptive in almost all instances, with the possible exception of self-destructive or self-injurious behavior, maladaptive responses can occur in all realms of behavior, including the autonomic where fear or anger may occur under inappropriate circumstances.

Whether a psychological disorder represents deficient or maladaptive behavior, corrective action must involve learning. The child must be helped to acquire the missing responses in the case of behavior deficit, or he must be helped to modify his responses in the case of maladaptive behavior so that these responses will be elicited or emitted only under the appropriate circumstances. All of this involves learning, unlearning, or relearning, and this corrective action has come to be known as behavior therapy.

The behavior therapist operates on the assumption that he can modify deficient and maladaptive behavior without necessarily understanding or knowing why this behavior is deficient or originally became maladaptive. Although all present behavior and behavior deficits undoubtedly have historical antecedents, these antecedents need not be reconstructed in order to undertake corrective action. On the other hand, the behavior therapist must seek to know as much as he can possibly ascertain about the *current* conditions under which the behavior in question occurs or fails to occur. Assessment for behavior therapy must seek to answer such questions as what responses the child is currently capable of making, what stimuli he is currently capable of perceiving, and what reinforcements are currently capable of maintaining behavior. "How can I teach this child to behave more adaptively?" is a far more relevant question than, "How did this child come to behave so maladaptively?" since the latter question can never lead to a conclusive answer and rarely helps in providing clues to corrective action.

The focus of behavior therapy is on behavior, and the first task of the behavior therapist is to decide which of a given child's behaviors he should attempt to modify. Since parents usually bring their child for treatment with a specific complaint, this complaint is a logical starting point in selecting a target behavior. Frequently, however, the complaint is vague or general and must be refined or redefined before the therapist can plan his corrective action. This is particularly true where complaints take the form of attributed emotional states such as, "He is unhappy" or "He is jealous." Redirecting the focus from how the child presumably feels to what he does, from the parents' inferences to the observable behavioral referents on which these inferences are based, permits the behavior therapist to define a target behavior he can try to modify.

Once a target behavior or behaviors have been defined, the treatment goal can be specified to the child and his parents as the modification of this behavior in the adaptive direction. With an explicit treatment goal, treatment outcome can be readily assessed for when deficient behavior is no longer lacking or when maladaptive behavior has become adaptive, treatment is considered successful and termination can be prompt and decisive.

Theoretical Principles

Since the establishment or modification of behavior involves learning, behavior therapy must be based on principles of learning, as these are currently understood. Most behavior therapists find it useful to work within the theoretical framework which holds that learning takes place through either respondent or operant conditioning, depending on the nature of the response in question. If the response is in the vascular-visceral-autonomic realm, the respondent conditioning paradigm seems to hold the greatest explanatory power. If the response is in the muscular-skeletal-voluntary realm, the framework of operant conditioning appears most relevant. The pragmatic behavior therapist bases his work on the principles derived from respondent and operant conditioning without much concern as to the adequacy of currently held formulations or the epistemologic soundness of a two-factor theory of learning. As basic learning research continues, the formulations will no doubt be modified and applied work will change accordingly, but for the present the following represents an overview of the most widely accepted theoretical principles on which behavior therapy rests.

Respondent Conditioning

Also known as classical or Pavlovian conditioning, this paradigm states that certain responses which are a part of the innate repertoire of the organism are reflectively *elicited* by specific stimuli. When a neutral stimulus, that is, one previously not capable of eliciting this particular response, is repeatedly paired with the innate elicitor, that stimulus acquires the capacity to elicit the response even in the absence of the original, innate stimulus. The well-known example of repeatedly pairing the presentation of food, which innately elicits salivation, with the presentation of a ringing bell, so that the bell acquires the capacity to elicit salivation illustrates this procedure. The technical terminology according to which salivation is called the unconditioned response (UR), food the unconditioned stimulus (US), the bell the conditioned stimulus (CS), and salivation elicited by the bell the conditioned response (CR) is also widely familiar. The distinctive features of respondent conditioning are that it involves an innate response that is elicited by a stimulus which *precedes* the response, and that the subject is *passively responding* to the presentation of the stimulus.

Several phenomena that have been intensively studied in laboratory experiments on respondent conditioning are of relevance to the behavior therapist. *Stimulus generalization* refers to the fact that after a specific stimulus has acquired the potentiality of eliciting a particular response, stimuli that are similar to the original stimulus will also be capable of eliciting the conditioned response. The frequency, intensity, or duration of the CR is a function of the degree of similarity of the generalized CS to the original CS and this function is reflected in the *generalization gradient.*

Repeated presentation of the conditioned stimulus without at least occasional pairing with the unconditioned stimulus results in *extinction,* the progressive weakening of the conditioned stimulus. If on those occasions when the CS is *not* paired with the US a distinct, different stimulus is also presented, this latter stimulus, the *conditioned inhibitor,* will come to suppress the CR, a state referred to as *conditioned inhibition* that differs from extinction in that the CS will elicit the CR whenever it is not paired with the conditioned inhibitor. Conditioned inhibition is related to *differential inhibition,* which involves the establishment of nonresponsiveness to stimuli that are somewhat similar to the conditioned stimulus and it is thus the opposite of stimulus generalization and can be used to correct overgeneralization by conditioning the organism to respond selectively.

Counterconditioning, a term not usually found in the traditional experimental literature, denotes a procedure of major importance in behavior therapy, where it is also known as *reciprocal inhibition* (Wolpe, 1958). It basically involves the production of a decrement of a conditioned response by the elicitation of an incompatible response to the same conditioned stimulus. When counterconditioning is completed, the original CR has been displaced by a new conditioned response.

The importance of respondent conditioning in the treatment of individuals with psychological disorders derives from the fact that many of these disorders entail the emotions of fear or anger which, since they involve endocrine secretions, represent responses of the vascular-visceral-autonomic realm. The individual is innately capable of the particular response but many, previously neutral stimuli apparently come to elicit the emotion as a result of experiences analogous to respondent conditioning. Once such conditioning and subsequent generalization has taken place, treatment of maladaptive emotional behavior will logically follow the respondent conditioning paradigm.

Operant Conditioning

In respondent conditioning, an event in the environment elicits a response from the organism; the environment "does something" to the organism and the organism reacts. In operant conditioning, on the other hand, the organism "does something" to the environment and the environment reacts. The important distinction between the two forms of learning is that in the former, the stimulus precedes and elicits the response, while in the latter, the response is *emitted* by the organism and the *consequence* of the response serves to increase or decrease the likelihood of that response's recurrence under similar circumstances. If the particular consequences to the response occur only under distinct and identifiable circumstances, these circumstances will come to represent the *conditions* under which the response will be emitted (hence, "conditioning").

The sequence of events in operant conditioning is the presence of a discriminative stimulus (S^D), the emission of an operant response (R_{op}) and the presentation of a reinforcing stimulus (S_R). The presentation of S_R is followed by a consummatory response (R_{cons}) on the part of the organism (ingestion where the S_R is food), but this important step is usually subsumed under the term reinforcement and implied in the definition of the reinforcing stimulus. Once operant behavior is well-established it seems to the casual observer that the stimulus elicits a response (the ringing of the telephone "makes" a man pick up the receiver), but more careful analysis reveals that the behavior occurs because of what follows (someone with a message is at the other end of the telephone). It must be stressed that operant behavior is a function of its consequences. Modification of operant behavior thus requires a manipulation of the contingencies under which the consequences are to occur.

Because the operant response must be emitted before it can be reinforced and its emission thus conditioned to a specific discriminative stimulus, the response must be in the person's repertoire in the first place. Where this is not the case, the teacher, parent, or therapist must select a similar response that is already established and *shape* the desired final response by *successive approximations*, that is, by selectively reinforcing responses that are increasingly like the response being taught.

As in respondent conditioning, one finds stimulus generalization in that an operant learned to one S^D is also emitted in the presence of a range of similar S^Ds, the response rate being a function of the degree of similarity. Extinction is also a phenomenon found in both types of conditioning; an operant is progressively weakened if it has no effect on the environment, that is, if no consequences are forthcoming. Under certain circumstances a distinctive stimulus may signal the contingency of "no consequences." This stimulus is technically referred to as an S^Δ (S-Delta) and the subject gradually learns *not* to emit his response when that stimulus is present.

The consequences of an operant response can be positive, negative, or neutral. Positive consequences will strengthen the response, that is, increase the probability of its occurrence; negative consequences will weaken the response, decreasing the probability of its occurrence; while neutral consequences, having no reinforcing effect, will result in extinction, i.e., weakening of the response. Positive consequences can consist of the presentation of satisfying stimulation or of the termination or avoidance of a noxious stimulation (negative reinforcement). Both of these consequences reinforce behavior and can be considered rewards. In both instances conditions must exist in order for the consequence to be introduced. In the case of the presentation of satisfying stimulation, the subject must be in a state of deprivation for that particular kind of stimulation. In the case of the removal of noxious stimulation it is obvious that such stimulation must be present before it can be removed.

Negative consequences of a response that will weaken the operant can consist of the presentation of noxious stimulation, i.e., the delivery of punishment, or it can take the form of the removal of satisfying stimulation, a "time-out from positive reinforcement." Again it is obvious that a condition of positive reinforcement must exist before "time-out" can take place.

When a given neutral event is repeatedly paired with a reinforcing stimulus, the pairing being such that the neutral event precedes the S_R, this neutral event can take on reinforcing properties and thus become a reinforcer in its own right. This phenomenon, called *conditioned* or *secondary* or *acquired reinforcement*, permits a wide range of stimuli to become reinforcing stimuli. A child's responses can thus be reinforced not only by such primary reinforcers as food, but also by such secondary reinforcers as praise, tokens, and grades on report cards. It has also been found (Premack, 1959) that a response with high probability of occurrence will reinforce a response of lower probability of occurrence so that, in the case of children, play behavior will reinforce work behavior, running about will reinforce sitting still, etc.

Positive reinforcement requires a preexisting state of deprivation, negative reinforcement requires the preexistence of an aversive condition that can be terminated, and time-out depends for its effectiveness on an on-going positive reinforcement that can be interrupted. The only consequence that is not dependent on a preexisting state and can thus be presented without preparation is punishment but this manipulation is fraught with complications.

Despite its ready availability and apparent effectiveness in reducing the probability of a response, punishment that takes the form of the delivery of noxious stimulation is complex, both in its effect and its theoretical status in learning research. Punishment appears to carry both respondent and operant implications (Rescorla & Solomon, 1967) because it elicits a physiologic arousal the reduction of which appears to reinforce an emitted operant response of avoidance or escape (Baum, 1966). The physiologic arousal state (fear/anxiety) will become conditioned to whatever stimuli are present when punishment is administered. These stimuli may be relevant to the specific behavior that is being punished to the effect that this behavior will come to be avoided or suppressed by incompatible responses. At the same time, however, stimuli relevant to the punishment situation and to the person who delivers the noxious stimulation may become conditioned stimuli for such emotional responses as fear and anxiety with the result that this situation or person will become the occasion for avoidance or escape responses.

An important consideration in the use of punishment is that it does not actually eliminate a given behavior from the response repertoire; it simply serves to suppress the behavior because of the arousal of incompatible emotional reactions and their respondent consequences. As long as the conditioned aversive stimuli are present, the punished behavior will remain suppressed, but the behavior will reappear when these stimuli are absent. This, as Skinner (1953) has pointed out, will be particularly true in instances where the behavior in question carries its own reinforcement as, for instance, in stealing food. Here, stealing behavior will reemerge when punishment is discontinued, although the individual will go through a period where the stimuli for approach responses and the stimuli for avoidance responses are in relative equilibrium, a condition of conflict which tends to be disruptive of behavior.

Research on the effects of punishment on children is complicated by the ethical impossibility of administering strong aversive stimulation for experimental purposes. A review by Marshall (1965) reflects the prevalence in controlled research of such relatively impotent punishments as blame, reproof, the taking away of previously earned candy or trinkets, and the emission of the word "wrong" on the part of the experimenter. Punishment of this mild nature appears to have information value and to speed up discrimination learning when specific incorrect responses are followed by negative reinforcement. On the other hand, when a more general situation, as opposed to specific responses, is punished, the motivational effect depends on such factors as task complexity, intelligence, nature of instructions, and experimenter variables.

The presentation of aversive consequences (punishment) has been used in behavior therapy with children. Details of these reports will be discussed in a later context. Here it can be stated that in all instances punishment of undesirable responses was used as a supplement to the far more potent and less complicated positive reinforcement of incompatible, desirable responses.

Treatment Methods

The Interrelationship of Operant and Respondent Factors

The foregoing summary of theoretical principles suggests that the therapist wishing to modify the maladaptive behavior of a child can take recourse to a variety of specific treatment methods that alone or in combination meet the specific treatment needs of a particular child.

Where the psychological disorder takes the form of a behavioral deficit, the missing response or responses can be established through the use of conditioning. When the respondent conditioning paradigm guides the therapeutic strategy, the therapist presents stimuli intended to elicit specific responses or classes of responses. In that case, the child in treatment is essentially a passive respondent, the therapist the active initiator. Lest it be assumed that the therapist "manipulates" an unwitting child, it must be stressed that unlike the animal in a classical conditioning experiment, the child is not in a restraining harness, unable to escape the stimuli presented by the therapist. Unless the cooperation of the child is established, and this usually entails a motivation for getting help with a problem, no stimuli can be effectively presented and thus paired with responses. This circumstance makes respondent conditioning treatment best suited for nonresidential clinic settings where children usually recognize the need for getting help and are motivated for treatment.

Where the therapeutic strategy is based on the operant conditioning model, the child, by definition, engages in an operation—does something to the environment—and is thus a very active participant in the treatment process. The therapist's role is to arrange the contingencies so that the child's operant responses encounter certain consequences under particular stimulus conditions. In order to do this, the therapist must be able to exert some control over the stimulus and reinforcement conditions which the child encounters. Thus, the level of possible control largely determines the level of treatment effectiveness. The possible control is, of course, greatest in an institutional setting where a therapist, through the cooperation of institutional personnel, can exert influence over the delivery of both primary and secondary reinforcements. In order to conduct operant conditioning treatment effectively in nonresidential settings it is necessary to obtain the close cooperation of the child's parents or teachers who are in a better position to manage reinforcement contingencies than the therapist who has only intermittent contact with the child.

While the preceding discussion differentiated between respondent therapy and operant therapy, all treatment—as any other complex human learning—entails both respondent and operant factors. The therapist's strategy may be predominantly respondent or operant, depending on whether the behavior to be modified is predominantly mediated by the "voluntary" or "involuntary" nervous system, but it is rarely possible to identify the exact principles involved in the learning of a particular response constellation. For example, most children who have to learn age-appropriate toilet behavior will have acquired some conditioned anxiety to stimuli associated with soiling or wetting by the time treatment is instituted. It can be assumed that all enuretic and encopretic children, no matter how retarded or autistic, have undergone anxiety conditioning punishment in connection with toilet training. Treatment is thus unlikely ever to be purely operant as some writers have suggested

(Giles & Wolf, 1966; Hundziak, Maurer, & Watson, 1965). When a therapist introduces the delivery of a positive reinforcement contingent on appropriate toilet responses (e.g., Neale, 1963), anxiety that had become associated with soiling will come to be avoided each time an appropriate toilet response occurs. As the frequency of appropriate responses increase, toilet anxiety will ultimately be extinguished. The training sequence thus involves respondent factors and must be viewed as more than simple operant conditioning. This is particularly true if, as in the work by Giles and Wolf (1966), aversive stimuli are presented contingent on inappropriate behavior and negative reinforcement is used as one aspect of the training procedure.

At times, a specific case may indeed call for an explicit, planned combination of operant and respondent approaches. A discussion of such an instance is presented by Lazarus, Davison, and Polefka (1965) who treated a nine-year-old boy's school phobic behavior using both respondent (classical) and operant techniques when it became apparent that his behavior was controlled both by intense fear of the school situation itself and by various secondary reinforcers, such as attention from parents, siblings, and therapists.

At the time of referral, this boy had been absent from school for three weeks. He had begun to avoid the classroom situation three weeks after entering fourth grade, following the summer vacation. He had begun by hiding in the cloakroom and then started to spend less time in school each day. At that point, neither bribes, threat, nor punishment would persuade him to return to school.

There had been several episodes of school refusal in this child's history. He had run away from kindergarten on the first day there and in second grade, after initial reluctance to go to school, he eventually refused to attend. At that time, on the advice of a psychiatrist, he was "literally dragged screaming to school by a truant officer" (Lazarus, Davison, & Polefka, 1965, p. 226). The boy had seven siblings, a moody, punitive, and perfectionistic father, and an inconsistent mother. He had nearly drowned when he was five years old, undergone surgery followed by complications toward the end of his third grade, and witnessed a drowning shortly thereafter. The death of a close friend of his older sister had upset him and his family following his entry into fourth grade. He had apparently been intimidated by his oldest sister who had told him that work in fourth grade was particularly difficult.

Since the school refusal was the most disruptive response pattern of this generally bewildered and intimidated child, the therapists chose it as the focus of treatment, setting the short-range goal of reinstating normal school attendance. They recognized that the home situation in general, and parental mishandling, in particular, would also require therapeutic intervention.

The principal therapeutic strategy was *in vivo* desensitization in which the boy was exposed to increasingly difficult steps along the main dimensions of his school phobia. These steps, as reported by Lazarus et al. (1965), were as follows:

1. On the first day, a Sunday, the therapist accompanied the boy to the school during an afternoon walk. This initial exposure was relatively pleasant in that the therapist allayed the child's anxiety by means of distraction and humor.

2. On the next two days, the therapist walked with the child from his home to the schoolyard at the hour when he would ordinarily leave for school. Anxiety reduction was achieved by means of coaxing, encouragement, relaxation, and the deliberate picturing of pleasant events, such as Christmas, that were related to the school situation ("emotive imagery," to be discussed below). On these days, the child did not enter school but spent approximately 15 minutes roaming around the school yard before returning home.

3. After the end of the school day, therapist and child entered the classroom where the boy was persuaded to sit down at his desk. A playful enacting of normal school routine followed before child and therapist returned to the boy's home.

4. The therapist accompanied the boy into the classroom as the other pupils entered. They had a chat with the teacher and left immediately after the opening exercises.

5. A week after the start of this program, the child was able to spend the entire morning session in class. The therapist remained in the classroom and smiled approvingly at the boy whenever he interacted with his teacher or one of his classmates. After eating his lunch, the boy took part in an active ball game and then returned home in the company of the therapist. As it happened, no afternoon classes were held during that week for administrative reasons.

6. Two days later, the boy entered his classroom with the other students. He did not insist on having the therapist in constant view and allowed him to wait inside the classroom.

7. Starting on the next day, the therapist sat in the school library adjoining the classroom. (It should be noted that the therapist was a graduate student, hence his ability to invest that much time in one case. On the other hand, any well-trained therapeutic assistant could carry out these aspects of treatment, thus freeing the professional therapist for other work.)

8. At this point it was agreed that the therapist would leave the school at 2:30 P.M. while the child remained there for the last half hour of school.

9. On the next day, the therapist's departure was moved back a half hour.

10. Instead of picking him up at his home, the therapist now arranged to meet the child at the school gate ten minutes before class time. The boy also agreed to remain alone at school from 10:45 A.M. until noon provided the therapist return at noon and ate lunch with him. The therapist would then leave at 1:45 P.M., promising that he would visit the child at home in the evening and play guitar for him, provided the child remain in school until the end of classes.

11. Because of occasional setbacks, the boy's mother was instructed not to allow him into the house during school hours. In addition, the teacher agreed to provide special tasks for the boy in order to increase his active participation and to make school more attractive for him.

12. A mild tranquilizer was prescribed by the family physician. This was to be taken on awakening in order to reduce anticipatory anxieties, but seemed of limited therapeutic value (see Chapter Eight).

13. After meeting the boy at school in the morning, the therapist left the boy at school for progressively longer periods and after 6 days of this, the therapist was able to depart at 10 A.M.

14. The therapist now assured the child that he would be in the faculty room until 10 A.M., in case he was needed. The boy thus came to school knowing the therapist was present, but he did not actually see him.

15. With the boy's consent, the therapist now arrived at the school shortly after the students had entered the classroom.

The rest of the treatment of this child's school phobia is described as follows.

16. School attendance independent of the therapist's presence was achieved by means of specific rewards (a comic book, and variously colored tokens which would eventually procure a baseball glove) contingent upon his entering school and remaining there alone. He was at liberty to telephone the therapist in the morning if he wanted him at school, in which event he would forfeit his rewards for that day.

17. Since the therapist's presence seemed to have at least as much reward value as the comic books and tokens, it was necessary to enlist the mother's cooperation to effect the therapist's final withdrawal. The overall diminution of the boy's anxieties, together with general gains which had accrued to his home situation, made it therapeutically feasible for the mother to emphasize the fact that school attendance

was compulsory, and that social agencies beyond the control of both therapist and parents would enforce this requirement eventually.

18. Approximately three weeks later, [the boy] had accumulated enough tokens to procure his baseball glove. He then agreed with his parents that rewards of this kind were no longer necessary (Lazarus et al., 1965, p. 227).

The treatment program had extended over 4½ months and while during that time there had been numerous setbacks of varying degrees of severity, the boy's school refusal abated and at follow-up ten months after termination of therapy, he had not only maintained his gains but had made further progress in school attendance as well as in other areas of behavior.

This case has been presented in some detail in order to illustrate that in actual practice, operant and respondent principles come into play, often in complex interaction. In the initial phases of treatment, the boy's high level of anxiety was dealt with by classical counterconditioning techniques; in the later phases, when anxiety was minimal, operant strategies were introduced with various reinforcements made contingent on school attendance. The authors stress that the choice and timing of the specific technique are crucial factors in treatment effectiveness. As an example, they cite the situation in which the boy left the classroom and came to the library where his therapist had stationed himself at this stage of treatment.

At this point the choice of strategy became crucial. In strict operant terms, active attempts to reduce anxiety by means of attention and reassurance would reinforce classroom-leaving behavior. On the other hand, the classical paradigm would predict that to withhold immediate attention and make it contingent upon returning to the classroom would augment the child's anxiety and thus reinforce avoidance behavior. The critical factor in determining the appropriate procedure was the degree of anxiety as judged by the therapist (p. 228).

The risk involved in the inappropriate use of the operant model is summarized by Lazarus, et al. (1965) as follows: "If the level of anxiety is very high, a premature re-exposure to the feared situation will probably lead to increased sensitivity. Moreover, if this heightened level of anxiety leads to another escape response, the resultant anxiety-reduction will strengthen the avoidance responses . . . ." On the other hand, an inappropriate use of the classical model would also impede treatment progress, for the very acts of inducing relaxation and giving reassurance may provide positive reinforcement for dependent behavior. The therapist must thus weight the relative advantages and disadvantages of his techniques and attempt to maximize therapeutic effectiveness while minimizing antitherapeutic risk. The apparent simplicity of behavior therapy that derives from its easily understood principles should not mislead anyone into believing that it is without risk and that it can be carried out by untrained or poorly trained individuals. This fact was recognized by Mary Cover Jones (1924) in her pioneering paper more than four decades ago. In describing her well-known work with Peter whose fear of rabbits had been treated by the application of a respondent conditioning paradigm, she wrote:

> This method obviously requires delicate handling. Two response systems are being dealt with: food leading to a positive reaction, and fear-object leading to a negative reaction. The desired conditioning should result in transforming the fear-object into a source of positive response (substitute stimulus). But a careless manipulator could readily produce the reverse result, attaching a fear reaction to the sight of food (p. 388).

The Ambiguous Theoretical Base of Sphincter Training

Not only is it often difficult to determine whether a particular behavioral approach to the treatment of a psychological disorder is based on respondent or operant factors, but it is also frequently uncertain just what mechanism of conditioning is responsible for the effects found in behavior therapy. The best example of this theoretical ambiguity is found in the treatment of enuresis for which conditioning methods, introduced by Mowrer and Mowrer (1938), have been applied for many years.

Empirically, the child sleeps on a special pad which is wired in such a way that a single drop of urine will close a circuit and activate a bell or buzzer that continues to sound until turned off manually by either the child or an attendant. A review of 20 studies of conditioning treatment of enuresis (Werry, 1966; see also Chapter Four) leads to the conclusion that it is an effective technique, and a carefully controlled study by De Leon and Mandell (1966) shows it to be superior to the traditional psychotherapeutic approach. Theoretically, however, it is not at all clear what is involved in learning bladder control and thus, why the treatment works. Following the analysis by Mowrer and Mowrer (1938), the usual formulation is that bladder distension serves as the CS, the buzzer as the US, and waking up as the response that is conditioned to the bladder distension. Viewed in this form, nothing is said about how the ultimate behavior pattern of sleeping through the night without wetting comes to be learned. Martin and Kubly (1955) gloss over the complication by stating that, "As time goes by, it is also hoped that the somewhat more temporally removed response of sphincter control will become associated with bladder tension, thus allowing the child to sleep through the night dry" (p. 71).

In addition to the question of how the "response of waking up" leads to the "response of sphincter control," there is the issue, as Lovibond (1963) points out, whether treatment follows the classical conditioning model, as in the formulation mentioned above, or whether it entails avoidance learning. In other words, the problem is whether the child learns to control the sphincter muscle and as a result does not wet, or whether he learns to avoid the noxious stimulus of the loud and waking noise by conditioned sphincter contraction. On a technical level, this amounts to the question whether the CS is the distension of the bladder or the micturition response.

The question of what is learned is not unique to the treatment of enuresis. In any instance where undesirable behavior is eliminated, one can ask whether the child learns to make the desirable response or to suppress the undesirable response. This is particularly true when the desirable response is the reciprocal of the undesirable response so that not emitting the undesirable response ipso facto produces the former. For example, if a child is treated because he refuses to go to school ("school phobia"), does he learn to go to school or does he learn not to stay away from school? It is, of course, likely that both are being learned at the same time so that it would seem good therapeutic strategy to make the simultaneous strengthening and weakening of antagonistic behaviors an explicit aspect of the treatment plan.

Such strengthening of adaptive behavior and simultaneous weakening of its maladaptive reciprocal seems to be operating in cases where enuresis is treated by behavior therapy. Regardless of the therapist's avowed theoretical basis, a combination of classical, avoidance, and operant factors would seem to be at work, operant aspects being involved in the many secondary reinforcements that the child receives once he no longer wets his bed. In fact, Lovibond (1964) suggests that the child be an active partner in the treatment program, helping with the record keeping and receiving praise for his progress.

In Lovibond's (1964) research on conditioning treatment with enuretic children, the pad and bell apparatus based on the classical conditioning model was compared with an instrument, the Twin Signal device, whose operation is based on the avoidance conditioning paradigm. The results favored Lovibond's avoidance conditioning hypothesis. The Twin Signal device was significantly more efficient than devices constructed on the assumption that bladder distension is the CS. However, treatment with either device resulted in a high relapse rate.

The high relapse rate in the treatment of enuresis might be viewed as a support for the view that this treatment follows the classical conditioning model and that the relapse represents extinction of the CR after the permanent withdrawal of the US (the buzzer or bell). Lovibond believes that his results argue against this view but the results are anything but conclusive with respect to this theoretical issue. Another explanation of relapse on the part of some children treated for enuresis by conditioning methods might be that maintenance of the response involved in staying dry requires at least intermittent secondary reinforcement after it has been established through the use of the pad-and-signal method. That is, whether dryness is originally established by classical or operant means, it can be maintained as an operant by reinforcing dry nights either by social reinforcement (e.g., praise by the parents) or self-reinforcement (feeling pleased with oneself). Where such reinforcement is absent, the child may well incur a relapse on the basis of extinction.

De Leon and Mandell (1966) who report a high relapse rate, using the extremely rigorous definition of a single wet night following treatment, point out that relapsed children can be retrained with a second course of treatment in significantly less time than was required for the first conditioning series. If there is indeed a competing response that regains prepotency, then repeated series of conditioning may well be required before the "dry" response is sufficiently well-established to resist relapse. Therapists would do well to prepare themselves and their clients for the possible need for repeated treatment series and it would also seem that efforts should be made to maintain intermittent reinforcement of dry nights instead of taking these for granted too soon after treatment.

Children who had once been toilet trained but regress to wetting, are probably cases where the adaptive response became extinguished or the competing response of wetting was reacquired. This consideration leads to the third possible explanation of relapse in the treatment of enuretics. Enuretic children as a group contain two identifiable categories; one composed of children who had never been dry at night and the other containing those who had once acquired the capacity to sleep through the night without wetting but who regressed to the immature pattern in later years. Since in the case of the first group, treatment consists of establishing a new response, while in the case of the latter it entails the reestablishment of a previously learned response or the elimination of a competing response, it would seem to follow that there should be a difference in acquisition rate as well as a difference in resistance to extinction of the newly established response.

A study by Novick (1966) seems to lend support to this speculation. He treated 22 persistent and 23 acquired (regressed) enuretics by symptom-focused supportive treatment. Those who failed to improve (80%) were then treated with a wetting-alarm apparatus, whereupon all but four of the subjects reached the cure-criterion of 14 consecutive dry nights. Comparing the persistent with the acquired cases, it was found that the acquired enuretics had reached the cure criterion sooner and with more rapid decrease in wetting. It thus seems that the group that merely had to reestablish a previously learned response did better than the group that had to learn an entirely new response. On the other hand, follow-up interviews over a period of one year revealed that significantly more children in the regressed than in the persistent group had relapsed or developed new symptoms. Cases who relapse after treatment thus seem to be those for whom enuresis represented a regression from previously established mature behavior. It may be that the reinforcement contingencies which operate in the child's environment are such that the response of wetting or other maladaptive behavior is strengthened while the responses involved in staying dry are weakened. This would explain why these children regress in the first place and then relapse after successful treatment and it would suggest that the therapist should work not only with the child but also with the parents who manage the crucial contingencies and whose relevant behavior must be modified if the child's treatment is to have lasting success.

Novick's report that 21 of the 23 acquired and 12 of the 22 persistent enuretics developed new symptoms is difficult to evaluate in the absence of a no-treatment control group that might have answered the question whether any group of children with a psychological disorder develops a certain number of new problems over a period of one year. Nor is this study particularly relevant to the question of symptom substitution in behavior therapy since supportive treatment and conditioning treatment were confounded by selecting for conditioning only those cases that had failed to benefit from prior supportive work. Since most of the cases that were successfully treated by supportive therapy were in the acquired group that also displayed the greater proportion of new symptoms, it is impossible to determine whether supportive therapy or conditioning treatment was responsible for the new problems, if there is indeed a causal relationship between treatment and the development of new problems.

Novick's discovery of new symptoms following symptomatic treatment, stands in marked contrast to the findings of Baker (1967) who treated ten enuretic children with a conditioning device and compared outcome with equal numbers of children in a no-treatment, waiting list control and a control group that received wake-up treatment which duplicated all features of the conditioning treatment except the conditioning procedure itself. The conditioning group improved significantly more than either control group. Most of the children in the wake-up group eventually shifted to conditioning, and the overall cure rate was 74% with another 15% showing very marked improvement. During a six-month follow-up, four cured subjects relapsed but when two of these underwent a second treatment program, they became dry again. Baker was particularly interested in the questions of symptom substitution and generalization of improvement to other, not treated areas of behavior. Measures of the child's adjustment were therefore obtained at home, from the parents, and in school from both teachers and children. These measures of adjustment were taken by a second investigator who did not know to which group a particular child had been assigned. In general, the cured children showed improvements in areas such as peer relations, school behavior, and general adjustment even though none of these had been subjects of direct treatment. In no instance was there a worsening of the child's general adjustment.

In the above discussion the relative contributions of the respondent and operant conditioning paradigms to behavior therapy were explored and the arbitrary nature of a classification of treatment techniques along lines of this dichotomy was stressed. In the following, a similarly arbitrary distinction has been made for the sake of exposition between the treatment of behavior deficit and the modification of maladaptive behavior. Not only will any individual case usually present aspects of both types of psychological disorder, but even in a behavior deficit per se, as in the case of enuresis, it is often difficult to decide whether the child lacks a response (control) or maladaptively makes a response (wetting) under inappropriate stimulus conditions (bed).

The Improvement of Deficient Behavior

Lack of sphincter control over bowel or bladder elimination seems one of the most obvious behavioral deficits that can be corrected through the application of principles of learning. In addition to the use of bell-and-pad devices which, as pointed out, are largely based on the classical conditioning paradigm, a number of studies report training methods that explicitly apply operant principles. Thus, Hundziak, Maurer, and Watson (1965) trained 8 mentally retarded boys between the ages of 7 and 14 whose IQs ranged from 8 to 33 by systematically dispensing candy, paired with light and tone stimuli, contingent on defecation or urination in the commode. The children so treated showed a significant increase in appropriate toilet use compared to a group trained by conventional techniques and the newly established behavior generalized from the special training cottage to the boys' original living unit. Giles and Wolf (1966) report similar success with 5 severely retarded males. Their study points to the importance of finding suitable reinforcers for each subject. Although such reinforcers as candy are effective with many children, one should not assume that this is true for all. Giles and Wolf found one boy who refused candy but accepted baby food, while for others a ride in a wheelchair, taking a shower, or being permitted to return to bed had greater effectiveness. One important aspect of assessment is a careful and systematic analysis of reinforcer effectiveness. Unfortunately, behavior therapists often overlook this point and operate on the assumption that one standard reinforcer will be effective with all. Giles and Wolf (1966) also point out that training can be improved if, in addition to the positive reinforcement of desired responses, inappropriate behavior is followed by aversive stimuli.

They introduced punishment when exhaustive use of positive reinforcers produced no results. Punishment consisted of physical restraint, the removal of which contingent on appropriate toileting behavior also served as a negative reinforcer. With this combination of techniques, all 5 subjects consistently eliminated in the toilet.

In cases of mental retardation, an absence of toilet training is merely one aspect of pervasive lack of learning and the introduction of behavioral techniques thus largely represents an attempt to teach the retardate one socially highly desirable behavioral unit. The situation was somewhat different in the case reported by Gelber and Meyer (1965) who treated an almost 14-year-old boy with an IQ of 117 whose chronic encopresis represented the only area of behavioral deficit. The problem presumably dated from unsuccessful attempts at toilet training when the boy was 8 months old and was complicated by the fact that he appeared to enjoy handling his feces. Not using the toilet thus seemed to receive some reinforcement from what these writers call his "perversion." The boy was hospitalized in order to permit greater contingency control than would have been possible had he remained at home. In this case too it was necessary to find a suitable reinforcer, which turned out to be time off the ward, contingent on appropriate toilet behavior. It should be noted that this method represents a form of negative reinforcement in that an aversive condition (being confined to a hospital ward) is introduced, but terminated following a desired response. Conversely, reduction in time off the ward and loss of the privilege to have the freedom of the hospital grounds can serve as a form of punishment in a subject whose symbolic capacity is sufficient to relate cause and effect.

The case reported by Gelber and Meyer (1965) also serves to illustrate some of the complications that can arise during treatment and that require modifications of the procedures on an ad hoc basis. Having learned that defecation in the toilet resulted in being permitted to leave the ward, the boy would store feces in order to deposit them in the lavatory bowl when he wanted to obtain permission to leave the ward. This behavior was eliminated by permitting the boy to use earned time off the ward whenever he wished, thus introducing delay in reinforcement, a procedure possible only with a subject who can handle such abstractions as "credits earned" and "later in the day."

A behavioral deficit in many ways more crucial to social adaptation than lack of sphincter control is the absence of speech or gross deficiency in language as is frequently found in autistic children. Techniques based on the operant paradigm have been used by a number of therapists to establish speech in nonverbal or echolalic children. While speech is a highly complex behavior, it can be analyzed in operant terms in that the child emits a word or words and the social environment presents a reinforcing stimulus that can be made contingent on the verbal response. As in all operant behavior, the response must occur before it can be reinforced; the therapist can do little to elicit a word and the child must thus actively participate in the training process. When a child is totally nonverbal speech must be *shaped* by beginning with any vocalization and developing words by successive approximations. In a case reported by Hewett (1965) training in social imitation preceded speech training while Risley and Wolf (1967) were able to use the child's echolalic behavior as a starting point.

Children with as gross a disorder as absence of speech will usually also manifest other forms of deviant behavior that can interfere with attempts to develop language. Peter, the 4½-year-old boy described by Hewett (1965), was so highly distractible and had such a low attention span that it was necessary to train him in a specially constructed booth that reduced extraneous stimuli to a minimum and permitted the administration of isolation and darkness contingent on inappropriate responses. Candy and light served as reinforcers for appropriate responses. After 6 months of speech training Peter had acquired a 32-word vocabulary and after a further 8 months, during which generalization from the training booth to the outside environment was stressed, his speaking vocabulary had grown to 150, words which represented the beginnings of spoken language. What is of particular significance in this as in many similar treatment programs is that the initial, artificial reinforcement contingency is soon supplemented by the natural reinforcers dispensed by the social environment to a child whose behavior is acceptable and non-aversive. Thus, Peter's change in behavior altered the reactions of others toward him. The nursing staff sought him out for verbal interaction, gave him cues for imitation, and insisted on speech before granting requests. Similarly, the boy's family responded favorably to the newly acquired speech with his parents participating in the later phases of the training program. Because of the natural reinforcers the social environment provides for adaptive behavior, such artificial rewards as candy can gradually be phased out without bringing about extinction of the newly established behavior. Risley and Wolf (1967) point out that the generalization of appropriate speech from the therapy setting to the child's wider environment can be increased and enhanced if the therapist systematically reinforces speech under a variety of conditions. The child might thus be trained to respond appropriately to a variety of individuals, including members of his family, and in a variety of situations, such as his home or the family car.

Some Technical Considerations

Behavior that disrupts the acquisition of adaptive responses because it is incompatible with learning or with the response to be acquired, such as attending to stimuli other than those presented by the therapist (distractibility) or making repetitive responses (hyperactivity) must be eliminated before treatment can progress. In the summary of their research on the development of speech in echolalic children, Risley and Wolf (1967) illustrate the use of *time-out from positive reinforcement* (TO) in eliminating such disruptive behavior. Simply looking away until the child once again sits quietly in his chair is sufficient for bringing mildly disruptive behavior under control while more severe forms of incompatible responses can be dealt with by having the therapist leave the room for a set period, reentering only after the child has not engaged in the disruptive behavior for a short length of time. Reentering thus serves as a negative reinforcer for desired behavior since the child's isolation represents an aversive condition that is being terminated.

As was pointed out earlier, when the absence of a response is the desired behavior pattern, as in the case of hyperactivity, it is somewhat difficult to decide whether one is establishing missing behavior or reducing surplus behavior inasmuch as one is the reciprocal of the other. In studies reported by Patterson, Jones, Whittier, and Wright (1965) and by Patterson (1965) treatment of hyperactive children led to a decrease of such nonattending behaviors as arm and leg movements, shuffling of chair, looking out of window, fiddling, talking to self, and wiggling of feet. The method used, differential reinforcement of other behavior (DRO), called for the delivery of candy contingent on the "nonoccurrence of nonattending behavior." This somewhat awkward formulation is dictated by the focus on behavior that can be observed. Since it is possible to keep an objective and reliable record of such behaviors as fingering a box of crayons, while "paying attention" is not directly observable (although "eye contact" [Quay, Sprague, Werry, & McQueen, 1967] is), treatment can focus on the absence of the observable behavior and reinforcement is made contingent on the nonoccurrence of the defined event.

Patterson (1965) makes the important observation that reinforcement not only takes the form of such concrete objects as candy, pennies, or plastic soldiers, but that social reinforcement on the part of the teacher and peer groups who become more accepting toward the previously disruptive child also support treatment. This point is related to Ferster's (1967) distinction between arbitrary and natural reinforcers whereby natural reinforcement meets the current response repertoire of the child who thus continues to perform in a variety of situations from which his behavior receives reinforcement. The hypothesis has been advanced "that the importance of any change in behavior lies in the effect which it produces upon the reactions of the social culture" (Patterson et al., 1965). It is this reaction that serves to maintain socially desirable behavior after the reinforcements used during actual training have been withdrawn, and in the study just cited, this may account for the persistence of the positive effects of treatment throughout a four-week extinction phase (that is, a period during which the experimenter did not deliver any reinforcements).

Another feature of the Patterson studies that carries wider implications is that the reinforcement contingency was announced to the child and to the entire class. The child "was told that the apparatus was being used in an effort to teach him to sit still so that he could study better" while the announcement to the class stressed that when the boy sat still he would earn candy for himself and the rest of them. The latter reduced the amount of distraction offered by the peers and, in the earlier Patterson (1965) study, led to clapping and cheers at the end of a trial.

Doubros and Daniels (1966) take issue with Patterson's approach of announcing the contingencies to the child because it introduces uncontrolled social reinforcement and awareness, a point to which we shall return in a later section. In their own study on the reduction of hyperactive behavior in six mentally retarded boys, Doubros and Daniels attempted to control these awareness factors. Thanks to their controlled experiment, it is now possible to state that differential reinforcement of other behavior (DRO) is an effective method of reducing hyperactivity and increasing constructive play. On the other hand, Doubros and Daniels conducted their treatment in a playroom where each child was by himself and it is not known whether the responses learned there generalized to other settings. If treatment is conducted in the more immediately relevant, natural settings, such as the home or the classroom, generalization is greatly enhanced.

It should be emphasized that the behavioral approach to the treatment of hyperactive children does not inquire into the etiology of hyperactivity. If the aim is to reduce this undesirable, disruptive behavior, it is not necessary to ask whether its "cause" is "organic" or "functional." Doubros and Daniels (1966) state that their "results strongly indicate that irrespective of the origin or etiology of retarded mental growth, psychological treatment by operant techniques is not only possible within the playroom setting, but it can be very effective in reducing those obnoxious behavior patterns that have been traditionally thought of as an exclusively medical problem" (p. 257).

A clear-cut behavioral deficit, where the establishment of missing responses is the obvious approach to treatment, occurs in children who are nonreaders. Staats and Butterfield (1965) applied reinforcement principles in the treatment of a 14-year-old boy with a long history of school failures and delinquencies. At the beginning of treatment this boy was reading at the second grade level. Following 40 hours of training, he not only read at the 4.3 grade level, but he passed all of his courses for the first time and his misbehaviors in school decreased to zero. This not only demonstrates generalization of improvement to areas not specifically designated as treatment targets, but it also underscores that extrinsic reinforcers (in this boy's case, money) can be gradually decreased as reading itself becomes reinforcing and other sources of reinforcement take over to maintain the behavior.

Covert events are, by definition, not observable. This makes it difficult to ascertain whether a child who, as in the case of the Patterson (1965) studies, has learned not to engage in attention-incompatible behavior is actually attending when he is observed to be sitting still. Marr, Miller, and Straub (1966), for example, assumed they had conditioned "attention" with a psychotic girl when she spent increasing amounts of time in a marked-off floor area where her presence had been reinforced with tape recorded music. The assumption that she was attending to the sounds was supported by the fact that she made appropriate responses to their content. Increased attention can certainly be inferred from this behavior but it remains an inference. Similarly, the boy in the Staats and Butterfield (1965) study, was reinforced for silent reading, a behavior that cannot be directly monitored but inferred by subsequent changes in performance. As these authors point out, there is a danger in reinforcing the behavior of just looking at a printed page since the child may be doing nothing else. An attempt was made to overcome this possibility by use of a double contingency. There were several levels of reinforcers (tokens of different colors representing different monetary values of back-up reinforcers). For looking at the page a low-value reinforcer was presented while greater amounts of reinforcement were made contingent on answering questions related to the content of the reading material. Even here one cannot be entirely certain that the boy was indeed attending to and not merely staring at the printed words because the story used for silent reading, on which the questions were based, had previously been used for oral reading. It is thus barely conceivable that the boy had learned the answers to the questions during the readily monitored oral reading and then did no more than sit and look at the story during the silent reading phase.

In order to consider learning to read as operant discrimination learning, the learning task must be viewed as having the child emit the correct verbal response while looking at the written stimulus, with the response followed by reinforcement. No assumptions about the nature of cognitive processes are required. Using this frame of reference, Hewett, Mayhew, and Rabb (1967) taught basic reading skills to mentally retarded, neurologically impaired, emotionally disturbed, and autistic children. Their report illustrates the flexible use of reinforcement schedules as training progresses. For the first three lessions, reinforcement was on a continuous basis with one unit of reinforcement for each correct response. After these initial sessions, each subject went on a 1:5 schedule, having to make five correct responses before receiving one unit of reinforcement. At this point, reinforcements were tangibles (candy or money) but in addition, the experimenters began to phase in a token reward in the form of marks on a card which were given on a 1:1 ratio. Tangible reinforcers were later placed on a 1:10 schedule and ultimately, 200 check marks could be exchanged for one tangible reinforcer so that a 1:200 schedule with a delay until the end of the session was in operation.

The establishment of deficient behavior through the application of operant methods is obviously not limited to the behaviors discussed thus far. Lovaas et al. (1967) established nonverbal imitative behavior in schizophrenic children for whom the ability to imitate an adult was a necessary first step in the later acquisition of socially and intellectually useful behavior, such as personal hygiene, games, and appropriate sex-role behavior. A similar approach has been reported by Metz (1965) who found that imitation generalized to related tasks where specific imitation training had not been given. One of the most ambitious attempts to apply operant methods in the establishment of socially desirable behavior is found in the well-controlled study by Schwitzgebel (1967) who recruited 48 male adolescent delinquents from street corners and differentially reinforced positive statements, prompt arrival at work and "general employability." Positive consequences consisted of verbal praise and small gifts, delivered on a variable ratio schedule while the subject was talking into a tape recorder. The procedure resulted in significant improvements in the number of positive statements and arrival time in the subjects who had been specifically reinforced for these behaviors. The author concludes his presentation by pointing out that a series of interviews with an operant-conditioning orientation was capable of developing dependable and prompt attendance and certain other prosocial behaviors in juvenile delinquents and asks why this knowledge is not being put to systematic use in the large majority of treatment programs.

The Use of Social Reinforcement

The gross behavior deficits of autistic children have been treated by a number of therapists who succeeded in establishing previously missing response patterns in addition to language, which has already been discussed. Because children with severe psychological disorders not only lack adaptive responses but often also have not learned the secondary reinforcement value of such social stimuli as praise, therapists wishing to strengthen desirable behaviors must, initially, resort to the use of food as a primary reinforcer. This has two obvious disadvantages. It limits the situations in which learning can take place to those where the therapist can readily deliver food rewards and it requires that the child be in a state of relative deprivation so that food is an effective reinforcer. One of the therapeutic tasks is thus to establish the effectiveness of generalized social reinforcers which are ultimately the most frequently encountered reinforcers in a child's social environment. As was discussed in Chapter Five, Ferster (1961) developed the thesis that autistic children are not responsive to secondary and generalized reinforcers because of their parents' erratic reinforcement schedules. Presumably, the child has not been rewarded consistently with primary reinforcements to endow stimuli such as adult attention and praise with reinforcing properties. This formulation differs from that of Rimland (1964) who postulates a dysfunction of the central nervous system that interferes with the child's ability to associate primary reinforcements with accompanying social stimuli. Whichever formulation is correct, the therapist will have to address himself to the behavioral deficit in social reinforcer effectiveness and the question why the deficit exists becomes of secondary, largely theoretical interest.

The establishment of social reinforcers was the focus of a study by Lovaas, Freitag, Kinder, Rubinstein, Schaeffer, and Simmons (1966) who worked with two four-year-old identical twins, schizophrenics with marked autistic features. It is of considerable interest that for these children a social stimulus (the word "good") did not acquire reinforcer characteristics by its mere pairing with the delivery of food, the classical conditioning paradigm. In spite of several hundred trials of such pairing, there was no change in the child's behavior when that behavior was accompanied by the word "good"; it had failed to acquire secondary reinforcement properties. The child seemed oblivious to the stimulus, that is, he did not attend to it. The authors suggest that failure to attend to social stimuli may be a basic problem of autistic children. Since the organism must attend to, or orient toward a conditioned stimulus if learning is to occur, the failure of autistic children to learn may well be based on their deficient orienting behavior. If this assumption is correct, it would support Rimland's thesis according to which infantile autism is a cognitive defect based on dysfunction of the reticular formation. Contrary to Davison's (1965) conclusion, such an organic hypothesis does not lead to a pessimistic prognosis, it merely challenges the therapist to find a method of teaching the child despite his constitutional deficiency. Such a method may well take the form pioneered by Lovaas et al. (1966) who, after finding the classical paradigm to be ineffective in establishing a social reinforcer, successfully used the operant model to establish a discriminative social stimulus for the primary reinforcer. That is, the child learned that the presence of the social stimulus signaled the availability of food; the discriminative stimulus training thus forced the child to attend to the social stimulus, an attention that seemed impossible when the social stimulus had been merely paired with food. Once this discrimination had been established, it was possible to use the social stimulus alone (as an acquired reinforcer) to maintain a bar-pressing response. By using intermittent reinforcement these investigators were able to show that the social stimulus retained its acquired reinforcement property over extended sessions as long as it continued to be discriminative for food.

This careful study by Lovaas et al. (1966) not only lends strong support to the assumption that the basic problem of autistic children centers on their deficient attending behavior but it also explains why any treatment that does not remedy this deficit is unlikely to succeed. Conversely it strengthens the theoretical rationale underlying the successful attempts at treating autistic children with operant techniques which have been reported by Davison (1964; 1965), Wetzel, Baker, Roney, and Martin (1966), Wolf, Risley, Johnston, Harris, and Allen (1967), and Wolf, Risley, and Mees (1964).

The Modification of Maladaptive Behavior

When one wishes to establish previously deficient behavior, the techniques are limited to teaching the new response by respondent or operant conditioning. In the case of the modification of maladaptive behavior, the methods of treatment are many and they can be used alone or in combination. Behavior that is incompatible with the maladaptive responses can be strengthened (counterconditioning); the maladaptive response can be extinguished by changing the reinforcement contingencies; suppression of the target behavior can be established by introducing aversive consequences (punishment); the stimuli preceding the behavior in question can be eliminated or greatly increased (stimulus deprivation or satiation).

Avoidance Behavior

The treatment of children's fears through the use of conditioning methods dates to the pioneering study of Mary Cover Jones (1924) who gradually strengthened a response incompatible with fear, a method that has come to be known as counterconditioning or therapy by reciprocal inhibition. The work of Wolpe (1958) is best known in the field of adult disorders, while A. A. Lazarus (1960) has written extensively on eliminating children's phobias. The fear-incompatible response most frequently used in work with adults, relaxation, is rarely used in work with children, possibly because training in deep muscle relaxation is difficult with young subjects, whose cooperation and ability to make accurate verbal reports of their condition is essential. In view of this difficulty, Lazarus and Abramovitz (1965) explored the use of "emotive imagery," the induction of anxiety-inhibiting imagery with positive emotional content. These are classes of images that presumably arouse feelings of self-assertion, pride, affection, mirth, and fearlessness—feelings that would be incompatible with anxiety. The child is instructed to imagine such a fear-incompatible state which would vary in content from child to child and thus has to be ascertained through prior interviews. Once such imagery is aroused, the therapist presents mildly anxiety-eliciting images, working his way up the previously established anxiety hierarchy until the pleasant imagery is paired with the most highly anxiety-arousing stimulus. When treatment is successful, the child should then be making his "pleasant" response to the previously anxiety-producing situation, presented in imagery. While Lazarus and Abramovitz (1965) report success with this method, no systematic research on this approach is yet available and there remain many untested assumptions. For example, it is unknown whether the positive imagery is accompanied by an autonomic state that is indeed incompatible with fear as the concept of reciprocal inhibition would suppose, nor is it known whether the verbally presented imaginal stimuli really succeed in a CS pairing as the respondent conditioning paradigm, that is presumably operating, would demand. Until relevant autonomic measures can be brought to bear on studies of "emotive imagery" it must continue to be viewed as an interesting possibility.

The child who refuses to go to school engages in maladaptive, surplus behavior that must be eliminated. Such behavior is frequently labeled "school phobia" although either fear of school or fear of leaving the home can be manifested in school refusal, only the former being, strictly speaking, a phobia. Desensitization techniques have been used in cases labeled school phobia (Chapel, 1967; Garvey & Hegrenes, 1966) although, as Lazarus, Davison, and Polefka (1965) have pointed out, both respondent and operant factors enter into such treatment. This is particularly true when, as is usually the case, treatment takes place not in the consulting room, but in the real-life situation itself. Thus, Garvey and Hegrenes (1966) had the therapist and the child approach the school in a series of graded steps from the least anxiety-evoking situation (sitting in a car in front of the school) to the most powerful fear stimulus (being in the classroom with teacher and other students present). The authors refer to this procedure as desensitization, view it as similar to Wolpe's work, and describe it in terms of the respondent conditioning paradigm. What this clearly overlooks is the operant aspect of this approach whereby the therapist's implicit and explicit approval reinforces the approach behavior of the patient. Whether a particular approach to treatment follows the respondent or the operant paradigm might seem an esoteric theoretical issue, but as Lazarus, Davison, and Polefka (1965) have noticed, the systematic and deliberate application of both approaches enhances treatment and avoids antitherapeutic interventions.

It is most likely that cases of so-called school phobia, even when they originally were genuine fear-reducing avoidance responses to the stimulus complex of school, are later maintained and complicated by the reinforcements available to a child who is not in school. As a result, many school phobia cases become chronic and difficult to treat. On the basis of this reasoning, Kennedy (1965) developed a rapid treatment procedure lasting three days and involving immediate intervention and forced school attendance in carefully selected, acute cases. All 50 cases so treated over a period of 8 years responded with complete remission and follow-up failed to produce evidence for the emergence of other problems.

Secondary gains in the form of social reinforcement for avoidance behavior can complicate school refusal but, conversely, it is possible to use social reinforcement in the treatment of avoidance behavior. Thus, Hallsten (1965), in treating a 12-year-old girl who refused most foods for fear of gaining weight, not only desensitized this fear using relaxation but also made visits by the family to this hospitalized patient contingent on weight gain.

An interesting variation of desensitization therapy is reported by Straughan (1964) who treated an 8-year-old girl whose mother was concerned because the child "was not as happy as she should be." Further investigation revealed that the girl had learned to inhibit much of the age-appropriate spontaneous emotional expression in the presence of her mother. Treatment was thus directed at desensitizing the child's anxiety responses to her mother and took the form of introducing the mother into the child's presence while the child was playing happily and enthusiastically in the playroom. Over a period of 5 play sessions the child did indeed become relaxed in the mother's presence and the mother was able to learn to interact with the child in a spontaneous manner.

Avoidance behavior can also be reduced without exposing the subject to the feared stimulus either directly, as in in vivo desensitization, or in terms of imagery, by having the child observe another child making approach responses to the fear-arousing object. Bandura, Grusec, and Menlove (1967) showed that children who displayed fearful and avoidant behavior toward dogs would show stable and generalized reduction in avoidance behavior after having observed a peer model who fearlessly made progressively stronger approach responses toward a dog. While the existence of vicarious extinction is now supported by strong experimental evidence, the nature of the mechanism by which such extinction occurs is not yet established. While cognitive factors may play a role, this is probably minimal inasmuch as verbal reassurance about the harmlessness of a feared object did not serve to reduce the fears of the children in the control groups of the Bandura study. These authors speculate that the reduction in avoidance behavior is partly mediated by the elimination of conditioned emotionality, particularly in view of the fact that emotional responses can also be vicariously aroused by observing models in relevant situations.

When it is possible to ascertain the immediate consequences of a particular kind of maladaptive behavior, the operant paradigm suggests that this behavior is maintained by these consequences. Modification of the behavior can thus be brought about by removing or changing the consequences. Since by its very nature, maladaptive behavior tends to call attention to itself, this attention often appears to be the consequence that serves as a reinforcement. This contingency has been repeatedly demonstrated in nursery school settings where withdrawal of social attention on the part of adults successfully modified such problem behaviors as regressed crawling (Harris, Johnston, Kelley, & Wolf, 1965), socially isolate behavior (Allen, Hart, Buell, Harris, & Wolf, 1965), excessive crying and whining (Hart et al., 1965), and deficient motor skills (Johnston, Kelley, Harris, & Wolf, 1966). In each of these studies, adult attention was withdrawn from the target behavior and selectively given to behavior that was incompatible with it. Thus, the child who spent a great deal of time isolated from other children, was ignored when engaged in this behavior but was given adult attention when the child approached and joined the group. By experimentally reversing the contingencies and again strengthening isolate behavior after having established interaction with other children, these experimenters were able to show that adult attention was indeed the independent variable that was responsible for the behavior modification. This method makes it possible to evaluate the effectiveness of a particular reinforcement technique by using a subject as his own control and permits research in clinical situations where group data are difficult to obtain because of heterogeneous and limited populations.

Complex Behavior Patterns

The relatively benign problems of children enrolled in a university nursery school may be said to be easier to modify than the more serious and disruptive difficulties of children coming to the attention of therapists in clinics and hospitals. Yet the reinforcement principles used in the simpler cases have also been successfully applied with complex multiple problem behaviors (Patterson & Brodsky, 1966), in the treatment of stuttering (Browning, 1967; Rickard & Mundy, 1965), and in such difficult situations as the case of an autistic child (Wolf, Risley, & Mees, 1964) or of a child whose excessive scratching had resulted in large sores and scabs (Allen & Harris, 1966). In clinical work conducted under this writer's direction, operant methods have been applied to cases of "parent-child conflict," passive-dependent immaturity, refusal to do homework, poor school achievement, and school behavior problems, cases largely typical of those referred for help to child guidance clinics.

In cases where only one specific maladaptive behavior is the target of attempts at modification, the manipulation of one reinforcement contingency may be sufficient to bring about the desired improvement. Where several complex behavior patterns are to be modified, a more complex combination of treatment methods may be required but the basic principles involved remain the same. Thus, in the case of Dicky, a variety of contingencies had to be manipulated and not only conditioning and extinction procedures but also a form of aversive control had to be brought to bear (Wolf, Risley, & Mees, 1964; Wolf, Risley, Johnston, Harris, & Allen, 1967). Dicky was a 3½-year-old boy with the diagnosis of childhood schizophrenia who engaged in self-destructive behavior such as head-banging, face-slapping, hair-pulling, and face-scratching. He refused to sleep alone, did not eat normally, and lacked adaptive social and verbal repertoires. Because of cataracts, he had to have the lenses of both eyes removed and since he refused to wear his glasses, he was in danger of incurring permanent retinal damage. Beginning with the most immediately serious problem, the refusal to wear and throwing of his eye glasses, the therapists worked with this child's various problems over a period of 3 years and succeeded in modifying his behavior to the point where he was able to attend a special education class in public school where he made a good adjustment and learned to read at the primary level.

The wearing of Dicky's glasses was established by reinforcing this behavior initially with food and later with walks, rides, play, and snacks. In order to control the boy's frequent throwing of his glasses on the floor, the therapists devised a mild form of punishment consisting of putting Dicky in his room for 10 minutes following each glasses-throw. The same method was used to eliminate tantrums, self-slapping, and pinching of other children and teachers in nursery school. This particular form of punishment is actually a time-out from positive reinforcement if being in the company of others is viewed as positively reinforcing. Wolf, Risley, and Mees (1964) clearly demonstrated the effectiveness of this technique in the case of Dicky by the experimental test of reversing contingencies. After the time-out procedure was instituted, glasses-throwing, which had occurred at the rate of approximately twice a day, decreased to zero within 5 days. When the contingencies were reversed, that is, when he was no longer put in his room for throwing the glasses, the rate resumed its earlier high level after about 3 weeks. When he was once again put in his room for this behavior, it quickly declined and 6 days later, virtually disappeared. Wolf and Risley (1967) pointed out that these data represent a design for analyzing the reliability of a treatment procedure. First, a base line for the frequency, intensity, or duration of the particular target behavior is established. Reinforcement contingencies are then changed and when the occurrence of the target behavior has been modified as reflected in continued quantitative recordings, the reinforcement contingencies that had existed before the intervention are reinstituted. If the observed change resulted from the variable being manipulated, the behavior should become reinstated at or near the base rate level. Finally, inasmuch as the aim of the treatment procedure is to modify the behavior in the desired direction, the therapeutic contingencies are once again introduced and maintained until the adaptive behavior has reached a stable level.

It is obvious that the ABAB design described above can only be carried out if a careful quantitative record of the incidence of the target behavior is maintained. That the need for careful recording goes beyond the requirements of testing the efficacy of a procedure is illustrated in the report by Wolf, Risley, Johnston, Harris, and Allen (1967), which deals with further work with the boy, Dicky. Shortly after Dicky had been enrolled in nursery school following the hospitalization during which some of the more bizarre behavior had been modified, he developed a high rate of pinching other children and teachers. When ignoring this behavior failed to change its rate, Dicky was sent to "his room," a small room made available for this special purpose, whenever he engaged in pinching. The rate of pinching drastically declined after the first use of this time-out procedure, there being only four more instances of it over the next 74 class sessions. During an earlier class session and before the introduction of the time-out procedure, a teacher had attempted to deal with the pinching by reinforcing an incompatible behavior, patting. This consisted of a combination of patting and stroking and the teacher encouraged and praised Dicky for doing this instead of pinching. Patting behavior stabilized at a moderate rate within a few sessions and the teachers reported that they were succeeding in substituting patting for pinching. Contrary to this impression, the record maintained by an observer who scored each ten-second interval containing patting as well as pinching, clearly showed that there was no decrease in pinching and that, in fact, this did not decline in rate until the time-out procedure was instituted some 13 sessions later. Had it not been for the quantified observer record, the teachers would have erroneously concluded that the decrease of the undesirable behavior was a function of the development of a substitute response. Such an erroneous conclusion would be particularly harmful when, as was the case with Dicky, parents are to be instructed in carrying out aspects of the treatment regime at home.

One of the unique attributes of behavior therapy based on operant techniques is that the actual treatment can be conducted by lay people working under the direction of a professional person who has expert knowledge of the theoretical basis and can devise the details of the treatment program. Thus, ward attendants, nursery school teachers, and parents were involved in the treatment of Dicky. Hawkins, Peterson, Schweid, and Bijou (1966) used the mother in the role of therapist treating her own child, a four-year-old who was extremely difficult to manage and control. He would kick objects and people, tear at his clothing, hit himself, and generally demand almost constant attention. The mother was instructed in the differential use of verbal commands to stop; praise, attention, and affectionate physical contact; and placing the boy in his room. Gestural signals by the professional therapist were used to indicate to the mother when she was to display what kind of behavior, inasmuch as the mother seemed to find it difficult, at least initially, to recognize incipient stages of undesirable behavior and to respond to it in a consistent manner. A similar approach to using mothers as behavior therapists for their own children was reported by Wahler, Winkel, Peterson, and Morrison (1965) and O'Leary, O'Leary, and Becker (1967) report on work involving deviant interaction between two siblings. In the latter case, treatment involved the reinforcement of desirable interaction between the two boys and a time-out (TO) procedure (isolation in the bathroom) for defined deviant behavior.

The O'Leary, O'Leary, and Becker report (1967) makes the important point that human subjects in a treatment situation can be instructed about the contingencies. Thus, the two boys were told that they would receive candy or tokens which could be exchanged for back-up reinforcers, "if they said 'Please' and 'Thank you,' if they answered each other's questions, and if they played nicely together." Similarly, the TO was spelled out as being the consequence of kicking, hitting, pushing, name-calling, and throwing objects at each other. Verbal instructions of this nature were also used in the Patterson (1965) study discussed earlier. This would seem an obvious procedure when working therapeutically with a child but to the psychologist trained in laboratory conditioning techniques, they represent a novel departure because in laboratory work with human subjects, such instructions would confound the experiment, making it impossible to tell whether a newly established response is the function of the independent variable used during conditioning or the result of the subject's attempt to comply with the experimenter's expressed intention. As long as it is necessary to test the effectiveness of a specific therapeutic procedure, a verbal explication of the contingencies will indeed confound the experiment, but where a therapeutic program has progressed beyond the experimental stage, anything that will enhance treatment process, such as verbal instructions, should certainly not be shunned.

Aversive Control

The self-injurious behavior found in such grossly disordered children as Dicky represents a challenge to reinforcement theory because it consists of responses that are consistently and immediately followed by an aversive condition (pain) and should thus become quickly suppressed. Yet, in an apparent paradox, the behavior continues, interfering with the production of responses that might receive positive reinforcement, and often leading to the real risk of severe and permanent physical damage, such as injury to the head and eyes. The paradox has led some to assume that the child "enjoys" hurting himself, or that he has a "need" to punish himself. But this attempt at an explanation is vitiated by reports of Wolf, Risley, and Mees (1964); Lovaas, Freitag, Gold, and Kassorla (1965); and Tate and Baroff (1966) who were able to reduce the incidence of self-injurious behavior by aversive control, that is by the administration of consequences that would be viewed as punishment. If the self-injurious child indeed sought punishment, then the administration of punishment contingent on his hurting himself, should increase, instead of decrease such behavior.

Lovaas, Freitag, Gold, and Kassorla (1965) analyzed self-injurious behavior and concluded that it is maintained not by the "pleasure" the child gets out of hurting himself, but by the reinforcement inherent in the social attention that is almost invariably the consequence of such behavior. They showed that self-injurious behavior is decreased when it is ignored but increased when it is followed by some "interpretive" comments such as "I don't think you are bad." The extinction procedure involved in ignoring self-injurious behavior, while effective, is a slow process requiring more time than the risk of permanent physical harm tends to allow, particularly in view of the fact that response rate increases in the initial phase of extinction. For this reason, both Lovaas and his co-workers (1965) and Tate and Baroff (1966) stress the effectiveness of the rapid response suppression possible through the use of electric shock contingent on self-injurious responses and combined with positive reinforcement of adaptive behavior. Because of the previously discussed complications inherent in the use of physical punishment, it is obvious that such procedures should be used only when the alternatives are permanent physical damage, such as retinal detachment as with the boy treated by Tate and Baroff, or gross interference with attempts to teach adaptive behavior, as was the case with Dicky and the children treated by Lovaas and his colleagues.

In most instances where particular responses in a child's repertoire are to be weakened, the negative consequences involved in social isolation or deprivation of privileges (time-out from positive reinforcement) appears to be a potent manipulation. Even the behavior of institutionalized adolescent delinquents, usually so intractable, can be modified by the use of a 15-minute period of isolation, when it is introduced immediately and consistently following every instance of clearly defined undesirable acts (Tyler & Brown, 1967). The antisocial behavior of a 13-year-old institutionalized delinquent boy was reduced through the use of isolation combined with positive reinforcement delivered for specified periods that he did not have to spend in isolation (Burchard & Tyler, 1965). Stealing would seem to be a behavior that is particularly difficult to treat because it carries its own inherent reinforcement, yet Wetzel (1966) succeeded in eliminating stealing behavior in an institutionalized boy through the use of a time-out procedure. In that case, it was first necessary to create a condition of positive reinforcement (the privilege of visiting the institution cook) in order to have something that could be withdrawn contingent on the boy's stealing small objects from other children or staff.

The fact that such relatively mild punishment as being sent to an empty room for 15 minutes is effective with delinquents with whom far more severe forms of punishment have usually failed, represents an apparent paradox. The boy treated by Burchard and Tyler (1965), for example, had spent a total of 200 days in an individual isolation room during the year prior to the onset of the reported study, yet his behavior had become increasingly more unmanageable. The answer to this apparent paradox seems to lie in the fact that a systematic application of operant principles stresses the *immediate* introduction of the negative consequence *whenever* unacceptable behavior occurs. In an unsystematic use of punishment, the unacceptable behavior usually has to reach a certain magnitude before the adult environment intervenes and even then intervention is usually such that punishment is introduced "as a last resort." What occurs between the incipient onset of the unacceptable behavior and the ultimate introduction of the negative consequences by and large tends to reinforce rather than suppress the behavior. This seems to have been the case with Donny where Burchard and Tyler (1965) describe the temporal sequence of staff reactions to his increasingly more disruptive behavior as follows: At first there were efforts to ignore the behavior for as long as possible during which time peer approval and attention tend to act as reinforcers. Staff would then turn to attempts at supportive persuasion to desist, followed by frustration, ambivalence, expression of anger, and—finally—the administration of punishment which was, in turn, followed by guilt reactions manifesting themselves in sympathy and visits to the boy in isolation. In view of the fact that the unacceptable behavior increased under these conditions, it would seem that they served as reinforcers largely because the staff and peer attention occurred immediately after the response while punishment was delayed. In contrast, the approach instituted by Burchard and Tyler involved having Donny immediately and perfunctorily placed in his isolation room upon displaying any unacceptable behavior. The instructions to the staff stressed the importance of a matter-of-fact approach without becoming emotionally involved and pointed out that isolation had to be on an all-or-none basis, that it should never be used as a threat. There is every reason to believe that it is the difference between this approach and the usual behavior of mothers or attendants that spells the difference between successful use of punishment and its failure.

Contingency Control

Most of the reports on behavior therapy with children emanate from institutional settings. This is at least in part, a function of the fact that therapists working in institutions have better control over the contingencies of reinforcement and more complete access to the variety of responses a child emits in the course of a day. Therapists or their surrogates among the institution staff can observe the child almost all of the time and they are able to give or withhold food, privileges, and activities depending on the child's behavior. Since none of this is available in a clinic situation where a child comes for only brief periods of time, the therapist working in such a setting must count on the child's parents to manage the contingencies, that is, to be the actual therapists. This requires that he first train the parents in the essential techniques, as was done by Hawkins et al. (1966) and O'Leary, O'Leary, and Becker (1967), but inasmuch as the basic principles of the operant approach are easily understood, this is often easier than one might at first suppose. An important aspect of using the parents as contingency managers is that they keep a detailed and accurate, quantifiable record of the child's behavior since this not only permits supervision of the program by the therapist but also tends to reinforce the parents' therapeutic behavior by demonstrating their progress.

Contingency control exerted during most of the child's day is of particular importance where behavior of relatively low frequency, such as stealing, fighting, or fire-setting is to be brought under control. In cases where a behavior that is deficient is to be established, as in the case of language or social cooperation, intermittent treatment sessions by the therapist in the clinic setting is more feasible. The same is true of responses that can be evoked at will by the therapist's verbal instructions so that treatment based on the respondent conditioning paradigm is more easily carried out in a consulting room.

Evaluative Research

Although the behavioral approach to the treatment of psychological disorders in adults has been tested by several well-controlled experimental studies that demonstrate its effectiveness (Lang, Lazovik, & Reynolds, 1965; Paul, 1966a, 1967; Paul & Shannon, 1966), most of the experimental support for behavior therapy with children comes from using the ABAB design where the subject is his own control (e.g., Hart et al., 1965; Hawkins et al., 1966; Wolf & Risley, 1967). This research design demonstrates the effectiveness of a particular intervention procedure, but it does not permit one to answer the question whether the procedure is more effective than some other, more traditional approach or, for that matter, no intervention at all. Some reports, such as that published by Burchard and Tyler (1965), show that a given child's behavior did not improve, or, in fact, deteriorated under different forms of treatment, but that positive changes occurred when a behavioral approach was instituted. Other reports such as that by Patterson, Jones,

Whittier, and Wright (1965) compare one experimental child with one control child, thus illustrating the effectiveness of an intervention. Case studies of this nature are often dramatic, but since they may well represent a selected and biased sample from the total population of treated cases, they cannot be adduced as evidence for the effectiveness of behavior therapy, let alone for its superiority over other techniques.

The reasons for the dearth of well-controlled outcome studies are well-known. As Bergin (1966) and Paul (1967b) have pointed out, the requirements of meaningful outcome research are difficult to meet. Relevant control groups are hard to find, therapies and therapists are difficult to equate, a sufficient number of subjects with the same problem behavior is rarely available, and objective criterion measures are often unacceptable or irrelevant to therapists of a different theoretical orientation.

Enuresis is a problem behavior that is readily operationalized and objectively measured. It has a sufficient frequency in the child population to permit a researcher to obtain a reasonably large number of subjects. Withholding treatment for enuresis from a child for a period of months in order to have him in a control group does not endanger him or others and thus does not raise major ethical qualms. Finally, the behavioral treatment of enuresis entails a well-developed conditioning technique that requires minimal activity on the part of the therapist so that he can treat a relatively large number of children during a reasonably limited period of time. For all these reasons, the best outcome research available deals with the conditioning treatment of bedwetting.

De Leon and Mandell (1966), Baker (1967), and Lovibond (1964) are among those who compared conditioning treatment with other modes of therapy for enuresis, and in all instances the children treated by the bell-and-buzzer conditioning method reached the cure criterion earlier than those treated by other methods or held in a no-treatment control group. Details of these studies have been presented earlier and will not be repeated here.

The effectiveness of an approach based on the operant paradigm compared to more traditional treatment and no treatment was reported by Clement and Milne (1967). By asking all third-grade teachers in a school district to refer boys who were socially withdrawn, nonspontaneous, and friendless, these authors were able to obtain 11 children who were assigned to one of three conditions: A Token group, a Therapist group, and a Control group. The children in the Token group participated in one weekly 50-minute group play session for 14 weeks and received token reinforcements for social-approach behavior. The Therapist group received the same treatment as the Token group but no tangible reinforcers were used. The Control group met in the playroom without a therapist but was observed through a one-way mirror.

The dependent variables were measures of productivity, anxiety, social adjustment, general psychological adjustment, and discrete problem behaviors. Some of these measures were based on observations, others on tests and mothers' reports. The analysis of the results showed the Token group to have improved on four measures, while the Therapist group improved on two and worsened on one. The Control group did not show any improvement. The measure on which the Therapist group decreased while the Token group increased was Social Play, the amount of time the children spent playing with each other. Since this was one of the behaviors that had been specifically reinforced, this finding strengthens the authors' conclusion that operant reinforcement is effective in treating shy, withdrawn eight-year-old boys in a group situation. At the same time, it should be recalled that the study had several weaknesses that the authors readily acknowledge. The therapist was the same for both groups and he was aware of the hypotheses being tested. Furthermore, the sample size was small and represented only one type of problem so that generalization to other problems is limited.

The only study that systematically compared behavior therapy with traditional psychotherapy and a no-treatment condition is one conducted by James Humphrey and cited by Eysenck (1967). Subjects were 71 children who had been referred to child guidance clinics for a variety of disorders, except brain damage and psychosis. A control group of 34 of these children was evaluated at the beginning and again at the end of the study, but received no treatment of any kind. Of the remaining children, one group was treated by behavior therapy, using a desensitization approach, while the other group received traditional psychotherapy. The children were evaluated for severity of disorder using a five-point rating scale which served as the criterion measure. "Cure" was defined as a rise of two or more points on this scale, the evaluation being conducted by clinicians who did not know to which group a given child had been assigned.

In each case treatment was terminated when the therapist and a consulting psychiatrist decided that the child had received maximum benefit. On this basis, the children in psychotherapy were in treatment for 21 sessions spread over 31 weeks, while those receiving behavior therapy required nine sessions during 18 weeks. On the basis of the criterion measure used, 75% of the children in behavior therapy were rated cured at the close of treatment, as compared to 35% of those who received psychotherapy. At follow-up ten months later, the percentage of those rated cured was 85% for the behavior therapy group, while among those who had received psychotherapy only 29% were still considered cured. Of the children in the no-treatment control group, 18% were found to be cured when they were reevaluated at the ten-month follow-up.

While this unpublished study appears to favor behavior therapy, its several flaws detract from the validity of the conclusions. A bias in the sampling had served to assign a larger population of the more seriously disturbed children to the behavior therapy group than to the psychotherapy group. The latter group thus began treatment with a higher clinical status rating, so that a ceiling effect made it less likely for them to achieve the two-point rise necessary to meet the cure criterion. Furthermore, a five-point rating scale would seem to lack the sensitivity necessary to detect changes in a child's behavior and the unusually brief time devoted to psychotherapy makes one wonder whether this form of treatment was represented in its most typical form.

A definitive experimental comparison of behavior therapy and psychotherapy with children thus remains to be carried out. At the same time, one might question the necessity of proving the superiority of one form of treatment over another. Available studies would seem to attest to the effectiveness of behavior therapy with the kind of problems on which it has been tried. Rather than spending research effort on the question whether one form of treatment is superior to another, it would seem more efficient to investigate what kinds of problems are best treated by which kind of therapy. It is unlikely that behavior therapy, as presently conceived and practiced, is the treatment of choice for every conceivable form of psychological disorder and it is to be hoped that, in addition to the conditioning and social learning paradigms now applied in treatment, other aspects of psychology, such as the study of cognitive processes, modeling procedures (Bandura, 1965), developmental phenomena, physiological correlates, and group dynamics, will eventually be brought to bear on clinical problems.

As we have seen in Chapter Six, another area in which research efforts would be well spent is the development of assessment techniques relevant to behavior therapy with children. As Goodkin (1967) has noted, there is a dearth of methods designed to select appropriate target behaviors, appropriate treatment methods, and suitable reinforcers. Objective measures for the evaluation of behavior changes must be developed and means must be devised to permit the assessment of the generalization of treatment effects. At present, each therapist is reduced to discovering appropriate techniques for each individual case. Giles and Wolf (1966), as pointed out earlier, had to discover specific reinforcers for each of the children in their study. Premack (1959) has pointed out that responses with high probability serve to reinforce responses with lower probability. It is thus necessary to find some means by which the relative probability of responses can be assessed.

Since the reactions of the social environment are an important source of reinforcement, adequate assessment for behavior therapy should also include data on the kind of reactions being elicited from others and the kind of behaviors that elicit these reactions. This point was stressed by Patterson, Jones, Whittier, and Wright (1965), who suggest that if it were possible to select for modification that response which is most likely to effect a change in the reactions of the peer group, treatment might be enhanced through the generalization of its effects. Instead of devising a treatment procedure to modify each of the child's responses singly and separately, the therapist could maximize his effectiveness by selecting for treatment that response which holds the most crucial position in the response hierarchy.

References

Allen, K. E., & Harris, F. R. Elimination of a child's excessive scratching by training the mother in reinforcement procedures. *Behaviour Research and Therapy,* 1966, **4**, 79–84.

Allen, K. E., Hart, B. M., Buell, J. S., Harris, F. R., & Wolf, M. M. Effects of social reinforcement on isolate behavior of a nursery school child. In L. P. Ullmann & L. Krasner (Eds.), 1965, pp. 307–312.

Baker, B. L. Symptom treatment and symptom substitution in enuresis. Paper presented at the 1st annual meeting of the Association for Advancement of the Behavioral Therapies, Washington, D.C., 1967.

Bandura, A. Behavioral modification through modeling procedures. In L. Krasner and L. P. Ullmann (Eds.), 1965, pp. 310–340.

Bandura, A., Grusec, J. E., & Menlove, F. L. Vicarious extinction of avoidance behavior. *Journal of Personality and Social Psychology,* 1967, **5**, 16–23.

Baum, M. Rapid extinction of an avoidance response following a period of response prevention on the avoidance apparatus. *Psychological Reports,* 1966, **18**, 59–64.

Bergin, A. E. Some implications of psychotherapy research for therapeutic practice. *Journal of Abnormal Psychology,* 1966, **71**, 235–246.

Browning, R. M. Behavior therapy for stuttering, in a schizophrenic child. *Behaviour Research and Therapy,* 1967, **5**, 27–35.

Burchard, J., & Tyler, V., Jr. The modification of delinquent behavior through operant conditioning. *Behaviour Research and Therapy,* 1965, **2**, 245–250.

Chapel, J. L. Treatment of a case of school phobia by reciprocal inhibition. *Canadian Psychiatric Association Journal,* 1967, **21**, 25–28.

Clement, P. W., & Milne, D. C. Group play therapy and tangible reinforcers used to modify the behavior of eight-year-old boys. *Proceedings of the 75th Annual Convention of the APA,* 1967, **2**, 241–242.

Davison, G. C. A social learning therapy programme with an autistic child. *Behaviour Research and Therapy,* 1964, **2**, 149–159.

Davison, G. C. An intensive long-term social-learning treatment program with an accurately diagnosed autistic child. In American Psychological Association, *Proceedings of the 73rd Annual Convention,* 1965.

De Leon, G., & Mandell, W. A comparison of conditioning and psychotherapy in the treatment of functional enuresis. *Journal of Clinical Psychology,* 1966, **22,** 326–330.

Doubros, S. C., & Daniels, G. J. An experimental approach to the reduction of over-active behavior. *Behaviour Research and Therapy,* 1966, **4,** 251–258.

Eysenck, H. J. New ways in psychotherapy. *Psychology Today,* 1967, **1,** 39–47.

Ferster, C. B. Positive reinforcement and behavioral deficits of autistic children. *Child Development,* 1961, **32,** 437–456.

Ferster, C. B. Arbitrary and natural reinforcement. *Psychological Record,* 1967, **17,** 341–347.

Garvey, W. P., & Hegrenes, J. R. Desensitization techniques in the treatment of school phobia. *American Journal of Orthopsychiatry,* 1966, **36,** 147–152.

Gelber, H., & Meyer, V. Behaviour therapy and encopresis: The complexities involved in treatment. *Behaviour Research and Therapy,* 1965, **2,** 227–231.

Giles, D. K., & Wolf, M. M. Toilet training institutionalized severe retardates: An application of operant behavior modification techniques. *American Journal of Mental Deficiency,* 1966, **70,** 766–780.

Goodkin, R. Some neglected issues in the literature on behavior therapy. *Psychological Reports,* 1967, **20,** 415–420.

Hallsten, E. A., Jr. Adolescent anorexia nervosa treated by desensitization. *Behaviour Research and Therapy,* 1965, **3,** 87–91.

Harris, F. R., Johnston, M. K., Kelley, C. S., & Wolf, M. M. Effects of positive social-reinforcement on regressed crawling of a nursery school child. In L. P. Ullmann & L. Krasner (Eds.), 1965, pp. 313–319.

Hart, B. M., Allen, K. E., Buell, J. S., Harris, F. R., & Wolf, M. M. Effects of social reinforcement on operant crying. In L. P. Ullmann & L. Krasner (Eds.), 1965, pp. 320–325.

Hawkins, R. P., Peterson, R. F., Schweid, E., & Bijou, S. W. Behavior therapy in the home: Amelioration of problem parent-child relations with the parent in a therapeutic role. *Journal of Experimental Child Psychology,* 1966, **4,** 99–107.

Hewett, F. M. Teaching speech to an autistic child through operant conditioning. *American Journal of Orthopsychiatry,* 1965, **35,** 927–936.

Hewett, F. M., Mayhew, D., & Rabb, E. An experimental reading program for neurologically impaired, mentally retarded, and severely emotionally disturbed children. *American Journal of Orthopsychiatry,* 1967, **37,** 35–48.

Hundziak, M., Maurer, R. A., & Watson, L. S., Jr. Operant conditioning in toilet training of severely mentally retarded boys. *American Journal of Mental Deficiency,* 1965, **70,** 120–124.

Johnston, M. K., Kelley, C. S., Harris, F. R., & Wolf, M. M. An application of reinforcement principles to development of motor skills of a young child. *Child Development,* 1966, **37,** 379–387.

Jones, M. C. A laboratory study of fear: The case of Peter. *Journal of Genetic Psychology,* 1924, **31,** 308–315.

Kennedy, W. A. School phobia: Rapid treatment of fifty cases. *Journal of Abnormal Psychology,* 1965, **70,** 285–289.

Krasner, L., & Ullmann, L. P. (Eds.). *Research in Behavior Modification.* New York: Holt, Rinehart, and Winston, 1965.

Lang, P. J., Lazovik, A. D., & Reynolds, D. J. Desensitization, suggestibility, and pseudotherapy. *Journal of Abnormal Psychology,* 1965, **70,** 395–402.

Lazarus, A. The elimination of children's phobias by deconditioning. In H. J. Eysenck (Ed.) *Behavior Therapy and the Neuroses.* New York: Pergamon Press, 1960.

Lazarus, A. A., & Abramovitz, A. The use of "emotive imagery" in the treatment of children's phobias. In L. P. Ullmann & L. Krasner (Eds.), 1965, pp. 300–304.

Lazarus, A. A., Davison, G. C., & Polefka, D. A. Classical and operant factors in the treatment of a school phobia. *Journal of Abnormal Psychology,* 1965, **70,** 225–229.

Lovaas, O. I., Freitag, G., Gold, V. J., & Kassorla, I. C. Experimental studies in childhood schizophrenia: Analysis of self-destructive behavior. *Journal of Experimental Child Psychology,* 1965, **2,** 67–84.

Lovaas, O. I., Freitag, G., Kinder, M. I., Rubenstein, B. D., Schaeffer, B., & Simmons, J. Q. Establishment of social reinforcers in two schizophrenic children on the basis of food. *Journal of Experimental Child Psychology,* 1966, **4,** 109–125.

Lovaas, O. I., Freitas, L., Nelson, K., & Whalen, C. The establishment of imitation and its use for the development of complex behavior in schizophrenic children. *Behaviour Research and Therapy,* 1967, **5,** 171–181.

Lovibond, S. H. The mechanism of conditioning treatment of enuresis. *Behaviour Research and Therapy,* 1963, **1,** 17–21.

Lovibond, S. H. *Conditioning and Enuresis.* Oxford: Pergamon Press, 1964.

Marr, J. N., Miller, E. R., & Straub, R. R. Operant conditioning of attention with a psychotic girl. *Behaviour Research and Therapy,* 1966, **4,** 85–87.

Marshall, H. H. The effect of punishment on children: A review of the literature and a suggested hypothesis. *Journal of Genetic Psychology,* 1965, **106,** 23–33.

Martin, B., & Kubly, D. Results of treatment of enuresis by a conditioned response method. *Journal of Consulting Psychology,* 1955, **19,** 71–73.

Metz, J. R. Conditioning generalized imitation in autistic children. *Journal of Experimental Child Psychology,* 1965, **2,** 389–399.

Mowrer, O. H., & Mowrer, W. M. Enuresis—a method for its study and treatment. *American Journal of Orthopsychiatry,* 1938, **8,** 436–459.

Neale, D. H. Behaviour research and encopresis in children. *Behaviour Research and Therapy,* 1963, **1,** 139–149.

Novick, J. Symptomatic treatment of acquired and persistent enuresis. *Journal of Abnormal Psychology,* 1966, **71,** 363–368.

O'Leary, K. D., O'Leary, S., & Becker, W. C. Modification of a deviant sibling interaction pattern in the home. *Behaviour Research and Therapy,* 1967, **5,** 113–120.

Patterson, G. An application of conditioning techniques to the control of a hyperactive child. In L. P. Ullmann & L. Krasner (Eds.), *Case Studies in Behavior Modification.* New York: Holt, Rinehart, and Winston, 1965, pp. 370–375.

Patterson, G. R., & Brodsky, G. A behavior modification programme for a child with multiple problem behaviors. *Journal of Child Psychology and Psychiatry,* 1966, **7,** 277–295.

Patterson, G. R., Jones, R., Whittier, J., & Wright, M. A. A behaviour modification technique for the hyperactive child. *Behaviour Research and Therapy*, 1965, **2**, 217–226.

Paul, G. L. *Insight vs. Desensitization in Psychotherapy.* Stanford, California: Stanford University Press, 1966.

Paul, G. L. Insight versus desensitization in psychotherapy two years after termination. *Journal of Consulting Psychology*, 1967a, **31**, 333–348.

Paul, G. L. Strategy of outcome research in psychotherapy. *Journal of Consulting Psychology*, 1967b, **31**, 109–118.

Paul, G. L., & Shannon, D. T. Treatment of anxiety through systematic desensitization in therapy groups. *Journal of Abnormal Psychology*, 1966, **71**, 124–135.

Premack, D. Toward empirical behavior laws: I. Positive reinforcement. *Psychological Review*, 1959, **66**, 219–233.

Quay, H. C., Sprague, R. L., Werry, J. S., & McQueen, M. Conditioning visual orientation of conduct problem children in the classroom. *Journal of Experimental Child Psychology*, 1967, **5**, 512–517.

Rescorla, R. A., & Solomon, R. L. Two-process learning theory: Relationships between Pavlovian conditioning and instrumental learning. *Psychological Review*, 1967, **74**, 151–182.

Rickard, H. C., & Mundy, M. B. Direct manipulation of stuttering behavior: An experimental-clinical approach. In L. P. Ullmann & L. Krasner (Eds.), *Case Studies in Behavior Modification.* New York: Holt, Rinehart, and Winston, 1966.

Rimland, B. *Infantile Autism; The syndrome and Its Implications for a Neural Theory of Behavior.* New York: Appleton-Century-Crofts, 1964.

Risley, T., & Wolf, M. Establishing functional speech in echolalic children. *Behaviour Research and Therapy*, 1967, **5**, 73–88.

Schwitzgebel, R. L. Short-term operant conditioning of adolescent offenders on socially relevant variables. *Journal of Abnormal Psychology*, 1967, **72**, 134–142.

Skinner, B. F. *Science and Human Behavior.* New York: Free Press, 1953 (paperback, 1965).

Staats, A. W., & Butterfield, W. H. Treatment of nonreading in a culturally deprived juvenile delinquent: An application of reinforcement principles. *Child Development*, 1965, **36**, 925–942.

Straughan, J. H. Treatment with child and mother in the playroom. *Behaviour Research and Therapy*, 1964, **2**, 37–41.

Tate, B. G., & Baroff, G. S. Aversive control of self-injurious behavior in a psychotic boy. *Behaviour Research and Therapy*, 1966, **4**, 281–287.

Tyler, V. O., Jr., & Brown, G. D. The use of swift, brief isolation as a group control device for institutionalized delinquents. *Behaviour Research and Therapy*, 1967, **5**, 1–9.

Ullmann, L. P., & Krasner, L. (Eds.). *Case Studies in Behavior Modification.* New York: Holt, Rinehart, and Winston, 1965.

Wahler, R. G., Winkel, G. H., Peterson, R. F., & Morrison, D. C. Mothers as behavior therapists for their own children. *Behaviour Research and Therapy*, 1965, **3**, 113–124.

Werry, J. S. The conditioning treatment of enuresis. *American Journal of Psychiatry*, 1966, **123**, 226–229.

Wetzel, R. Use of behavioral techniques in a case of compulsive stealing. *Journal of Consulting Psychology*, 1966, **30**, 367–374.

Wetzel, R. J., Baker, J., Roney, M., & Martin, M. Outpatient treatment of autistic behavior. *Behaviour Research and Therapy*, 1966, **4**, 169–177.

Wolf, M., & Risley, T. Analysis and modification of deviant child behavior. Paper presented at American Psychological Association meeting, Washington, D.C.: 1967.

Wolf, M., Risley, T., Johnston, M., Harris, F., & Allen, E. Application of operant conditioning procedures to the behavior problems of an autistic child: A follow-up and extension. *Behaviour Research and Therapy*, 1967, **5**, 103–111.

Wolf, M., Risley, T., & Mees, H. Application of operant conditioning procedures to the behaviour problems of an autistic child. *Behaviour Research and Therapy*, 1964, **1**, 305, 312.

Wolpe, J. *Psychotherapy by Reciprocal Inhibition.* Stanford: Stanford University Press, 1958.

Chapter Eight

Pharmacotherapy of Psychopathology in Children
C. Keith Conners

Introduction

Psychoactive agents have been used in the treatment of children with a variety of labels: brain damage, minimal brain dysfunction, behavior disorders, psychosis, delinquency, emotional disturbance—to name but a few. The use of these descriptive categories reflects the fact that psychopharmacology of children has been developed within a psychiatric treatment framework in which the basic phenomena of interest are clinical-pathological characteristics of children referred for therapy. Unlike the situation for adults, the use of drugs with children is, quite properly, restricted to clinical settings in which experimental and scientific tactics must be subjugated to the primary task of healing. Unfortunately, the primitive state of classification in child psychiatry (see Chapter One), the preoccupation with treatment of symptoms, and the limitations of therapeutic settings for research have resulted in a lack of information about variables that affect or are affected by various drugs.

The basic dimensions underlying two different psychopathological states may be qualitatively similar, differing only in degree or by the introduction of some other variable such as age; and conversely, two qualitatively different underlying dimensions might give rise to seemingly similar observable symptomatic pictures. To take an example from Cattell (1957) in psychological testing, if one finds such tests as vocabulary, verbal analogies, and verbal

316

comprehension clustering together, and showing regular increments with age, one might conclude that variation in an underlying variable (verbal intelligence) is causing the individual differences in performance levels, *provided* educational opportunity were held constant. On the other hand, if intelligence is controlled or held constant, such variations between individuals might result from variations in educational opportunity. Thus, the overt symptom cluster or pattern by itself cannot give information about the organismic variables influencing the behavior. Deviant behaviors, then, become relatively uninformative dependent variables in drug studies, although therapeutically they may be the essential variables.

Some diagnostic labels, such as "brain damage," are based on a presumed (sometimes verifiable) neuropathology; while others, such as "delinquency," are based on external social or legal criteria. Since these two labels are not based on common frames of reference, there is usually no way to compare drug effects in a group defined in one way with those defined in the other, nor can we be certain whether there is a real difference in some organismic or environmental variables which affect the outcome of treatment with a psychoactive agent. If, however, it were possible to show that both groups could be characterized by some common parameters (such as arousal level, degree of inhibitory capacity, amount of environmental stimulation, etc.), one could then develop a rational therapeutic program utilizing target functions instead of target symptoms (Fish, 1967; Irwin, 1968).

Many of the contradictions in the literature may be because of the focus on psychiatric labels or symptoms instead of on underlying variables. One author, for example, maintains that benzedrine is contraindicated in psychopathic personalities (Bender & Cottington, 1942; Bender & Nichtern, 1956), while another finds it useful (Korey, 1944). It is possible that these two sets of findings are based on samples differing in some important function and hence are not really comparable. The disagreement in the literature about the value of amphetamine for organic versus nonorganic hyperactive children may be because these "diagnostic" groups differ *quantitatively* on an underlying dimension of inhibitory control. The source of this difference (e.g., exogenous trauma or developmental delay) may be entirely irrelevant to the kind and degree of drug response. On the other hand, there may indeed be *qualitative* variations in brain function as a result of different kinds of injury, genetic variation, or early environmental input which, however, lead to similar overt phenotypic behavior, but are critical in determining the response to psychoactive agents. In either case, the symptom pattern itself cannot form an adequate base from which to build a rational psychopharmacology.

This chapter does not attempt an exhaustive review of the use of psychoactive agents with children. Recent reviews are available summarizing much of the literature (Baker, 1968; Eveloff, 1966; Fish, 1960a; Freeman, 1966,

1970; Millichap & Fowler, 1967; Sprague & Werry, 1968, 1971; Werry, Sprague, Weiss, & Minde, 1970). We shall discuss the effect of stimulants, tranquilizers, antidepressant and anticonvulsant drugs, attempting where possible to point out the effect of drugs on functions that may be important in understanding drug responses in children.

Methodologic Considerations

It is becoming commonplace in the recent literature to begin a paper with the indictment that "most studies prior to the one being presented suffer from gross methodologic deficiencies." Although it is perhaps a healthy sign that some concern about methodology is evident, it is doubtful whether there have been real advances in the state of the art over the past 15 years. The principal methodological problems stem from the intrinsic difficulty of gaining control over relevant stimulus, response, and organismic variables within a clinical setting. Careful selection of homogeneous samples, randomization of assignments to drug and placebo, counterbalancing of treatment or test conditions, objective, valid, and reliable measurements, and a number of other common scientific considerations may be desirable but impractical within the treatment context. Moreover, it is likely that some degree of control is actually sacrificed in drug trials when these considerations are met.

For example, the effort to use groups large enough for statistical analyses, with randomized assignments to treatment conditions, may well lead to a trial conducted on a heterogeneous sample, with some real drug effects being canceled by negative effects, or washed out by a certain number of nonreactors included in the sample. In this regard, a careful "clinical" trial which is "uncontrolled" may in fact be superior to an ostensibly tighter design. The clinician may be able to group patients in small but homogeneous groups and he may detect improvement or change in areas that would be insensitive to "objective" measurement. This principle is analogous to the type of experimental control often achieved in operant analysis of behavior.

A good example of meaningful drug findings on a well-controlled study of a single individual is the paper by Hutt, Jackson, and Level (1961), which describes a 2½-year study of a hyperactive, autistic child treated with trifluoperazine, thioridazine, sultiame, and no drug. The stimulus environment was carefully controlled by using 5 toys and a novel object on each occasion of observation. A fixed period of 12 minutes observation with time-sampling for 10 minutes and filming for 2 minutes provided the source of data. Easily definable categories of visual exploration, locomotion, toy-directed responses, gestures, and investigatory responses were recorded. The interesting findings were that there were differential changes in these parameters due to the different drugs. The behavior was clearly under the control of the drugs used, but in specific ways for each drug (except trifluoperazine, which had no effects). This is a useful and surprising finding in view of the presumed efficacy of the latter drug for this type of child (Beaudry & Gibson, 1960; Fish, 1960a; Fish, Shapiro, & Campbell, 1966).

It is our contention, therefore, that the practice of dividing studies into "controlled" and "uncontrolled" trials and believing only the former is sometimes misleading. The use of the word "control" should not be restricted to the classical experimental designs, but should refer to real as opposed to formal control over the variables involved. Those studies with formal control may or may not exert real control over relevant variables, while some careful studies of a clinical nature may have real control without formal designs. The danger of ignoring an "uncontrolled" trial of a drug is equivalent to minimizing a Type I statistical error at the expense of maximizing a Type II error; that is, a real and significant drug effect might be missed in the effort to maintain pristine formal designs. For this reason careful consideration should be given to clinical drug trials, without premature rejection of findings that could be very useful.

Other methodologic problems sometimes neglected by nonclinically trained researchers include the use of fixed dosage schedules that ignore idiosyncratic responses of patients (which may be very significant with children); psychosocial variables such as the family attitude toward drugs and the child's unique personality trends; symptoms that fluctuate markedly from one setting to another or with rapid alterations of developmental status; subtle "internal" changes that occur and that only sensitive methods may detect (e.g., a change in mood or change in "inner" distractibility).

Stimulant Drug Treatment of Behavior Disorders in Children

Effects on General Behavior and Symptomatology

Charles Bradley's earliest report (1937–1938) of the use of benzedrine for treatment of behavior disorders in children described effects of the drug on 30 children of normal intelligence between 5 and 14 years of age. He noted a "striking change" in school activities of many of the patients during the week of benzedrine therapy. A great increase of interest in school material was noted immediately, with a "definite drive to accomplish as much as possible during the school period." He also noted an increased sense of well-being, decrease of mood swings, mild euphoria, and less self-preoccupation. Arithmetic performance was most strikingly improved. Many of the children became calmer, but a few became more active and irritable, with one child developing marked fearfulness.

A later report of observations on 100 children from the same residential inpatient setting (Bradley & Bowen, 1941) reported that 54 children became subdued, 21 showed no change in behavior, 19 appeared generally stimulated, and 6 showed improved school behavior without other changes. Only children with demonstrable neurological deficits failed to show improvement. Bradley's (1950) summary of 275 children, reflecting over a decade of observations with benzedrine and dexedrine, indicated that 60 to 75% were clinically improved, 15 to 25% showed no change, and 10 to 15% showed unfavorable effects. School adjustment, academic performance, readiness for testing, enuresis, subdued behavior, stimulation of shy and seclusive children, increased drive for achievement, increase in attention span were all described as effects of these stimulants.

These early studies merit careful consideration since they were carried out in a well-controlled environment in which detailed observations by staff members was possible over a long period of time. The children were under intensive observation by people who knew them well, and the reports themselves show a conservative, critical approach that gives the reader confidence in the final results despite the limitations in experimental design. These findings are in accord with most subsequent work, and anticipate most of the effects described in rather different settings and with different methods in later research. To be sure, placebo controls and double-blind conditions were not usually established, but the findings are in many respects superior to studies done on patients in less controlled settings.

Bender and Cottington (1942) reported the effects of benzedrine on 40 children with psychoneuroses, neurotic behavior disorders, psychopathic personality, organic brain disease, and schizophrenia. Among the changes observed were "feelings of well-being," stimulation of drive in learning, relief of fear, depression and sexual tension, integration of activity, more sociability, and ability to relate in therapy. The authors attempt to explain results in individual children by considering the dynamics of the child in relation to the effects of the drug. For example, psychopathic personalities were adversely affected and this was presumed to occur because "the personalities became overwhelmed by the sudden awareness of affects which led to a breakdown of a superficial integration overlying the disorganization in the emotional sphere." They noted that although the aggression in these children decreased, sensitivity to criticism increased and they retired into corners, to sit and cry for prolonged periods. Although this study used small samples, was impressionistic and uncontrolled, the above observations are worth noting; in particular, the negative mood changes that occur are of interest and will be discussed more fully below.

The paucity of systematic investigation of the type of effects described in these clinical studies is partially a function of the difficulty of operationaliz-ing the clinical concepts, but also undoubtedly results from a tendency among researchers to focus on easily observable symptom changes without regard to more complex aspects of personality functioning. It seems reasonable to expect that, given in adequate dosages, most drugs will have *some* effects on behavior; but the more interesting question of why certain effects appear in one child and not in another has seldom been attacked except in clinical studies, such as the ones mentioned here. Other clinicians have also reported observations indicating that the personality of the child may be importantly related to the type of outcome with stimulant drugs. Fish (1960b) found that amphetamine "was markedly effective only in children with behavior disorders. In this group it was most effective in the more mature, better organized children with more neurotic features. Some of the most dramatic responses occurred in children with school phobias and sexual preoccupations."

A number of clinical reports and controlled studies have reported changes in a variety of behaviors through the use of rating scales or checklists of behavior. In general, these reports show that disruptive behavior is most noticeably affected by the stimulants. In an early study, Lindsley and Henry (1941) used a list of undesirable behavior traits, with a total score derived by summing across all items, thus giving a sort of general undesirability index of behavior. The overall reduction in disturbing symptoms was at least 10% in all subjects with benzedrine therapy, but they do not report the specific symp-toms that changed. However, since their study involved an EEG analysis, they had the opportunity to note that in taking the recordings during the period of benzedrine administration "sociability, cooperation, attention and alertness all seemed to be improved."

Knobel, Wolman, and Mason (1959) used a checklist of behavior traits (such as temper tantrums, fighting, irritability, etc.) and also developed a Guttman scale of hyperkinesis. The effect of methylphenidate in one study with 20 children was felt to be unrelated to whether the child was hyper- or hypokinetic. Burks' rating scale of symptoms showed over a 35% overall re-duction in symptom score, but again no details of individual symptom change were given. In another report, Knobel (1962) reported on 150 patients treated with Ritalin over a period of 8 months. The symptoms most modified in this uncontrolled study were a decrease in hyperactivity, an increase in frustration tolerance, less aggressivity and destructiveness, diminished impulsivity, class-room performance improvement, better peer relationships, and a marked de-crease in hostility and resentment to authority figures.

Korey (1944) carried out a controlled study with benzedrine on severe juvenile delinquent cases at the National Training School for Boys. He used a checklist that included work-effort and efficiency, school performance, manifest sociability, misconducts, evenness of mood, and responsiveness during interviews. He reported improvement in all categories for the benzedrine group as compared with controls, although specific scores were not detailed.

Levy, in two papers (1959, 1966) described 225 cases of children with hyperkinetic behavior patterns thought to resemble the postencephalitic behavior disorders. Of the children, 219 tolerated the drug well and "all showed remarkable lasting improvement in their outward behavior-restlessness, hyperactivity, unpredictability and temper outbursts . . . concentration and attention spans . . . general attitudes . . . less sensitive and more cooperative."

Ginn and Hohman (1953) reported that the symptoms they found most responsive to dextroamphetamine were excessive restlessness, short attention, impulsiveness, and moderately severe emotional variability.

Burks (1964) devised a 28-item rating scale divided into three classes of symptomatology: Perceptual discriminative, social-emotional, and vegetative-autonomic. The effects of amphetamine seemed to differ in children according to their EEG status, with those children having normal EEG's showing most improvement with amphetamine, particularly in "vegetative-autonomic" symptoms (hyperactivity and restlessness, cyclic behavior, variability in work quality, daydreaming alternating with hyperactivity, erratic, flighty or scattered behavior, easy distractibility and lack of continuity and persistence, explosive and unpredictable behavior, and self-control). Unfortunately, the data in this study are so poorly analyzed that it is not possible to be sure they support the author's conclusions. The role of EEG status will be discussed in another section of this chapter.

Eisenberg, Lachman, Molling, Lockner, Mizelle, and Conners (1963), in a well-controlled study, found a significant decrease in disruptive symptoms in juvenile delinquents treated with dextroamphetamine, and Conners and Eisenberg (1963) found that in a group of severely disturbed and deprived children treated with methylphenidate, the following symptoms significantly improved: Leading others into trouble, demanding, disobedient, lying, listless and apathetic, childish or immature, quarrelsome. Interestingly, nailbiting was significantly *increased*. This might appear to be an isolated and chance phenomenon, although recently, Knights and Hinton (1968) found an increase in "fiddling" behavior at meals as reported by parents of children treated with methylphenidate. They also found a reduction in symptoms of laziness, distractibility, restlessness, disobedience, fluctuating performance, restlessness while shopping, wiggling during homework, and periods of quiet play.

Conners and Rothschild (1968) found an overall reduction in ratings of activity level in specific situations using the Werry-Weiss-Peters scale (Werry, 1968b), as rated by parents of children treated with dextroamphetamine. A factor analysis of a 93-item symptom scale used by parents to rate their children produced two factors, which Conners, Rothschild, Eisenberg, Stone, and Robinson employed in a double-blind study with dexedrine. One cluster of symptoms consisted of symptoms of restlessness, disruptive behavior, short attention span, and the like, and showed marked (18%) improvement in the dextroamphetamine group, but the symptoms of seclusiveness, anxiety and inhibited behavior failed to improve significantly more than in the placebo group. Two other studies by this author (Conners, Eisenberg, & Barcai, 1967; Conners, 1969) employed ratings by teachers. A factor analysis of the scale produced five factors, all of which showed significant improvement with dextroamphetamine treatment over a one-month period. Factor I consisted of items reflecting disturbing, disruptive behavior (selfish, disturbs others, quarrelsome, defiant, impudent, etc.). Factor II included poor concentration, poor motor coordination, daydreaming, inattentiveness, and being easily led by others. Factor III consisted of oversensitivity, overly serious or sad, fearfulness, shyness, and anxiety to please. Factor IV included restless and overactive behavior, but unlike Factor I it lacked the aggressive content (excitable, making odd noises, fiddling with small objects, excessive demands for teacher's attention, etc.). Factor V appeared to reflect sociable, cooperative behavior. These ratings were highly reliable as separate scales over a one-month period, with the test-retest reliability for placebo subjects being between .72 and .91 for the five scales.

However, the difficulty with such rating studies is the possibility that raters may exert a strong "halo" effect, rating a child who shows *any* improvement as improved across all areas. The presumed specific changes may, therefore, be spurious. Other studies, however, tend to support these general findings with stimulants. Moreover, in perhaps the best study of its kind, using time sampling of specific individual behaviors, Werry (1968a; Sprague, Barnes, & Werry, 1970) showed that certain deviant classroom behaviors, attention to work, nontask related activity, and points earned for "good" behavior were improved by methylphenidate as compared with placebo. Recent studies (Alexandris & Lundell, 1968; Conners, 1970a, 1970c; Weiss, Minde, Douglas, Werry, & Sykes, 1971; Werry, et al., 1970) have tended to be better controlled and to substitute methylphenidate (Ritalin[R]) for the older dextroamphetamine (Dexedrine[R]) since the former is reputed to have fewer side effects. These studies have confirmed the superiority of the stimulants over placebo in the treatment of hyperactive-aggressive behavior.

In summary, many clinical reports have appeared to support the view that stimulant drugs (amphetamine, dextroamphetamine, methylphenidate) have positive effects on symptoms of a disturbing, uncontrolled, impulsive nature. These reports are mostly based on children in whom such symptoms represent the basis of the original sample selection; that is, these are children who have been seen in clinical settings precisely because of presenting complaints of a disturbing nature at home or in school. Therefore, the degree of severity of these symptoms is probably in general above that of a normal sample and more apparent than for other types of disturbance of development. The occasional reports of stimulation of the shy-seclusive child to more active, outgoing behavior are less frequently seen in the literature, possibly because such behavior is less likely to come to the attention of adults. In careful studies such as those by Bradley and his co-workers, where such improvement was noted, the children were sufficient problems to warrant residential treatment. It may be the case, then, that the action of these drugs is not so paradoxical as is usually assumed. Instead, they *may* produce behavior changes in either overcontrolled or undercontrolled children, depending on which symptoms are of sufficient severity to show detectable changes.

Effects on Activity Level and Motor Performance

Perhaps because of the disruptive behavior patterns that are frequently seen by clinicians as responding to stimulant drugs, and because of the similarity, in many respects, of these behavior patterns to those of the organically driven, hyperkinetic syndrome described by Kahn and Cohen (1934), a good deal of attention has been focused on the effects of drugs on activity level. Some authors have felt that psychomotor excitement is the main criterion for the use of psychotropic drugs with children (Fish, 1960b; Werry, 1967). It has already been noted that Bradley's studies found that many children became quieter and calmer when treated with stimulants. Molitch and Eccles (1937) found improvement in form-board tasks, with strength of grip and a form-board test being among those showing improvement after amphetamine treatment. Similarly, Zimmerman and Burgermeister (1958) found faster speeds of performance of several performance tasks such as block designs, Seguin form board, building a tower, etc. In some respects these alterations in simple motor speed and performance levels are contrary to findings with adults treated with amphetamines. Blum, Stern, and Melville (1964) found no effects on tapping speed and reaction time, although performance was improved if the task required concentrated attention. These findings are similar to those of others (Holliday & Devery, 1962; Kleemeier & Kleemeier, 1947) with adults.

Connors (1966) found no effects of amphetamine on a Luria-type tremorgraph, but visual discriminations performed during the motor task showed significant changes. In other studies from the same laboratory (Epstein, Lasagna, Conners, & Rodriguez, 1968; Conners, 1970c) it was found that motor steadiness was significantly improved by dexedrine. In a more complete study, Knights and Hinton (1969) also found improvement of steadiness using a similar apparatus requiring holding a stylus in progressively smaller holes, and a maze tracing task.

Millichap and Boldrey (1967) reported a significant *increase* in activity measured by an actometer (an activity-watch that counts as a function of locomotion in the horizontal plane); and at the same time teachers and parents reported impressions of more motor coordination and less impulsivity. In a subsequent study, Millichap, Aymat, Sturgis, Larsen, and Whittle (1968) measured actometer changes and keytapping speed, and found significant improvement (less actometer activity and faster keytapping) in a Ritalin-treated group compared with control levels, but neither test improved more than placebo.

In the best study dealing specifically with motor behavior and stimulants, Sprague, Barnes, and Werry (1970) found that Ritalin reduced reaction times, improved accuracy, lowered seat activity (measured with an activity cushion), and reduced troublesome behavior in the classroom. Interestingly, dosage level did not influence the results, either suggesting an all-or-none type of effect or too narrow a range of dosages. It should be recalled that a dose-response effect did seem to appear in the early study by Molitch and Eccles (1937).

Werry (1968a; Sprague et al., 1970), using a time-sampling observational method, found that noisy behavior and nontask-oriented activity were reduced by Ritalin in a classroom setting. This study is one of the few that attempts to use a molecular analysis of activity instead of global judgments. Such measurements are both more meaningful in terms of relevance to molar behavior, and less likely to be confounded with halo or attitudinal variables that impinge on ratings of a more global type.

The effects of the stimulants on motor activity in children are, in general, contradictory—at least from a superficial point of view. A similar apparent divergence of findings may be found in the literature on amphetamine and activity level in animals (Dews & Morse, 1961). Part of the difficulty lies in inexact terminology. As Werry (1968b) and others have remarked, it is important to distinguish between modal activity level and situationally appropriate motor behavior. Lytton and Knobel (1958) noted that "The administration of methylphenidate . . . resulted (not only) in a decrease in the absolute amount of motoric activity but in an increase in the amount of motoric activity devoted to goal-directed behavior." Knobel et al. (1959) also made a useful distinction between a *related* type of hyperactivity: "that is, the child even though disorganized shows an interpersonal relatedness which can be easily differentiated from the *unrelated* type of hyperactivity, which is seen in some schizophrenic children who show the autistic, apparently meaningless, personally uninvolved type of hyperactivity."

Clinical reports on stimulant effects, frequently point to *a better integrated or more controlled performance,* and not simple alteration of activity level per se (Knobel, 1959, 1962; Knobel et al., 1959; Werry et al., 1970). Moreover, it seems that with both animals and humans, the starting level of activity is an important factor in determining whether a drug will alter the level. In the rat, cortical lesions do not alter activity level itself, but sensitize the animals to amphetamine-induced hyperkinesis (Adler, 1961); and animal studies generally show that the animals with the most active predrug condition display the greatest response to drugs (Irwin, 1961).

Some of the divergent findings with children almost certainly result from varying levels within a heterogeneous population of activity level and degree of motor control.

The literature indicates that in the child (within the dose ranges used therapeutically) the stimulants facilitate motor performance by either increasing speed or giving more selective control over motor response. This type of effect is well illustrated by findings reported by Conners and Rothschild (1968) for a continuous performance test: The drug-treated group showed a decreased latency of response on trials in which no signal occurred, but an *increased* latency when a target signal appeared, while the placebo group had significantly faster latencies on trials on which errors occurred. These data suggest that the drug group becomes slower when it is more appropriate to do so in terms of the demands of the particular task.

As will be discussed below, motivational factors enter into most controlled motor tasks, and consequently may account for changes in level of performance, rather than direct drug action on activity or motor behavior per se. An interesting study by Schickedanze (1967; Sprague & Werry 1971) illustrates this problem. Using a sample of institutionalized retarded boys, treated with both methylphenidate and thioridazine, he found that the children performed longer at a task requiring persistence (marble dropping) when treated with methylphenidate. (An activity cushion also showed some changes in the direction of diminution of irrelevant seat activity, though not significantly different from placebo.) While such tests have a motor component, they almost certainly measure motivational traits of persistence or psychological satiation, as may be seen from loading of such tests on personality factors (Hundleby, Pawlik, & Cattell, 1965).

Effects on Mood and Personality

Although a "blue ribbon" committee of experts convened by the Office of Child Development to look at the use of stimulant drugs in children concluded that stimulants do not cause a euphoriant effect in children (Office of Child Development, 1971) in fact, there has been very little systematic work on the effects of psychotropic drugs of any kind on mood and personality in children. It has already been noted that Bradley remarked on a generalized euphoria and positive attitude in his patients, and Bender and Cottington (1942) described some improvements in mood. The zestful, energetic approach to tasks described by Bradley was confirmed in a study by Conners, Eisenberg, and Barcai (1967) using a very large battery of objective personality tests devised by Cattell and his co-workers. The factor showing the largest effect of dexedrine consisted of a number of tests reflecting vigorous and energetic approach to the tasks. The results were interpreted in terms of an enhanced need for achievement, in the sense described by McClelland, Atkinson, Clark, and Lowell (1953). A study specifically designed to test this effect of amphetamine in adults also showed enhanced "n Ach" (Evans & Smith, 1964).

Another study by Conners, Eisenberg, and Sharpe (1965) used parents' Clyde Mood Scale descriptions of their children who were being treated with dexedrine. Two factors, named "friendliness" and "concentration" showed significant improvements over placebo. An examination of the items involved in these factors suggests that the children were judged as being happier, more cooperative, and as showing enhanced concentration and attention span. A similar effect on sociability was reported by Eisenberg et al. (1963) in a study of delinquent boys using a sociometric device. The children were asked to nominate cottage mates for roles in a fictitious class play. The roles were then scored according to positive and negative characteristics (e.g., the good prince versus the wicked king). The dexedrine treated subjects showed an increase in the number of positive roles assigned to them over the drug treatment period as compared with the placebo treated subjects.

Turner and Carl (1939) administered benzedrine to a group of normals and concluded that

> it is reasonably clear that in a majority of individuals benzedrine sulfate produces a definite heightening of mood, a fairly generalized optimism and interest together with an increased willingness to work for extended periods of time. In other individuals the same dosage had none of these effects, in still others, the opposite effects.

Livingston, Kajdi, Bridge (1948) found similar effects in epileptic children being treated with benzedrine; they concluded that the effects were direct effects on mood rather than secondary to control of the seizures. These effects on optimism perhaps account for changes in the risk-taking and gambling strategies of persons taking the drug (Hurst, 1962).

A less frequently reported effect of the stimulants is the production of sadness and depression. Ounstead (1955), in a study of hyperkinetic children with epilepsy, found that two-thirds responded with a depressive reaction including crying, withdrawn and motionless behavior, while only 9% showed the more frequently described positive responses of decreased hypermotility, reduced aggression, and improved attention. This is no doubt a somewhat different sample of children from most of the behavior disorders described by others, but the hyperkinesis, poor impulse control, destructive behavior, and labile moods and attention fit a syndrome of behavior frequently noted by others, even in the absence of demonstrable neuropathology.

Conners (1965) used the Holtzman Inkblot Test and found no effect of dexedrine on scoring factors usually associated with mood and affect, such as the color and shading responses that are usually presumed in clinical literature to reflect responsiveness to the blots and emotionality.

Effects on Cognition, Attention, and Perception

A number of studies have shown that stimulants have facilitatory effects on complex intellectual performances. However, these effects are frequently difficult to interpret because they can either represent direct changes in the higher cognitive functioning of the individual or more limited changes in specific aspects of the information-processing sequence. For example, there is good reason to suppose that the stimulants alter the child's ability to attend to the task at hand; and given such alterations almost any task will show enhanced performance unless the specific attending component has been controlled. The process of attending is itself complex, involving aspects of arousal, orienting reaction, cessation of distracting motor movements, and internal processes such as filtering or sensory gating. Any or all of these processes are conceivably altered by psychoactive agents.

Mention has been made of the first controlled study by Molitch and Eccles (1937) who found apparent improvement on intelligence tests for young delinquent boys treated with benzedrine. Most of the change in that study appears to be in those tests with a motor performance component. But "Morgan's Intelligence Test" showed about 18% improvement with benzedrine and 5% with placebo, while changes in the Kuhlmann-Anderson test were approximately the same for drug and placebo groups.

Bradley and Bowen (1941) secured data on school performance over a one-month period prior to and after benzedrine sulfate administration. Before medication only 6 of 19 children were making normal progress. While on drug 17 of the 19 produced more work than before drug. Spelling was not noticeably improved. In another study, Bradley and Green (1941) found that "In general there was no striking change in intelligence quotient when amphetamine sulfate was used." That study also found no noticeable change on psychomotor tasks. These results led Bradley to conclude that positive effects to be found in testing of this type result mainly from a change in the emotional attitude of the child instead of in any intrinsic elevation of intellectual capability.

Zimmerman and Burgemeister (1958) found no effects of ritalin on verbal IQ measures, although they did find a significant benefit on performance IQ (as compared with a reserpine comparison group). In a pilot study, Sprague, Werry, and Scott (1967) found decreased latencies of response in a two-choice discrimination learning task, but no changes in level of correct performance, possibly because of a low ceiling of the test. The dexedrine-treated Ss also showed decreases over placebo levels in activity, but the designs of the study did not permit a separation of effects of practice and drug. In a more carefully designed study, Sprague, Barnes, and Werry (1970) treated 12 underachieving boys in a special classroom with methylphenidate, thioridazine, and placebo. Methylphenidate significantly increased correct responding, decreased reaction times and hyperactivity, and significantly increased attention and cooperative behavior in the classroom.

Knights and Hinton (1969) found a significant positive effect on performance IQ with ritalin, as did Epstein et al. (1968) with dexedrine. Conners and Rothschild (1968) found no significant effects of dexedrine on the WISC IQ scores, though performance IQs were consistently higher than placebo after treatment. Millichap and co-workers (1968) found improvements in the Draw-A-Man IQ and a figure-ground subtest from the Frostig Test of Developmental Perception in a study of 30 children with learning disorders treated with ritalin. Similar results were found by Conners (1971) and Conners and Rothschild (1968) as well as significant effects on the Spatial Relations subtest and the overall Perceptual Quotient of the Frostig. Significant improvement was also found on tests of continuous attention, reading and arithmetic, auditory synthesis, and paired-associate learning.

In a series of studies Conners et al., 1965, 1967; Conners, Eisenberg, & Sharpe, 1964; Conners & Eisenberg, 1963; Conners et al., 1969; and Conners & Rothschild, 1968), we have found consistently significant drug-induced improvements in children with learning or behavior problems in the Porteus Maze Test (Porteus, 1968). This test requires the subject to trace his way through a pencil maze at his own rate, penalizing impulsive darting into blind alleys, and thus placing a premium on planned, controlled responding. The improvements have often been striking, being as much as 16 to 25 IQ points over the placebo controls. It is our belief that much of the change seen in many intellectual and performance tests results from this change in the more basic capacity selectively to inhibit, plan, and control response.

Weiss, Werry, Minde, Douglas, and Sykes (1968) used a battery of intelligence tests on 26 hyperactive children treated with dextroamphetamine and chlorpromazine, and found no individual test effects. As a whole the dexedrine group showed more improvement than either placebo or chlorpromazine. Conners (1966) used a mild stress situation and found better performance on a test of visual discrimination for drug-treated patients, especially under the more stressful conditions.

In a well-controlled study, Creager and Van Riper (1967) documented an oft-noted clinical response to stimulants: They found that the total number of words spoken and number of verbal responses were significantly increased by methylphenidate in a group of 30 children. In seems plausible that an increase in available verbal production together with more controlled or selective responding should lead to enhanced performance in children in a number of situations.

Effects on EEG and Other Direct Measures of Brain Function

Drug effects on the electroencephalogram (EEG) in children are of interest from two points of view: First, because of the implications such effects have on understanding the mechanism of action of the drugs; and second, because the presence of EEG abnormalities may shed light on the underlying nature of the behavior disorder in question. There is some evidence to indicate that EEG measures are tapping specific kinds of abnormality of function instead of being a general indication of brain damage. Werry (1968c) found EEG abnormalities to be a separate factor in a factor analysis of a number of variables thought to be related to minimal brain dysfunction. Many authors have reported high associations between EEG abnormalities and behavior disorders, though the range of the correlations is so broad as to cast doubt on any simple relationship (Ellingson, 1954). Jasper, Solomon, and Bradley (1938) found that over half of 71 children with behavior problems in the Bradley hospital showed "distinctly abnormal" EEGs. Cutts and Jasper (1939) later reported that "Benzedrine® did not appear to have a definite effect on any aspect of the electroencephalogram of these patients." However, they also found that "The electroencephalogram in all cases in which there was improvement with benzedrine® (amphetamine) was characterized by predominance of the 6 cycle pattern." Lindsley and Bradley (1939) gave five careful case studies in which the EEG abnormality, particularly 6 cycles per second bursts of large amplitude, appeared to underlie the behavior disorder. In a later study, Lindsley and Henry (1941) found that amphetamine improved the behavior of 13 problem children, but did not alter the EEG pattern. In a recent, large study, Klinkerfuss, Lange, Weinberg, and O'Leary (1965) examined EEG tracings from 353 hyperkinetic children (without gross brain damage, psychosis, severe psychoneurosis, mental deficiency, trauma, or encephalitis), and found that 60% showed mild abnormality of EEG, with 30% being clearly abnormal. However, it has been pointed out that these abnormalities may also be characteristic of other disturbed groups of children (Werry, 1968c). In a well-controlled investigation, Nuffield (1961) found that children with a temporal lobe focus of EEG abnormality tended to have a high incidence of aggressive manifestations and low neuroticism, while the reverse was true for those with

3 c/sec spike and wave responses ("petit mal" group). Children with "diffuse" abnormalities were also highly aggressive and the least neurotic.

The role of the stimulants in those children with abnormal EEGs is still moot. Gross, Wilson, and Ill (1964) studied 117 nonepileptic children with abnormal EEGs and found that "The medication found most useful by far was dextroamphetamine (Dexedrine®)." They found about 55% were significantly improved with drug treatment, often a dramatic kind of behavior change becoming immediately apparent. Pasamanick (1951) studied several drugs in 21 resident disturbed children with abnormal EEGs and found amphetamine to give the best results, although overall the drug effects were "disappointing." Knobel, Wolman, and Mason (1959) found no relationship between EEG abnormality in hyperkinesis and response to stimulant drugs.

Amphetamine has the property of decreasing the high amplitude, slow waves (3.5–7.5 cps) in adults (Fink, 1967) which has often been mentioned as the most frequent anomaly in the EEGs of behavior-problem children.

Although many authors have found an apparent high incidence of EEG anomalies among behavior problem children, particularly among hyperactive children, the relationship between the action of stimulant drugs and the EEG deficits is poorly understood at present.

Further light may be shed by the use of the average evoked response method. In this method averages of the EEG response to external stimuli (light, click, shock, etc.) are obtained by time-locking the stimulus to the sweep of a computer memory storage unit which stores the response immediately following the stimulus in memory, averaging out the random EEG "noise" and nonspecific background rhythms. I am currently collecting pre- and postdrug-evoked responses of children treated with dextroamphetamine, methylphenidate, or placebo. One preliminary analysis (Conners, 1970a; 1970b) of 25 completed cases showed an interesting differentiation in drug action: While methylphenidate produced a significant speeding of the late components of the evoked response, dextroamphetamine showed changes not significantly different from placebo. These late components, although of somewhat uncertain functional significance, are thought by many to reflect processes involving the arousal system and attentional factors. Further studies (Conners, 1970c) suggest that evoked response variables may show a relationship to the clinical typologies and to the type of drug response to be expected from a given child.

Summary

It has been found that stimulant drugs are a useful clinical tool for the management of disruptive symptoms and some psychoneurotic complaints. Effects on activity level and motor performance are generally in the direction of more controlled, skilled performances, particularly where goal-directed striving is an important component of the tasks. Various perceptual, intellective, and performance tasks have been enhanced by the stimulants in children with a variety of behavior disturbances, but usually those with poor impulse control and impulsivity. These changes are most likely a function of enhanced attention to the tasks or control over response. Effects on mood and personality are less well understood, though often the drugs appear to produce a slight euphoria and a more vigorous, zestful approach to the environment. Well-controlled studies on stimulant drugs other than methylphenidate and dextro-amphetamine (e.g., deanol) (Kugel & Alexander, 1963) have not been done.

Effects of Tranquilizers and Sedatives

A rather large literature on the tranquilizers and their use with children exists, but most of this literature is uncontrolled and contradictory in its findings. Carefully controlled studies usually show small effects (Molling, Lockner, Sauls, & Eisenberg, 1962). Bradley's summary of clinical findings (1958) shortly after the introduction of tranquilizers suggests a certain limited value of these drugs for control of symptoms. Little is to be gained by a detailed review of the extensive literature in view of the paucity of experimental findings. The best survey of findings on these drugs is to be found in a chapter by Karen Veazie Davis in a report compiled by Sprague and Werry (1968). Other useful reviews are those by Freeman (1970) and Sprague and Werry (1971).

In brief, the following conclusions seem warranted from the existing literature:

1. Thioridazine (mellaril) appears to be the most effective of the phenothiazine derivatives that have been tried, particularly in retarded-hyperactive, brain-injured, or highly excitable patients (Alexandris & Lundell, 1968; Baldwin & Kenny, 1966a, 1966b; Pavig, Deluca, & Ostenheld, 1961; and Vasoncellos, 1960). Chlorpromazine (thorazine) has been most widely used, with one or two well-controlled studies showing positive clinical benefits, again in those children with *severe* hypermotility (Brummit, 1968; Fish et al., 1966; Fish, 1969; Freed, 1961; Freed & Frignito, 1961; Hunt, Frank, & Krush, 1956; Lane, Huber, & Smith, 1958; Shaw, Lockett, Lucas, Lamontagne, & Grimm, 1963; Werry, Weiss, Douglas, & Martin, 1966).

2. Although the tranquilizers may be useful for symptom control, most evidence indicates that they have deleterious effects on cognitive functions and learning, making them contraindicated for children of normal intellectual endowment (Garfield, Helper, Wilcott, Muffly, 1962; Hartlage 1965). The conclusion that is sometimes drawn that the drugs are desirable for children of low intelligence, however, seems unwarranted, since it is precisely those

children who would stand to lose most from reduced intellectual capability. Reports of tranquilizing benefits for learning disturbances (Freed, Abrams, & Peifer, 1959) have not been confirmed by controlled studies and there is better reason to suspect depression of function (Hartlage 1965; Sprague et al., 1970; Werry et al., 1970).

3. Many of the studies, in the opinion of one of the most experienced clinicians in the field (Fish, 1967) have utilized dosages that are inappropriate for maximum clinical benefit.

4. Sedatives, such as phenobarbital, are generally contraindicated because of a tendency, except in very high doses, to produce hyperexcitement in many children, though many clinicians attest to the calmative effects of the antihistamine drug, benadryl (Effron & Freedman, 1953).

Antidepressant Drugs

A number of recent studies have suggested that antidepressant drugs may be useful in certain disorders (Campbell & Young, 1966; Mariuz & Walter, 1963; Meijer, 1965; Treffert, 1964). The use of the tricyclic amines (imipramine, nortryptiline, amytryptiline) with children is relatively recent, but it deserves mention because of promising reports on enuresis and behavior disorders. Two studies using hospitalized patients (Abrams, 1963; Fisher, Murray, Walley, & Kiloh, 1963) found no effects of imipramine on enuresis, while a number of studies have reported quite striking diminution of wetting in a variety of children in both inpatient and outpatient settings. The relapse rate when the drug is withdrawn is high, though apparently this may be reduced by gradual drug withdrawal (Poussaint & Ditman, 1965). The possible mechanism for this specific action is not known, though it may be a direct action on diuretic hormones or the sleep cycle. It is of interest, however, to note that other drugs such as dextroamphetamine and methylphenidate, which are essentially CNS stimulants, have occasionally been noted to reduce enuresis (Eisenberg et al., 1963). Whether this occurs because of a change in the sleep pattern, by direct autonomic effects, or otherwise is not known. One report (Abrahams, 1963) notes the effectiveness of imipramine in encopresis in a child.

A more interesting application of this drug is with emotionally disturbed or hyperkinetic children. Goldfarb and Venutolo (1963) conducted a controlled study in 100 "chronically allergic" children, of whom 54% improved (with a total of 66 patients improving altogether).

Krakowski (1965) studied 122 children from 2 to 18 years of age, of various diagnostic categories, and found sufficient improvement to warrant a controlled study. Fifty hyperkinetic children, with a mean age of approximately 10 years were followed over a six-month period or until symptoms disappeared. In general, improvement was excellent or good in 72 to 87% of the cases, with 8 of 10 enuretics showing complete remission of symptoms. When switched from placebo to drug 72 percent showed excellent or good response. This study is methodologically unsound in many respects, but suggests that more work with this drug might be worthwhile in children with hyperkinesis.

Rapoport (1965) reported results that are hard to believe, especially since no objective data are given, but he did find results that deserve further research: Approximately 80% of 41 children (ages 5 to 21) had complete or marked remission of all symptoms after periods ranging from 6 to 24 months. He makes the interesting observation that "It may be that the inability to concentrate is the most dynamic factor involved in compulsive behavior and learning difficulties," and that both depression and behavior disorders stem from reticular arousal defects which imiprimine should effect rather directly.

Similar reasoning regarding the antidepressant action of these drugs was used by Splitter and Kaufman (1966) who assumed that cholinergic mechanisms might be involved in activation level and hence in depression, which should be altered by nortriptyline. His patients were 23 children with school problems involving loss of interest, low grades, and failing marks, 4 children with schizoid trends, and 2 with marked depression. Using 2 independent raters, "excellent" or "good" results were found in 73%. Although no placebo was used, the authors claimed the results were sustained over many months.

One recent report, fairly well controlled (Frommer, 1967), suggests that antidepressants might be useful in childhood depressions.

In summary, the antidepressant drugs have little or no background of carefully controlled clinical investigation, though results reported seem to warrant further investigation in the application to control of behavior disorders.

Anticonvulsant Drug Therapy of Behavior Disorders

Few well-controlled studies of the use of anticonvulsants in behavior disorders of children have been carried out, but many clinicians use such drugs for these disorders, often being quite convinced of dramatic benefits in certain cases, regardless of whether the child also has accompanying EEG abnormalities. Undoubtedly the most serious neglect in the published studies is the tendency to use very heterogeneous samples that obscure any meaningful changes in smaller subgroups and the absence of placebo controls.

The most widely used and longest tested drug of this class is diphenylhydantoin (Dilantin, DPH). Pasamanick (1951) treated 21 boys, 6 to 13 years old with behavior patterns "not acceptable in the community or home," some of whom had abnormal EEG records. No improvement attributable to DPH was found. Cohn and Nardini (1958) treated children with unruly, violent behavior and abnormal slowing on EEG, with no change in either behavior or EEG pattern. Green (1961) found DPH ineffective for behavior disorders in children with an EEG focus, and Gross and Wilson (1964) found no improvement in disturbed children with abnormal EEG. Fish (1960b) stated that DPH is not recommended in psychiatric disorders of children. On the other hand, Walker and Kirkpatrick (1967) gave DPH to behavior-problem children with abnormal EEG records and they "appeared" improved. Lindsley and Henry's early study (1941) used behavior ratings of 13 problem children at the Bradley Home over a 6-week interval and found marked improvement in some patients, though less than was found for benzedrine. Brown and Solomon (1942) found that 3 of 7 boys with serious behavior difficulties in a training school setting and grossly abnormal EEGs of the psychomotor type showed definite improvement of hyperactivity, inattention, excitability, and temper tantrums. Zimmerman (1956) reported 200 cases of severe behavior disorders with 70% of the cases being treated with DPH showing "improvement." Putnam and Hood (1964) found the drug useful in a study of delinquents as have others working with delinquents (Lynk & Amidon, 1965). Chao, Sexton, and Davis (1964) studied the effect of DPH on the convulsive equivalent syndrome (paroxysmal cerebral disorder characterized by autonomic disturbances and dysfunction in behavior and communication), with good overall clinical results, often of a dramatic quality. Reasonably well-controlled studies with brain-injured children with behavior disorders show a high percentage of positive results (Baldwin & Kenney, 1966b). Resnick (1967) conducted a double-blind controlled study that included delinquents ranging in age from 12 to 15 years. This study carefully selected the subjects on the basis of symptoms thought by some to be particularly suitable for DPH treatment: Overthinking, sleep difficulties, depression, anger, and hostility, with chronic impatience and irritability being prominent features (Jonas, 1965). Significant positive benefits were described, although the study has serious flaws in the manner in which the data were obtained.

Two studies (Conners, Kramer, Rothschild, Schwartz, & Stone, 1971; Looker & Conners, 1970) using double-blind placebo control, with randomized group assignments, objective performance measures, behavioral ratings by trained observers, and naturalistic observations failed to show any benefit for children in a training school for delinquents, and children with severe temper outbursts. However, these studies also suffer from heterogeneity of the subject population, and from the necessity to use subjects who were only mildly disturbed.

Further studies with DPH and other anticonvulsants in behavior disorders of children need to be done, with major emphasis placed on careful selection of subjects, and with special attention to patients who fail to improve on safer medications such as the stimulants.

Factors That Affect the Outcome of Drug Treatment of Behavior Disorders and Hyperactivity in Children

Very little systematic work has been done to clarify the role of social, family, organismic, genetic, or ontogenetic variables that might influence the outcome of treatment. Kraft (1968) points out that treatment of children is always a treatment that involves parents and others such as teachers and peers. Clinical experience would seem to indicate that there are medication-accepting and medication-rejecting families that can significantly alter the impact of drug therapy (Knobel, 1962). Bradley (1950) had noted in his residential treatment setting the importance of the controlled, supportive environment for achieving maximum effects, and indicated that under deleterious family circumstances the positive benefits might disappear.

Organic factors have often been mentioned as playing a significant role in the type of response (Pincus & Glaser, 1966). Zrull, Patch, and Lahtinen (1966) claimed that "There was . . . a greater proportion of 'organic' children in the group that responded." The study by Epstein et al. (1968), which employed carefully documented organic and nonorganic hyperactives found that on *some* measures the organic children did better, and that their clinical response was more dramatic. Many other reports allude to the significance of organicity, but in general the concept itself is so poorly defined that until more specification is given it is unlikely that organicity can contribute to a clarification of responders and nonresponders.

An interesting finding on the role of both organic and emotional factors was reported by Conrad (1967). He classified 31 children treated with amphetamine into primarily organic, organic-emotional, and primarily emotional. None of the organic children (defined on the basis of history, EEG, and testing) showed a negative response to medication, but 67% of the emotional group showed a negative; 63% of the organics improved, and only 17% of the emotionals improved. Parents were classified as "grossly deviant," "socially incompetent," "poor," or "competent." When either parent was regarded as "grossly deviant" or "socially incompetent" the child was less likely to respond positively to medication than when parents were competent and stable. As might be expected, the social competency of parents was related to the presence of emotional psychopathology in the child, while a positive parent-child relationship was unrelated to the diagnostic classification but positively related to favorable drug response. Conrad found that those children who started taking medication between 5 and 10 years of age responded better than children either older or younger. Whether this effect results from severity of symptom, the fixity of the symptoms because of secondary neurotic complications, or other factors cannot be determined.

In general, the role of organismic and ontogenetic variables in drug response with children is poorly understood due to a paucity of systematic research. Most of the claims about organicity are merely opinions unsubstantiated by empirical data. A systematic approach to the subject would require a consideration of stimulus, organismic (including genetic, biochemical, neurophysiological), and response parameters.

As an example, one *stimulus* parameter of importance might be level of environmental stimulation (frequency and magnitude of physical stimuli, social stimuli). Clinical experience suggests that stimulant drug effects may depend somewhat on the extent to which the environment is chaotic or organized, as in Conrad's findings mentioned above. An important *organismic* variable might be the patient's level of arousal, or capability of returning to a base-line level of arousal following stimulation ("how excitable is the child?"), which could be measured with habituation or orienting response procedures employing autonomic measures of arousal. A number of testable hypotheses regarding level of arousal and response to stimulants are possible here. An important *response* variable might be the extent to which the patient's alterations of behavior lead to consequences in the family or school environment. That is, perhaps a child whose lowered activity level on drugs is reinforced by social reinforcements from the family will have a more profound effect than a child whose initially similar level of drug response is ignored or negatively reinforced.

Concluding Remarks

Most of this chapter was devoted to studies with stimulant drugs (specifically dextroamphetamine and methylphenidate), which partially reflects the longer use of these agents, the larger number of controlled studies and positive findings, and the author's own predilections. It is also fitting in view of recent public concern about the use of these drugs in children (House of Representatives, 1970). The large numbers of reports on other agents that have been tried with children are so poorly documented or restricted to limited populations or symptom conditions that they are not yet of sufficient generalizability to warrant extensive discussion. However, it is perhaps worth repeating that in a field where so little success in the management of behavior has been evident, that the Type II error may be the worst sin to commit.

Apart from clinical considerations of treatment and management of behavior, there is the profoundly important contribution that drugs can make in the understanding of the mechanisms of behavior, of personality and development in children. The effect of the stimulants, for example, in altering attentional behavior and drive level, while at the same time also altering the behavior disorder (hyperkinetic or impulsive behavior in particular), has important implications for the genesis of the behavior disorder in neurophysiologic disturbances of arousal and inhibitory mechanisms. Whether these occur because of delayed maturation of the cortices, as some have suggested (Knobel, et al., 1959) diencephalic disorders, or imbalance in cortico-reticular regulation of afferent input remains to be decided by much further work. This work must involve cooperative efforts of scientists *and* clinicians and be carried out with due attention to clinical obligations to the child and his family. These obligations have been succinctly formulated by Eisenberg as follows.

> No drug should be employed without firm indication for its use, without careful control of the patient to be treated, and without due precautions for toxicity. With any potent drug, toxicity is inevitable; to justify its use, the severity of the presenting condition and the likelihood of benefit must outweigh the risk of toxicity. Toxicity studies on adults cannot be safely extrapolated to children because of differences in the immature organism. Clinical decisions must be based upon data from pediatric studies.

> An old and familiar drug is to be preferred to a new unless evidence for superiority for the latter is preponderant. This principle of pharmacologic conservatism is based upon the fact that unexpected toxicity from a new agent may be apparent only after prolonged experience with its use . . . This is not a statement of pharmacologic nihilism. Drugs can make a decisive difference in treatment but their very potency commends us not to use them lightly.

> Despite these cautions, drugs can be useful agents in the management of pediatric psychiatric disorders when chosen appropriately and applied with discrimination . . . They can be effective in controlling symptoms not readily managed by other means and can facilitate other methods of psychiatric treatment by allaying symptoms that disrupt learning. If they are not the panaceas portrayed in advertisements, neither are they the poisons claimed by those wedded to exclusively psychological methods of treatment.

> Every drug study reveals the potency of placebo effects; that is, benefits

occurring from the relationship between physician and patient and from positive expectations in the patient . . . Skill in the use of drugs requires, in addition to knowledge of their pharmacologic properties, sensitivity to their psychologic implications.

Drugs should be used no longer than necessary. Dosage should be reduced periodically with the goal of cessation of treatment if symptoms do not return on lower dosage. Dosage must be individualized. Undertreatment, as well as overtreatment, can result in incorrect judgments about the appropriateness of particular drugs for the patient.

The use of drugs does not relieve the physician of the responsibility for seeking to identify and eliminate the factors causing or aggravating the psychiatric disorder. All of the currently available psychopharmacologic agents treat symptoms, not diseases. Clearly symptomatic relief is not to be disparaged; indeed it will remain a major part of medicine so long as causes are unknown and cures unattainable in many diseases. However, symptom suppression may also delay diagnosis and hence effective treatment. To prescribe drugs for a child whose symptoms stem from correctable social, familial, biological or intrapersonal disturbances without attempting to alter the factors causing the symptoms is poor medicine (Miller, 1968).

References

Abrahams, D. Treatment of encopresis with imipramine. *American Journal of Psychiatry*, 1963, **119**, 891–892.

Abrams, A. L. Imipramine in enuresis. *American Journal of Psychiatry*, 1963, **120**, 177–178.

Adler, M. W. Changes in sensitivity to amphetamine in rats with chronic brain lesions. *Journal of Pharmacology and Experimental Therapeutics*, 1961, **134**, 214–221.

Alexandris, A., & Lundell, F. Effect of thioridazine, amphetamine and placebo on the hyperkinetic syndrome and cognitive area in mentally deficient children. *The Canadian Medical Association Journal*, 1968, **98**, 92–96.

Baker, R. R. The effects of psychotropic drugs on psychological testing. *Psychological Bulletin*, 1968, **69**, 377–387.

Baldwin, R., & Kenny, T. Thioridazine in the management of organic behavior disturbances in children. *Current Therapeutic Research*, 1966a, **8**, 373–377.

Baldwin, R., & Kenny, T. Medical treatment of behavior disorders. In J. Hellmuth (Ed.), *Learning Disorders*, Volume II. Seattle, Washington: Special Child Publications, 1966b. Pp. 313–327.

Beaudry, P., & Gibson, D. Effect of trifluoperazine on the behavior disorders of children with malignant emotional disturbances. *American Journal of Mental Deficiency*, 1960, **64**, 823–826.

Bender, L., & Cottington, F. The use of amphetamine sulfate (benzedrine) in child psychiatry. *American Journal of Psychiatry*, 1942, **99**, 116–121.

Bender, L., & Nichtern, S. Chemotherapy in child psychiatry. *New York State Journal of Medicine*, 1956, **56**, 2791–2795.

Blum, B., Stern, M., & Melville, K. A comparative evaluation of the action of depressant and stimulant drugs on human performance. *Psychopharmacologia*, 1964, **6**, 173–177.

Bradley, C. The behavior of children receiving benzedrine. *American Journal of Orthopsychiatry*, 1937–1938, **94**, 577–585.

Bradley, C. Benzedrine and dexedrine in the treatment of children's behavior disorders. *Pediatrics*, 1950, **5**, 24–36.

Bradley, C. Tranquilizing drugs in pediatrics. *Pediatrics*, 1958, **21**, 325–336.

Bradley, C., & Bowen, M. Amphetamine (benzedrine) therapy of children's behavior disorders. *American Journal of Orthopsychiatry*, 1941, **11**, 92–103.

Bradley, C., & Green, E. Psychometric performance of children receiving amphetamine (benzedrine) sulfate. *American Journal of Orthopsychiatry*, 1940–1941, **97**, 388–394.

Brown, W. T., & Solomon, C. I. Delinquency and the electroencephalograph. *American Journal of Psychiatry*, 1942, **98**, 499–503.

Brummit, H. The use of long-acting tranquilizers with hyperactive children. *Psychosomatics*, 1968, **9**, 157–159.

Burks, H. F. Effects of amphetamine therapy on hyperkinetic children. *Archives of General Psychiatry*, 1964, **11**, 604–609.

Campbell, E. W., & Young, J. D. Enuresis and its relationship to encephalographic disturbances. *Journal of Urology*, 1966, **96**, 947–949.

Cattell, R. B. *Personality and motivation structure and measurement.* New York: World Book Co., 1957.

Chao, D., Sexton, J., & Davis, S. Convulsive equivalent syndrome of childhood. *Journal of Pediatrics*, 1964, **64**, 499–508.

Cohn, R., & Nardini, J. E. Bilateral occipital slow activity in the EEG. *American Journal of Psychiatry*, 1958, **115**, 44–48.

Conners, C. K. Effects of brief psychotherapy, drugs, and type of disturbance on Holtzman inkblot scores in children. Proceedings of American Psychiatric Association, 1965.

Conners, C. K. The effect of dexedrine on rapid discrimination and motor control of hyperkinetic children under mild stress. *Journal of Nervous and Mental Disease*, 1966, **142**, 429–433.

Conners, C. K. A teacher rating scale for use in drug studies with children. *American Journal of Psychiatry*, 1969, **126**, 152–156.

Conners, C. K. The use of stimulant drugs in enhancing performance and learning. In W. L. Smith (Ed.), *Drugs and Cerebral Function*, Springfield, Ill.: Charles C. Thomas, 1970a.

Conners, C. K. Stimulant drugs and cortical evoked responses in learning and behavior disorders in children. Paper presented at The Second Annual Cerebral Function Symposium, Denver, Colorado, June 24–27, 1970b.

Conners, C. K. A clinical comparison between magnesium pemoline, dextroamphetamine and placebo in hyperkinetic children. Paper presented at The Annual Meeting of the American College of Neuropsychopharmacology, San Juan, Puerto Rico, December 9–11, 1970c.

Conners, C. K. The effect of stimulant drugs on human figure drawings in children with minimal brain dysfunction. *Psychopharmacologia*, 1971, **19**, 329–333.

Conners, C. K., & Eisenberg, L. The effects of methylphenidate on symptomatology and learning in disturbed children. *American Journal of Psychiatry*, 1963, **120**, 458–464.

Conners, C. K., Eisenberg, L., & Barcai, A. Effect of dextroamphetamine in children. *Archives of General Psychiatry*, 1967, **17**, 478–485.

Conners, C. K., Eisenberg, L., & Sharpe, L. Effect of methylphenidate (ritalin) on paired-associate learning and Porteus Maze performance in emotionally disturbed children. *Journal of Consulting Psychiatry*, 1964, **28**, 14–22.

Conners, C. K., Eisenberg, L., & Sharpe, L. A controlled study of the differential application of outpatient psychiatric treatment for children. *Japanese Journal of Child Psychiatry*, 1965, **6**, 125–132.

Conners, C. K., Kramer, R., Rothschild, G., Schwartz, L., & Stone, A. Treatment of young delinquent boys with diphenylhydantoin sodium and methylphenidate—A controlled comparison. *Archives of General Psychiatry*, 1971, **24**, 156–160.

Conners, C. K., & Rothschild, G. H. Drugs and learning in children. In J. Hellmuth (Ed.), *Learning Disorders*, Volume III. Seattle, Washington: Special Child Publications, 1968. Pp. 191–224.

Conners, C. K., Rothschild, G. H., Eisenberg, L., Stone, L., & Robinson, E. Dextroamphetamine in children with learning disorders. *Archives of General Psychiatry*, 1969, **21**, 182–190.

Conrad, W. G. Anticipating the response to amphetamine therapy in the treatment of hyperkinetic children. *Pediatrics*, 1967, **40**, 96–98.

Creager, R. O., & Van Riper, C. The effect of methylphenidate on the verbal productivity of children with cerebral dysfunction. *Journal of Speech and Hearing Research*, 1967, **10**, 623–628.

Cutts, K. K., and Jasper, H. H. Effects of benzedrine sulfate and phenobarbital on behavior problem children with abnormal electroencephalograms. *Archives of Neurology and Psychiatry*, 1939, **41**, 1138–1145.

Dews, P. B., & Morse, W. H. Behavioral pharmacology. *Annual Review of Pharmacology*, 1961, **1**, 145–174.

Effron, A., & Freedman, A. The treatment of behavior disorders in children with benadryl. *Journal of Pediatrics*, 1953, **42**, 261–266.

Eisenberg, L., Lachman, R., Molling, P., Lockner, A., Mizelle, J., & Conners, C. K. A psychopharmacologic experiment in a training school for delinquent boys. *American Journal of Orthopsychiatry*, 1963, **33**, 431–447.

Ellingson, R. J. The incidence of EEG abnormality among patients with mental disorders of apparently nonorganic origin: A critical review. *American Journal of Psychiatry*, 1954, **111**, 263–274.

Epstein, L. C., Lasagna, L., Conners, C. K., & Rodriguez, A. Correlation of dextroamphetamine excretion and drug response in hyperkinetic children. *Journal of Nervous and Mental Disease*, 1968, **146**, 136–146.

Evans, W. O., & Smith, R. P. Some effects of morphine and amphetamine on intellectual functions and mood. *Psychopharmacologia*, 1964, **6**, 49–56.

Eveloff, H. H. Psychopharmacologic agents in child psychiatry. *Archives of General Psychiatry*, 1966, **14**, 472–481.

Fink, M. EEG patterns of common psychoactive compounds in man: Review and theory of behavioral associations: Paper presented at the meeting of the American College of Neuropsychopharmacology, San Juan, December 1967.

Fish, B. Drug therapy in child psychiatry: Pharmacological aspects. *Comprehensive Psychiatry*, 1960a, **1**, 212–227.

Fish, B. Drug therapy in child psychiatry: Psychological Aspects. *Comprehensive Psychiatry*, 1960b, **1**, 55–61.

Fish, B. Methodology in child psychopharmacology. Paper presented at the meeting of the American College of Neuropsychopharmacology, San Juan, December 1967.

Fish, B. Drug use in psychiatric disorders of children. *American Journal of Psychiatry*, 1969 Supplement, **124**, 31–36.

Fish, B., Shapiro, T., & Campbell, M. Long-term prognosis and the response of schizophrenic children to drug therapy: A controlled study of trifluoperazine. *American Journal of Psychiatry*, 1966, **123**, 32–39.

Fisher, G. W., Murray, F., Walley, M. R., & Kiloh, L. G. A controlled trial of imipramine in the treatment of nocturnal enuresis in mentally subnormal patients. *American Journal of Mental Deficiency*, 1963, **67**, 536–538.

Freed, H. The current status of the tranquilizers and of child analysis in child psychiatry. *Diseases of the Nervous System*, 1961, **22**, 434–437.

Freed, H., Abrams, J., & Peifer, C. A. Reading disability: A new therapeutic approach and its implications. *Journal of Clinical and Experimental Psychopathology and Quarterly Review of Psychiatry and Neurology*, 1959, **20**, 251–259.

Freed, H., & Frignito, N. Tranquilizers in child psychiatry: Current status on drugs, particularly phenothiazines. *Pennsylvania Psychiatric Quarterly*, 1961, **1**, 39–48.

Freeman, R. D. Drug effects on learning in children: A selective review of the past thirty years. *Journal of Special Education*, 1966, **1**, 17–44.

Freeman, R. D. Psychopharmacology and the retarded child. In F. Menolascino (Ed.) *Psychiatric Approaches to Mental Retardation*, New York: Basic Books, 1970.

Frommer, E. A. Treatment of childhood depression with antidepressant drugs. *British Medical Journal*, 1967, **1**, 729–732.

Garfield, S. L., Helper, M. M., Wilcott, R. C., & Muffly, R. Effects of chlorpromazine on behavior in emotionally disturbed children. *Journal of Nervous and Mental Disease*, 1962, **135**, 147–154.

Ginn, S., & Hohman, L. The use of dextroamphetamine in severe behavior problems of children. *Southern Medical Journal*, 1953, **46**, 1124–1127.

Goldfarb, A. A., & Venutolo, F. The use of an antidepressant drug in chronically allergic individuals: A double blind study. *Annals of Allergy*, 1963, **21**, 667–676.

Green, J. B. Association of behavior disorder with EEG focus in children without seizure. *Neurology*, 1961, **11**, 337–344.

Gross, M. D., Wilson, W. C., & Ill, E. Behavior disorders of children with cerebral dysrhythmias. *Archives of General Psychiatry*, 1964, **11**, 610–619.

Hartlage, L. C. Effects of chlorpromazine on learning. *Psychological Bulletin*, 1965, **64**, 235–245.

Holliday, A. P., & Devery, W. J. Effects of drugs on the performance of a task by fatigued subjects. *Clinical Pharmacology and Therapeutics*, 1962, **3**, 5–15.

House of Representatives. Federal involvement in the use of behavior modification drugs on grammar school children of the right to privacy inquiry. Hearing before a subcommittee of the Committee on Government Operations, House of Representatives, Washington, D.C. U.S. Government Printing Office, 1970.

Hundleby, J., Pawlik, K, & Cattell, R. *Personality factors in objective test devices: A critical integration of a quarter of a century's research.* San Diego, California: Robert R. Knapp, 1965.

Hunt, B. R., Frank, T., & Krush, T. P. Chlorpromazine in the treatment of severe emotional disorders of children. *American Medical Association Journal of Diseases of Children,* 1956, **91,** 268–277.

Hurst, P. M. The effects of d-amphetamine on risk taking. *Psychopharmacologia,* 1962, **3,** 283–290.

Hutt, C., Jackson, P. M., & Level, M. Behavioral parameters and drug effects: A study of a hyperkinetic epileptic child. *Epilepsia,* 1961, **7,** 250–259.

Irwin, S. The actions of drugs on psychomotor activity. *Revue Canadienne de Biologie,* 1961, **20,** 239–250.

Irwin, S. A rational framework for the development, evaluation, and use of psycho-active drugs. *American Journal of Psychiatry,* 1968 Supplement, **124,** 1–17.

Jasper, H. H., Solomon, P., & Bradley, C. Electroencephalographic analyses of behavior problem children. *American Journal of Psychiatry,* 1938, **95,** 641–657.

Jonas, A. *Ictal and subictal neurosis: Diagnosis and treatment.* Springfield, Ill.: Charles C Thomas, 1965.

Kahn, E., & Cohen, L. Organic driveness: A brain stem syndrome and an experience. *New England Journal of Medicine,* 1934, **210,** 748–756.

Kleemeier, L. B., & Kleemeier, R. W. Effects of benzedrine on psychomotor performance. *American Journal of Psychology,* 1947, **60,** 89–100.

Klinkerfuss, G. H., Lange, P. H., Weinberg, W. A., & O'Leary, J. L. Electroencephalographic abnormalities of children with hyperkinetic behavior. *Neurology,* 1965, **15,** 883–891.

Knights, R. M., & Hinton, G. The effects of methylphenidate (ritalin) on the motor skills and behavior of children with learning problems. *The Journal of Nervous and Mental Disease* 1969, **148,** 643–653.

Knobel, M. Diagnosis and treatment of psychiatric problems in children. *Journal of Neuropsychiatry,* 1959, **1,** 82–91.

Knobel, M. Psychopharmacology for the hyperkinetic child—Dynamic considerations. *Archives of General Psychiatry,* 1962, **6,** 198–202.

Knobel, M., Wolman, M. B., & Mason, E. Hyperkinesis and organicity in children. *Archives of General Psychiatry,* 1959, **1,** 310–321.

Korey, S. R. The effects of benzedrine sulfate on the behavior of psychopathic and neurotic juvenile delinquents. *Psychiatric Quarterly,* 1944, **18,** 127–137.

Kraft, I. A. The use of psychoactive drugs in the outpatient treatment of psychiatric disorders of children. *American Journal of Psychiatry,* 1968, **124,** 1401–1407.

Krakowski, A. J. Amitriptyline in treatment of hyperkinetic children: A double-blind study. *Psychosomatics,* 1965, **6,** 355–360.

Kugel, R. B., & Alexander, T. The effect of central nervous system stimulant (deanol) on behavior. *Pediatrics,* 1963, **31,** 651–655.

Lane, G. G., Huber, W. G., & Smith, F. L. The effect of chlorpromazine on the behavior of disturbed children. *American Journal of Psychiatry,* 1958, **114**, 937–938.

Levy, S. Post-encephalitic behavior disorder—A forgotten entity: A report of 100 cases. *American Journal of Psychiatry,* 1959, **115**, 1062–1067.

Levy, S. The hyperkinetic child—A forgotten entity: Its diagnosis and treatment. *International Journal of Neuropsychiatry,* 1966, **2**, 330–336.

Lindsley, C. B., & Bradley, C. Electroencephalography as an aid to understanding certain behavior disorders of childhood. *Ztscher. f. Kinderpsychiat.,* 1939, **6**, 33–37.

Lindsley, D. B., & Henry, C. E. The effect of drugs on behavior and the electro-encephalograms of children with behavior disorder. *Psychosomatic Medicine,* 1941, **4**, 140–149.

Livingston, S., Kajdi, L., & Bridge, E. M. The use of benzedrine and dexedrine sulfate in the treatment of epilepsy. *The Journal of Pediatrics,* 1948, **32**, 490–494.

Looker, A., & Conners, C. K. Diphenylhydantoin in children with severe temper tantrums. *Archives of General Psychiatry,* 1970, **23**, 80–89.

Lynk, S. M., & Amidon, E. Chemotherapy with delinquents. *Michigan Medicine,* 1965, **64**, 762–766.

Lytton, G. J., & Knobel, M. Diagnosis and treatment of behavior disorders in children. *Diseases of the Nervous System,* 1958, **20**, 1–7.

Mariuz, M. J., & Walter, C. J. Enuresis in non-psychotic boys treated with imipramine. *American Journal of Psychiatry,* 1963, **120**, 596–599.

McClelland, D. C., Atkinson, J. W., Clark, R. A., & Lowell, E. L. *The achievement motive.* New York: Appleton-Century, 1953.

Meijer, A. Value of imipramine for bedwetting children. *Diseases of the Nervous System,* 1965, **26**, 309–311.

Miller, E. Psychopharmacology in childhood: A critique. In E. Miller (Ed.), *Foundations of Child Psychiatry.* Oxford: Pergamon Press, 1968. Pp. 625–641.

Millichap, J. G., Aymat, F., Sturgis, L. H., Larsen, K., & Whittle, R. Hyperkinetic behavior and learning disorders III: Battery of neuropsychological tests in controlled trial of methylphenidate. *American Journal of Diseases of Children,* 1968, **116**, 235–244.

Millichap, J. G., & Boldrey, E. E. Studies in hyperkinetic behavior. *Neurology,* 1967, **17**, 467–471.

Millichap, J. G., & Fowler, G. Treatment of minimal brain dysfunction syndrome. In J. G. Millichap (Ed.), *The Pediatric Clinics of North America, Pediatric Neurology,* Volume 14. Philadelphia, Pennsylvania: W. B. Saunders, Co., 1967. Pp. 767–777.

Molitch, M., & Eccles, A. K. The effect of benzedrine sulfate on the intelligence scores of children. *American Journal of Psychiatry,* 1937, **94**, 587–590.

Molling, P. A., Lockner, A., Sauls, R. J., & Eisenberg, L. The impact of perphenazine and placebo in committed delinquent boys. *Archives of General Psychiatry,* 1962, **7**, 70–76.

Nuffield, E. J. Neurophysiology and behavior disorders in epileptic children. *Journal of Mental Science,* 1961, **107**, 438–458.

Office of Child Development, Department of HEW. Report of the conference on the use of stimulant drugs in the treatment of behaviorally disturbed young school children. Washington, D.C.: 1971.

Ounstead, C. The hyperkinetic syndrome in epileptic children. *The Lancet,* 1955. Pp. 303–311.

Pasamanick, B. Anticonvulsant drug therapy of behavior problem children with abnormal EEG. *Archives of Neurology and Psychiatry,* 1951, **65**, 752–766.

Pauig, P., Deluca, M. A., & Ostenheld, R. G. Thioridazine hydrochloride in the treatment of behavior disorders in epileptics. *American Journal of Psychiatry,* 1961, **117**, 832–833.

Pincus, J. H., & Glaser, G. H. The syndrome of minimal brain damage in children. *New England Journal of Medicine,* 1966, **275**, 27–35.

Porteus, S. D. New applications of the Porteus Maze Test. *Perceptual and Motor Skills,* 1968, **26**, 787–798.

Poussaint, A. F., & Ditman, K. S. A controlled study of imipramine (tofranil) in the treatment of childhood enuresis. *Journal of Pediatrics,* 1965, **67**, 283–290.

Putnam, T. J., & Hood, O. E. Project Illinois: A study of therapy in juvenile behavior problems. *Western Medicine,* 1964, **5**, 231–233.

Rapoport, J. Childhood behavior and learning problems treated with imipramine. *International Journal of Neuropsychiatry.* 1965, **1**, 635–642.

Resnick, O. The psychoactive properties of diphenylhydantoin: experiences with prisoners and juvenile delinquents. *International Journal of Neuropsychiatry,* 1967, **3**, S30–S48.

Schickedanze, D. Effects of thioridazine and methylphenidate on performance of a motor task and concurrent motor activity in retarded boys. M.A. thesis, University of Illinois, 1967.

Shaw, C. R., Lockett, H. J., Lucas, A. R., Lamontagne, C. H., & Grimm, F. Tranquilizer drugs in the treatment of emotionally disturbed children: I. Inpatients in a residential treatment center. *Journal of the American Academy of Child Psychiatry,* 1963, **2**, 725–741.

Splitter, S. R., & Kaufman, M. A new treatment for underachieving adolescents: Psychotherapy combined with nortriptyline medication. *Psychosomatics,* 1966, **1**, 171–174.

Sprague, R., Barnes, K., & Werry, J. Methylphenidate and thioridazine: Learning, activity, and behavior in emotionally disturbed boys. *American Journal of Orthopsychiatry,* 1970, **40**, 615–628.

Sprague, R., & Werry, J. Survey of research on psychopharmacology of children. Children's Research Center University of Illinois, 1968 (Mimeo).

Sprague, R., & Werry, J. Methodology of psychopharmacological studies with the retarded. In N. Ellis (Ed.), *International Review of Research in Mental Retardation,* vol. 5, New York: Academic Press, 1971.

Sprague, R., Werry, J., & Scott, K. Effects of dextroamphetamine on activity level and learning in retarded children. Paper presented at Midwestern Psychological Association, Chicago, May 5, 1967.

Treffert, D. A. Evaluation of imipramine in enuresis. *American Journal of Psychiatry*, 1964, **121**, 178–179.

Turner, W. D., & Carl, G. P. Temporary changes in affect and attitude following ingestion of various amounts of benzedrine sulfate (amphetamine sulfate). *The Journal of Psychology*, 1939, **8**, 415–482.

Vasoncellos, J. Clinical evaluations of trifluoperazine in maximum security brain damage patients with severe behavioral disorders. *Quarterly Review of Psychiatry*, 1960, **21**, 25–30.

Walker, C. F., & Kirkpatrick, B. B. Dilantin treatment for behavior problem children with abnormal electroencephalograms. *American Journal of Psychiatry*, 1947, **103**, 484–492.

Weiss, G., Minde, K., Douglas, V., Werry, J., & Sykes, D. Comparison of the effects of chlorpromazine, dextroamphetamine and methylphenidate on the behavior and intellectual function of hyperactive children. *Canadian Medical Association Journal*, 1971, **104**, 20–25.

Weiss, G., Werry, J., Minde, K., Douglas, V., & Sykes, D. Studies on the hyperactive child V: The effects of dextroamphetamine and chlorpromazine on behavior and intellectual functioning. *Journal of Child Psychology and Psychiatry*, 1968, **9**, 145–156.

Werry, J. The use of psychoactive drugs in children. *Illinois Medical Journal*, 1967, **131**, 785–787.

Werry, J. The effects of methylphenidate and phenobarbital on the behavior of hyperactive and aggressive children. Unpublished manuscript. University of Illinois, 1968a.

Werry, J. Developmental hyperactivity. *Pediatric Clinics of North America*, 1968b, **15**, 581–599.

Werry, J. Studies on the hyperactive child IV: An empirical analysis of the minimal brain dysfunction syndrome. *Archives of General Psychiatry*, 1968c, **19**, 9–16.

Werry, J. S., Sprague, R. L., Weiss, G., & Minde, K. Some clinical and laboratory studies of psychotropic drugs in children: An overview. In W. L. Smith (Ed.), Drugs & cerebral function. Springfield, Illinois: Charles C. Thomas, 1970.

Werry, J. S., Weiss, G., Douglas, V., & Martin, J. Studies on the hyperactive child III: The effect of chlorpromazine upon behavior and learning ability. *Journal of the American Academy of Child Psychiatry*, 1966, **5**, 292–312.

Zimmerman, F. T. Explosive behavior anomalies in children on an epileptic basis. *New York State Journal of Medicine*, 1956, **56**, 2537–2543.

Zimmerman, F. T., & Burgemeister, B. B. Action of methylphenidylacetate (ritalin) and reserpine in behavior disorders in children and adults. *American Journal of Psychiatry*, 1958, **115**, 323–328.

Zrull, J. P., Patch, D., & Lahtinen, P. Hyperkinetic children who respond to d-amphetamine. Scientific proceedings summary of American Psychiatric Association, Atlantic City, New Jersey, April 1966.

Chapter Nine

Community Programming for the Behaviorally Deviant Child

William C. Rhodes and Spencer Gibbins

Introduction

The first recommendation of the Joint Commission on Mental Health of Children, Inc. to the Congress, the state governors, the National Institute of Mental Health, and the Department of Health, Education and Welfare was for a "Child Advocacy System to Guarantee Mental Health." (Joint Commission, 1970). The importance of this recommendation lies in the recognition of the need for a unified organizational framework within major power structures at the national, state, and local level which would attempt to synthesize and control the independent actions of various organized systems of "care" represented, most especially, in the health, education, welfare and legal-correctional systems of the nation. The recommendation explicitly recognizes, first, that these systems of care have a profound effect on the lives of children (labeled either mentally ill or normal); also, that they are not being as effective as they might be:

> . . . they have been poorly coordinated with one another, meager in kind, and sometimes short lived. Often they have failed to reach those most in need. Too frequently they have been directed to special and separate problems rather than to the whole child and his family (Joint Commission, 1970, p. 22).

348

Implicitly, the full report seems also to imply that, at worst, these separate domains can be "iatrogenic" in their effects on children—that is, the "illness" may itself be created by the medicine and the doctors administering to the illness.

When a professional moves out of the role of direct care to the deviant and into the role of program planner for deviance he becomes cognizant of the overriding importance of dynamic community factors in the problem of behavioral deviance. He becomes acutely aware of the "politics of mental health" (Connery, 1968). He also becomes aware of the role of the collective dynamics of deviation in the community, the significance of public imagery around deviation, and the tremendous influence of past and present community circumstances, as well as the coercive and co-opting power exerted by "service hardware" (facilities, buildings, beds, etc.) on freedom-of-movement in attacking community problems of children.

"Models of Madness"

Even though scientific knowledge is not the most important factor in programming, it is one of the factors exerting influence on community activity in the field of child psychopathology. The program planner soon must come to grips with the fact that within the scientific fraternity there is conflicting data and sometimes strong disagreement over what constitutes psychopathology and how it is to be construed and managed. This divergence of theoretical models is explicitly recognized in the professional literature by several authors (Millon, 1967; Hall & Lindzey, 1965; Siegler & Osmond, 1966). The theoretical model that prevails in a particular locale at a particular time and the kinds of derived organizational structures and facilities that are dominating in that locale at a particular period of time will set the dimensions, directions, and limits of program actions and program development. The strength of a particular professional guild in that geographical area and the concentration of believers in a particular theoretical model of deviance will influence the direction in which a program will go.

These alternative scientific models, with their separate definitions, explanations, and interventions, are not mutually exclusive, nor do they necessarily deny the validity or legitimacy of other models. Nevertheless, they have a tendency to lead to separate dogma and to result in quite different types of programs or program emphases in community intervention into the problem of child disturbances.

There are at least four alternative theoretical models that are currently finding some expression in programs for behaviorally disordered children: (1) the psychodynamic model; (2) the biophysical or biogenetic model;

(3) the behavioral or learning theory model, and (4) the sociological or ecological model. Each represents a body of knowledge and each influences concrete operational facilities for problem children. Each model has its own adherents who clearly differentiate themselves from one or more of the other groups.

As was noted in the preface to this book, the psychodynamic model has exerted a dominant influence in programs for disturbed children in the United States over the past century. It has made us very conscious of the child's inner life and has built a vast theoretical body of knowledge about how this inner life unfolds. It has impressed us with those factors which lead to abnormal development (S. Freud, 1938; A. Freud, 1965; Klein, 1932). More recently, psychoanalytic theory has also begun to move beyond the necessity which seemed to impel it, in its earlier days, to establish the fact that moralistic and hypocritical social demands are apt to crush the adult and exploit the child (Hartman, 1958). Heinz Hartman criticized psychoanalysis for using the terms "outer world" and "environment" to designate an uncharted area said to be "outside" merely because it is not "inside" (Hartman, 1958). More recently, however, emphasis on intrinsic antagonisms between the individual and the society that has guided so much of the "treatment" programs, has given way to a concern for the interactions between the psychic life and the society in which it develops and is sustained (Erikson, 1959; Hartman, 1958). This concern is turning some psychodynamic theorists toward the community and community problems.

The application of psychodynamic theory to psychopathology in the community has seen movement from the distinctly clinical applications (Redl & Wineman, 1957; Bettleheim, 1950; Alt, 1960; Axline, 1947) to educationally oriented applications (Jones, 1968; Berkowitz & Rothman, 1967; Dreikurs & Dinkmeyer, 1963).

The concern of psychodynamic theory with psychopathology, with symptoms and etiology, and with diagnosis and treatment has caused this viewpoint to flourish in medical climates and has spawned community clinics, hospitals, and therapeutic services. This way of thinking about child behavior problems and the necessary interventions has made the psychodynamic model a favorite of medical schools and other university departments training clinically oriented professionals. This frame of reference has also intrigued and influenced legislators concerned with adequate funding for public medical care and has made the "mental health" of children an important program element in health-oriented agencies at national, state, and local levels. It has therefore become a very established part of the community and community care of children.

The biophysical or biogenetic model of psychopathology is an older theoretical view of child problems, but its history is closely interwoven with the psychodynamic model. Its adherents are found in the same agencies, university programs, and governmental bureaus as the psychodynamic proponents. Political figures rarely make a distinction between this model and psychodynamic conceptions. For most political figures both frames of reference are "medicine" and for them the politics of behavioral disorder are in a medical domain, with legal authority for the diagnosis and treatment of children being a medical responsibility. Theoretically, biogenetic or biophysical theorists are much more likely to concentrate on severe conditions such as infantile autism (Rimland, 1964) or childhood schizophrenia (Bender, 1968). However, many followers of this view translate the behaviors that might be seen as "emotional disturbance" by the psychodynamic theorist into minimal brain damage (Cruickshank, 1961), the hyperkinetic child (Burks, 1960; Reitan, 1964), learning disorders (Boshes & Myklebust, 1964), or the slow learner (Kephart, 1960).

The behavioral or learning theory model has not, until recently, had wide-scale influence on community programs. Even though the history of its application to child problems such as with phobias, fears, and sexual disturbances goes back to early learning theorists (Rhodes, 1962) the rapid proliferation of programs and large-scale applications of learning theory have occurred only within the last ten years.

Basic assumptions about psychopathology that are held by the behavioral proponents are frequently contrasted quite clearly with the assumptions of the psychodynamic school of thought (Eysenck, 1960; Ullmann & Krasner, 1969). Deviant behavior is viewed as learned behavior, which follows the normal, systematic course of any learning. Its problem-producing capacity lies in its incompatibility with the behavioral prescriptions of the particular environment in which it is occurring (see Chapters Six and Seven).

Since this point of view does not readily accept the illness paradigm and since it frequently rejects the concepts of "patient," "diagnosis," "symptom," and "etiology," it harbors inherent conflicts with the medical superstructure and the medical operational patterns typified by hospitals, clinics, and treatment units. Where it challenges the "medical model" of psychopathology it also falls outside the coalition between public imagery (about "sick" children) and the political and economic power structures which appropriate money and distribute legal responsibility and authority for public intervention into the problem of child disturbance.

However, where learning and behavioral theory have fused with clinical and therapeutic concepts (Wolpe, 1958; Wolpe & Lazarus, 1966; Franks, 1964; Phillips & Weiner, 1966), it is somewhat more compatible with those community systems that grow out of and support medicine public health. Conversely, since the philosophy, assumptions, and accumulated body of knowledge deal with behavior and learning, it is very compatible with the judicial-correctional and educational superstructures in the society. It is being widely employed within both institutionalized public bodies (Hewett, 1968; Cohen,

Filipczak, & Bis, 1967), and is very likely to enlarge its public-political-professional acceptance in dealing with both "delinquent" behavior and learning "disorders," thus playing an increasingly important role in the lives of children now called "emotionally disturbed."

The ecological and sociological models are grouped together in this section because of their overlaps. However, there are distinctive differences between them that will probably become more pronounced as they are elaborated and applied to research, theory, and community programming. The ecological theories of child disorder or deviation are concerned with the interacting environmental and biotic system to a greater degree than the sociological theories—or, more definitively, the ecological theories incorporate biotic concepts more deliberately than sociology. Furthermore, ecologists interested in deviant children are drawn from and integrate multiple fields (e.g., medicine, epidemiology, psychology, sociology) in their thinking. Sociologists who are interested in mental illness specifically are much more closely identified with their parent discipline (Scheff, 1966; Goffman, 1961; Clausen, 1959; Faris & Dunham, 1965). Other sociologists concerned with the general field of deviance in children, focus attention on society's implication in the problem. (Becker, 1964; Rubington & Weinberg, 1968). For them deviance is a socially created condition. They do not mean that the causes of deviance are located in the social situation of the deviant or in "social factors" that prompt his action; instead they mean that:

> social groups create deviance by making the rules whose infraction constitutes deviance, and by applying these rules to particular persons and labeling them as outsiders. From this point of view, deviance is not a quality of the act the person commits, but rather a consequence of the application by others of rules and sanctions to an offender. The deviant is one to whom that label has been successfully applied; deviant behavior is behavior people so label (Becker, 1964, p. 9).

The multidisciplinary group concerned more clearly with ecology (specifically the ecology of mental illness) treat organism and setting as mutually dependent systems (Faris & Dunham, 1965; Rausch, Dittman, & Taylor, 1960; Clausen, 1959; Fawl, 1963). They make a conscious attempt to study psychopathology as a function of the organization of the environment around the behaving organism (Calhoun, 1967; Gerard & Houston, 1955; Jordan, 1963).

Different disciplines or different scientists in different disciplinary settings give special emphases to ecology as seen from the perspective of their respective fields—that is, medicine, sociology, psychology. Their viewpoint reflects the more basic or generic ecological theory within these separate fields (e.g.,

Barker, 1963, 1968; Sells, 1969; Hawley, 1950, 1951; Duncan, 1964; Dubos, 1965).

Interventions growing out of these allied frameworks of sociology and ecology have been largely demonstration effects to date. Those specialists who are primarily sociological in orientation have paid particular attention to "juvenile delinquency" (Conger & Miller, 1966; Empey, 1967; McCorkle, Elias, & Bixby, 1958). They have also focused on other kinds of community deviancy (Mercer, 1965; Hooker, 1960). Some of the ecologically oriented have also been concerned with emotionally disturbed and normal children (Rausch, 1969; Hobbs, 1966; Lewis, 1967; Rhodes, 1967, 1970).

Even though the sociological and ecological theorists do not yet have operational patterns to translate their theory into community practice, their perspective is compatible with the philosophies, bodies of knowledge, and technologies of their multiple disciplines. Therefore, this general model has implications for interventions that could cross guild lines and integrate the efforts of community agencies allied to specific disciplines (medicine, social work, education, etc.) and that specialize in therapeutic, correctional, educational, or welfare approaches.

Contemporary Program Influences

National Level

Community programming involves much more than scientific knowledge and conceptions of the psychopathology of children. It is a composite of political operations, public threat, historical precedent, professional and scientific knowledge, and established community frameworks for forming and controlling social behavior.

Political operations interact most intimately with and are influenced most directly by, public anxiety over the threat of behaviors that depart from the community sanctioned patterns. Those behavioral patterns or traits that are most threatening to the community will differ somewhat from community to community and from time to time, but they are crucial to programming.

Anyone involved at the local, state, and national level in planning and implementing programs for children has discovered that those who make laws or appropriate funds will shift their programming emphasis according to shifting cycles in public concern over first one pattern of behavioral deviation and then another. Delinquency may receive high public and political priority one year and illegitimacy or drug abuse another. In 1958 there was strong legislative activity at the federal level in the area of delinquency. In 1970 the political concern revolved around drug abuse. Both national political concerns influenced programming for "emotionally disturbed" children at local and state levels because they made funds available and provided a national signal of high priority for a particular concern.

Delinquency.   The years 1957–1961 were the times in which youth gangs in urban areas had been attracting national attention for some time. There was increasing public anxiety over the phenomena as the news media reported one disturbing incident after another—a youth from a rival gang was killed in a school yard and another on the church steps; a well-known priest was mugged and left to die by a gang operating in a park—these kinds of incidents accelerated the sense of threat felt by the nation. This was the period in which professional studies of gangs (Miller, 1958, 1959; Block & Niederhoffer, 1958) were being reported in professional conventions and published in books (Cohen, 1961; Whyte, 1946).

The phenomenon of bopping or fighting gangs was well known. Civic groups conducted public programs on delinquency. Legislators in regions of the country and states with large urban populations were feeling tremendous public pressure to "do something." The sense of national psychological threat resulted in a buildup of pressure that then led to the passage of legislation which outlined national programs and provided national funds to "combat" delinquency.

During the period when the collective psychological dynamics of behavioral threat and public recoil focused on the phenomenon of delinquent gangs, two national agencies in the bureaucratic structure had major concern for programming from a social science or mental health point of view: The Children's Bureau and the National Institute of Mental Health. Each became involved in writing reports on the phenomenon of delinquency and in testifying before appropriate legislative committees.

Drug Abuse.   The year 1970 saw national concern raised to a fever pitch over drug abuse. It was no longer the gang phenomenon that produced patterns of psychological threat and recoil in collective groups throughout the United States. It was the youth drug culture and the widespread involvement of the middle class. The threat-vulnerable and politically influential public was, this time, finding threat from within.

The drug problem had been building since the quiescence over the bopping gangs. Many professionals had claimed that drugs were responsible for the quieting of the fighting-gang phenomenon. However, the public had a sense of relief and quiet. There was no threat and recoil associated with this new urban gang phenomenon. It was not until the drug culture moved across class lines and there was the mass phenomenon of drug-taking among youth, with the socially disturbing incidence of murder of well-known public figures (e.g., the Tate murder case in Los Angeles) under circumstances linked with the drug culture, and the phenomenon of massive rock and drug festivals that this focus of public threat produced collective recoil throughout the country, and political power structures began to feel the pressure of public anxiety to "do something."

Again, the phenomenon of the interaction between public anxiety in response to a behavioral threat created a wave of recoil, with increasing pressure on the legislative, judicial, and executive branches of the federal government for some type of action to meet or reduce anxiety over the threat. Also there are two major behavioral intervention systems within the federal bureaucratic structure that could be mandated by legislation to expend funds and to plan and implement programs. Which will be given major responsibility depends on the way in which public ambivalence over "disciplining" or "treating" the threat-provokers is resolved.

In both of these national threat-recoil cycles, the relevance to the problem of "emotional disturbance" is very direct. It affects funds for programs, professional salaries, operation of facilities, and university training stipends. The twin forces of political power and public pressure continually play major roles in the renewal of program funds and fresh impetus for new program development.

Local Level

When a national signal of the kind discussed above highlights one deviation pattern or another, regional and local culture dictate the form and emphasis of the program for deviant children that will function at those levels. It is easier in certain locales to obtain funds for a legal-correctional approach to children who fall under the particular rubric of concern (i.e., delinquency, drug-abuse, sexual deviancy) than for a mental health approach. In other locales of the country mental health intervention may be quite consonant with the patterns of "liberal" attitudes. For a variety of cultural reasons there are other striking regional differences in the way in which a community will permit a professional to move to plan programs for disturbed children. In certain racially dominated neighborhoods of heavily urbanized regions, the very labels "emotional disturbance" and "mental retardation" are threatening and tabooed, and community programs aimed at such children must find some other focus for their operational patterns and some other program access to such children.

The same type of urban political climate also influences who is allowed to intervene in the lives of the threat-provoking populations. The credentials of the established professionals are being challenged in unusual ways, and the authority of the governing bodies of agencies is under attack. The struggle over "community control" of the school system within the Ocean Hill-Brownsville area of New York is one example. In addition, the confrontation, which among other demands was for nonprofessionals to assume primary "treatment" roles in mental health agencies, which occurred in the Lincoln Hospital Mental Health Services and the Bronx State Hospital strike (Roman, 1969; Staff of Bronx State Hospital, 1968), is an example of such challenge. These challenges have a definite influence over what kinds of programs can be implemented in various locales.

Political considerations operate in programming for behavioral deviance in another way. Governors, or mayors (like Presidents), find it necessary not only to identify and capitalize on public behavioral "issues" or threats but they must also establish their own program identity, independent of previous holders of their office and distinctive from their political opponents. If one office holder has been identified with the "community mental health" programs approach to disturbed and disturbing children, another may have to capitalize on "day care" or "education." If the political figure involved has correctly identified the current focus of public threat over deviating children, he can also influence as well as detect what form of programming will best appeal to the nature of focus of the public threat.

The professional person interested in programming for deviant children must, then, have some understanding of the live context created by the structure and dynamics of behavioral threat, power, collective anxiety, and the culture of the geographical area in which he is functioning. He must know, too, that such a context is a shifting one and needs to be assayed from year to year. Although "program planning" should have a long-term reference, the dynamic aspect of the psychology of communities establishes the parameters of such planning. Behavioral threat varies from period to period and collective response is usually conditioned by the prevailing psychological climate at the time that a behavioral pattern or pattern of traits captures local or national concern.

Historical Program Influences

In addition to contemporary influences on community programs for deviant children, historical influences also play a part. Threatening behavioral patterns, collective reaction to these behavioral patterns, and institutionalized power structures, are carried over from the past to influence community action in current operating programs.

History can be detected both in the "conceptual" or deviance imagery residue and in the structural remains of the past which are still visible and operational within current community life.

The Child Savers.   A specific illustration of influences out of the past can be taken from the Child Saver Movement as reported by Platt (1969). These events took place at the end of the last century and the beginning of the current one. They occurred primarily in the city of Chicago, but their influence rapidly spread across the nation and influenced youth programming in other nations. Their conceptual and structural product are a major source of behavior regulation in today's communities.

According to Platt, the Child Saver Movement was a feminist movement which, at the end of the nineteenth century, helped to create special judicial and correctional institutions in society "for the labeling, processing, and management of 'troublesome youth'" (p. 3). In Platt's account of the psychosocial context out of which this movement was generated, there was broad public support for the idea that it was woman's business to be involved in regulating the welfare of children. The particular social circumstances behind this appreciation, even by antifeminists, were women's emancipation and accompanying changes in traditional family life. However, child saving was a reputable task for any woman who wanted to extend her housekeeping functions into the community without denying antifeminist stereotypes of women's nature and place. Platt says that:

> Although the child savers were bored at home and unhappy with their lack of participation in the "real world" they vigorously defended the virtue of traditional family life and emphasized the dependence of the social order on the proper socialization of children (p. 78).

According to Platt, the influential group who created the delinquency metaphor and the organizational or program paraphernalia that went with it came out of remarkably similar backgrounds, patterns of life, and interests. They were career women, social philanthropists, women's clubs, settlement houses, and politically important personages who were connected with these individuals and groups. Militant organizations saw child saving as a problem of women's rights, whereas their opponents seized on it to keep women "in their place."

As indicated, the center of the Child Saver Movement was Chicago. The women involved had direct access to political and financial resources. Louise Bowen and Ellen Henrotin were both married to bankers, Mrs. Potter Palmer's husband was an influential broker and hotel owner, the fathers of Jane Addams and Julia Lathrop were Republican Senators in the Illinois legislature.

Since the participation of the child savers in public affairs was justified as an extension of their housekeeping function, they were not regarded by others as competitors for jobs usually performed by men. In their own perception of themselves, they were housekeepers to the community. In a quotation offered in Platt's account, Mrs. Louise Bowen addressed the Friday Club of Chicago by exhorting women to find places on charity boards and give their opinion on garbage disposal, cleanliness of the streets, and care and education of children. "If a woman is a good housekeeper in her own home, she will be able to do well that larger housekeeping" (Platt, p. 79). Women also had another unique role in society, according to the child savers. They were urgently required to participate in public life because of their feminine capacity to act as custodians of public morality. The leaders of the movement saw the influences of city life as corrupting and as robbing children of their innocence.

Platt includes direct quotes from their speeches about the immorality of Chicago. Children were being "beguiled" into "all sorts of wickedness." Mrs. Bowen said that it was claimed that Chicago was becoming the largest and most beautiful city in the world ". . . but what is it going to profit us if our children lose their souls!" Unless conditions were remedied, "The children, in order to quench their thirst for joy, will take deep draughts of the poisonous stuff which is everywhere offered to them, and which ultimately will end in their complete demoralization."

In summary, Platt said the Child Saver Movement was heavily influenced by middle class women who extended their housewifely roles into public service and used their extensive political contacts and economic resources to advance their cause. They defended the home, family life, and parental supervision, since it was these institutions that had traditionally given purpose to a woman's life.

As a result of their efforts, in 1899, Illinois passed the Juvenile Court Act. This was the first such enactment to be acknowledged as a model statute by other states and counties. By 1917 juvenile court legislation had been passed in all but three states and by 1932 there were over 600 independent juvenile courts throughout the United States.

In this case study we see how the circumstances of a particular place and time created a conception, aroused public concern, mobilized economic and political power, and created a total institution. This internal public concern, the category of delinquent, and the vast machinery created in response to the concern are active parts of current community approaches to children today. A "program" devoted to this particular problem definition is a deposit of the past which, unlike an archaeological layer, still has a crucial influence on community life.

Platt saw this participation of politically conservative, socially prominent, middle class women as a regressive and nostalgic thrust to preserve and reinforce a code of values that were threatened by urban life, industrialization, and the influx of immigrant cultures.

The child saving movement was not so much a break with the past as an affirmation of faith in certain aspects of the past. Parental authority, home education, domesticity, and rural values were emphasized because they were in decline as institutions at this time (p. 176).

Platt concluded, in his book, that the Child Saver Movement had personalized the administration of justice by removing many aspects of due process and approaching "troublesome" youth in medical-therapeutic terms.

Child Guidance Clinics. Although not reported by Platt, this medical-therapeutic approach to delinquents paved the way for, and interacted with, another powerful child movement and another child program that took place shortly afterwards. This movement embraced psychodynamic views of, and psychotherapeutic approaches to, child problems in this country. It specifically helped to create and asure the success of the Child Guidance Movement and the rapid proliferation of child guidance clinics in the United States. This movement also originated in Chicago, close in time to the Child Saver Movement. Its first concrete operational pattern, the Chicago Juvenile Psychopathic Institute, was founded in collaboration with the newly established Chicago Juvenile Court. This Institute opened in 1909, under the sponsorship of Mrs. W. H. Drummer, and directed by Dr. William Healy, to establish another major institutional pattern and to concretize the medical imagery of child guidance. Here, we have a medical mechanism established to process the imagery of illness, diagnosis, and treatment—the new "scientific" response to threatening or troublesome youth. Then we had the category of "sick" youth coupled with the category of "delinquent" youth, with the twin behavioral management systems of judicial-correction and medical-mental health to protect the community.

Although Lightner Witmer's Psychological Clinic, established in 1896 at the University of Pennsylvania, was a forerunner of the child guidance clinic, the Child Guidance Movement did not capture national public attention until it was aligned with the medical superstructure and given the political push of the National Committee for Mental Hygiene, which was established in 1909.

Like all public conceptions of variant behavior and all community attempts to protect itself against behavioral threat, it flowered on the interlocking fields of threat of poverty and behavioral deviation. In the history of child guidance clinics Stevenson wrote in 1934, "Historically, however, it owes its existence to the broader concern of various groups with the age-old and overwhelming problems of delinquency, mental disease and dependency" (p. 9). In 1920, supported by the Commonwealth Fund, the National Committee for Mental Hygiene established a Division on the Prevention of Juvenile Delinquency. This Division set out to demonstrate that "psychiatric work in the diagnosis and treatment of children coming from the juvenile court" was the answer to the control of troubling tendencies in youth. Stevenson (1934) declared of the techniques used in the mental hygiene clinic: "This represents the latest of many attempts to meet a fundamental long recognized need for control of those tendencies in human beings which lead to delinquency, to dependency, and to mental illness" (p. 10). He claimed that ". . . many disturbing behaviors and personality reactions in childhood recorded in histories of psychotics were paralleled in histories of prisoners and in those of chronic dependents as well" (pp. 10 & 11). In fact, the Mental Hygiene Movement also promised to assist in normal child rearing.

> Many teachers and parents, concerned in the main with rearing and educating of normal children and only to a minor degree with pathological conditions and abnormal trends, likewise saw in the movement a response to needs which they felt (p. 11).

And so, backed by the medical superstructure and spurred on by the National Committee for Mental Hygiene, clinics spread across the United States. By 1932, only 21 years after the founding of the Chicago Psychopathic Institute, there were 232 child guidance clinics in the nation. This rapid proliferation is interesting. Stevenson noted that even though the clinics could not develop measures "to say definitely that it does prevent delinquency or prevent mental disease . . ." "Communities all over the country, by finding the money year after year to support clinical services, indicate that they value it" (p. 169).

The Legacy to Today

In these two examples, the convergence of a particular period, a threat, and a particular public reaction to that threat created two new social institutions. This total composition has been carried over from the past as a viable legacy to the present. The ways of thinking about the threat, the strategies of defense, and the structures for naming, processing, and managing threatening youth are all part of that legacy in today's community. Two of the major special settings for "disturbed" children in our current era are the mental health clinic and the correctional facilities and clinics. The concepts of delinquency and sickness are the two major frames through which we view children who differ behaviorally. Even though the research evidence for the effectiveness of these two composite child care systems is less than impressive, their influence is very much a part of community life today.

In different eras in the history of Western civilization, identical behavioral patterns have evoked quite different community responses. These live deposits from a succession of eras have accumulated in the culture to provide a current storehouse of alternative community response patterns which are immediately available when released by threatening variant behavior.

Older Influences

Prior to the fourteenth or fifteenth century, the prevailing and most widely held conception of behavioral disorder was a demonic one. The dominant belief was that disturbed individuals were possessed and in need of religious measures to cast out the devil that possessed them. Such possession was a direct threat to individuals around them. The possessed individual was capable of jeopardizing or corrupting all who related to him. This social responsibility for warding off evil, therefore, was ascribed to the church, which had its own highly trained specialists to perform the exorcising rites.

Later, when ecclesiastic power declined and monasteries fell on hard times, there was a shift in the conception of mental illness and in the body of knowledge and societal institution that had the power to deal with behavioral deviation. The church-state gave way to the municipal form of government, and the Elizabethan Poor Laws were enacted. The care of the demented was given over from the monasteries and the ecclesiastic order to the welfare care of municipal councils through the operational intervention of "indoor relief." Special asylums and institutions were established for the care and protection and incarceration of these wards of the state. The idea was both to care for them and to protect the community from them. Later, under the influence of men like Pinel and the Tukes, the medical conception of the problem began to gain preeminence in the society, and the problem began to be conceptualized as one of an illness or an illnesslike condition, which required diagnosis, treatment, and inpatient and outpatient care.

Even though this latter frame of reference has a high value in community thinking today, each of the other perceptions of the problem are still active within society and influence its programs with respect to such children. They can be observed to exist side-by-side in the community and to provide alternate routes for children whom we might call emotionally disturbed. A child who repeatedly attacks other people might be called delinquent, referred to a juvenile court, and placed in a correctional facility. He might be seen as sick, diagnosed as "acting-out" or "sociopathic," and hospitalized in a mental institution. He might be seen as socially maladjusted and he and his family referred to a child service agency or family agency for intensive casework. Conceivably, he can travel each route at different times or even be caught at some stage within each route simultaneously.

Brick and Mortar Influences

The shape and organization of programs for children are also very much influenced by the brick-and-mortar institutions carried over from past periods and past frames of reference. Any social institutional form that includes buildings and facilities has a tenacious capacity for maintaining itself within the social body. These edifices have a powerful influence on the way in which communities continue to handle human problems no matter what new discoveries or methods may evolve. Institutions have an uncanny ability to co-opt and absorb new discoveries of orientation and procedure into their old forms. Even when society makes a radical shift to a new major frame of reference about the human problem of "disturbance," the old institutional form persists. Under such conditions, even if new structures and edifices evolve to fit the new conceptions, the old institution may continue to exist side-by-side with the new operational pattern.

Society seems very reluctant to fully abandon either a frame of reference or a facility that it has brought into existence to handle a human problem. Most characteristically, the new dominating frame of reference is imposed on the old one, like a new archaeological layer on an older deposit. This can be seen, for instance, in some of the residential treatment centers for children. Many of them were originally "indoor-relief" types of facilities such as orphanages, which were transformed into medically modeled treatment institutions. For instance, Bellefaire, in Cleveland, was founded in 1868 as the Cleveland Jewish Orphan Home to take care of Civil War orphans. In 1924, Bellefaire incorporated psychiatric services and the facility took on a new role. Others were formerly correctional or incarcerational facilities and shifted to the medical frame of reference and the residential model (e.g., Wiltwick School, Hawthorne, Cedar Knolls). In such institutions one can see traces of the old orientation and functioning remnants of the old system.

One of the best examples of functional remnants of "archaeological" layering in old institutions is the Federal Narcotics Hospital in Lexington, Kentucky. One enters through a guarded gate and proceeds up a sweeping drive to a heavily barred, massive prison structure. Once inside, one finds a peculiar blending of the older correctional form and the newer psychiatric treatment form. There are uniformed guards on small platforms in the middle of corridor intersections. There are unused, heavy-doored, tiny-peepholed solitary cells; there are massive, iron-barred anachronistic and useless gates in hallways and the heads of stairways. And, in weird juxtaposition, side-by-side with this prison motif and appurtenances, the medical frame of reference is very much in evidence. It can be seen in the medical wards, beds, medical personnel, medical routines and atmosphere of "patient" care, which is also part of the "hospital." Although the medical model seems to have ascended to a dominant position in the culture of the old building, the correctional model is still strongly visible and very much a part of the institution.

Recapitulation

To summarize, programming for deviant children in the modern community has grown out of a very complex process of influences, both contemporary and historical, which can be relatively independent of specific scientific knowledge or a particular program planner. Even the scientific model that effects the program seems to be a product of a particular locale and its own "scientific" history. Thus far, in the history of programming, the scientific conception of the problem and its hard-data input has been only a small part of the larger complex of factors that bring a program into existence and that keep it functioning as a sustained segment of the community's history.

A large proportion of the current demonstration projects and intervention-research projects being conducted by social and behavioral scientists is not part of the mainstream community dynamics such as discussed earlier in this chapter. These are isolated community laboratory exercises which, in all probability, will cease to exist when a grant expires or a principal investigator moves on to a new job in a different locale. One need only review a five-year period of such governmental-funded projects to realize the high mortality rate of these social experiments.

On the other hand, major programs that have become institutionalized in the community usually have a history similar to that described in the Child Saver Movement or the Child Guidance Movement. What is the difference between a short-lived program exercise and an operational program for disturbed children that becomes an integral part of community life and a more permanent implant in the continuing body of the community?

Deviance Programming in the Community

First, community programming appears to be something more than the establishment and operation of an agency or unit to deal with "emotional disturbance." It seems to grow out of natural community processes and revolves around a state of collective readiness for intensive community response to certain forms of variant behavior in one or more collective members. The part of community activities that we now identify as its programs is only one functional aspect of a more complex collective process revolving around deviation. That collective process, for lack of a more descriptive term, might be called "deviance programming" on the part of the community. Such "deviance programming" appears to function in almost all forms of collective living and to be intrinsic to collective life. This aspect has been dealt with in other publications of Rhodes (Rhodes, 1968, Rhodes, in press) and is treated much more fully in a coming publication. The particular process that is being called "deviance programming" can be looked on as naturalistic, instead of as a contrived process, which has a particular cyclical nature in the on-going life of communities. The professional entry into the programming cycle and his professional messages about deviance (usually called program planning) can be looked at as merely a single phase in the total cycle.

To have an influence the professional must attempt to enter into and become a part of the "intrinsic" associational dynamics in communities that contribute to that cycle. He must understand that his entry does not create the necessary associational dynamics, but rather, that the dynamics are always there, and unless he realizes and makes use of them, he is very likely to be extruded along with his ideas, or have himself and his ideas well encapsulated and neutralized by elements and systems that are already an integral part of the community.

The following postulation of such a cycle of associational dynamics is drawn from case examples of programming such as presented in the previous section of this chapter. Those case descriptions referred to the birth, development, and historical carry-over of community programming around behavioral threat and community reactivity to that threat. It appears as though a pattern of threatening behavior either occurs (the outbreak of gang rumbles in the late 1950s and early 1960s) or is depicted by community members (delinquency is on the rise, youth is taking drugs, children are becoming sick). The threatening behavior is captured within some public metaphor or public image (hippie, disturbed, addict, etc.) The community recoils or reacts (they're dirty, they're dangerous, they have to be extruded, they need help). Spokesmen appear in the community (we must save our children, we must crack down, we must treat them). The collective distress moves outside a small circle and begins to have wider and wider effects on the populace (this is not a classroom problem, it is a school problem. It is more than a school problem, it is a community problem. This is a statewide crisis. We are in a state of national emergency). Public distress becomes a political or power issue in the society (we need a state mental health authority. Why doesn't the incumbent have his Welfare Director set up a program? If I am elected, I will move the power of my office behind a statewide program). Political action is taken (legislation is passed, special funds are allocated, program priorities are established).

It is at this phase in the "natural" cycle of community deviance programming that the public service agent or activity is engaged and either launched or reactivated. The public service aids most generally called on are the established mechanisms or bureaus that have responsibility for regulating behavior and behavioral exchanges in the community (education, social welfare, judicial-corrections, medical and mental health, etc.). These bureaus are actually part of a more complex behavioral system of society, which will be described later. However, they have an established armamentarium of strategies for intervening in the community deviance programming cycle, in an attempt to interrupt the particular threat-exchanges that are distressing the community.

Since the same variant behavioral pattern can be interpreted within several different frames of thought and systems of behavioral institutions (delinquent for correctional institutions, sick for mental health institutions, neglected and dependent for welfare institutions, etc.), a chain of competitive exchanges are instigated among local agencies. Since most of these systems are direct extensions and offices of the executive branch of national, state, county, and local government (Welfare Department, Mental Health Department, Judicial Department, etc.), the power of this office is transferred to the agency that is finally rewarded primary responsibility for intervention into the troubling exchanges.

The Behavioral System

When a particular agency or bureau is mobilized in a community cycle of deviance programming, a vast, complex system is engaged. This system is one of several domestic composite patterns of structures, activities, and organizations devoted to forming, controlling, and regulating community behavior and behavior exchanges. These huge composite systems have already been discussed many times in this chapter. In this section we shall take a closer look at their magnitude and their integration of major social institutions which are brought to bear on the troubling deviance exchanges.

Each system integrates major components of governmental and economic power, university training and research, professional guild bodies and university departments and their facilities. The major systems that intervene in community behavior are:

1. education
2. judicial-corrections
3. social welfare and rehabilitation
4. medical mental health

and to a lesser extent (because of separation of church and state in this nation), the religious system.

Each system, as a system, has evolved through lengthy historical developments in Western civilization. Each system consists of the live composite residues of such historical events as described in the Child Saver Movement. Within each is reflected the vicissitudes of social change and shifting focal concerns as different eras singled out different threatening behavioral patterns in communities and sanctioned different power complexes to come to bear on them. The composite network of each system amalgamates certain uniquely identifying elements. Most critical among these elements, as they apply to emotional disturbance, are:

1. A systematic philosophy, set of assumptions, and accumulated body of knowledge about normal and deviant child behavior.
2. A group of intervention techniques derived from the body of knowledge.
3. A guild that has learned the body of knowledge and techniques, along with its university or other educational programs.
4. Operational or action patterns through which the above components are brought to bear on the threat-excited situation.

The educational system has the operational pattern of schools and other facilities.

The judicial-correctional system has its correctional and incarceration facilities.

The social-welfare system has its operational patterns of community-centers, family-service agencies, child-protection agencies, etc.

The mental health system has clinics, hospitals, centers, etc.

In addition, these operational patterns have special subunits or "programs." The schools have guidance programs, special education programs, remedial programs, school-social work programs, school psychology programs, etc. The legal-correctional patterns have probation programs, friends of the court, big brothers programs, etc. The social-welfare patterns have marital counseling programs, aid-to-dependent children programs, child-neglect programs, etc. The mental health patterns have group-therapy programs, milieu-therapy programs, crisis-intervention programs, etc.

Intervention Strategies

Operational patterns and programs differ in their intervention strategies as they attempt to alleviate the disturbance that occurs between the child and his environment. However, programs within any one societal system are derived from that particular system's frame of reference concerning deviant behavior in children. Most of the strategies of change have historically concentrated unilaterally on the threat-exciter (i.e., "disturbed," "disturbing") child. This emphasis on correcting the defect within the child was a result of the dominance of the medical model of disturbance within professional guilds and also a result of the need of political forces within the community to identify a clearly delineated and recognizable target for intervention efforts. However, recently, we have seen the growing awareness of the importance of environmental factors and the consequent emphasis on changing the responding microenvironment or macroenvironment in which the threat-exciter child is embedded and in which the behavioral deviance is occurring. This search for new intervention strategies, which focuses less on changing the child than on changing the environment or the interaction of the child with the environment, has come about with the crushing overload of cases and lack of specialized personnel for the child-centered program. Prevention and environmental influence are playing greater roles in contemporary intervention strategies. These new strategies also take cognizance of the ecological nature of disturbance and attempt to change the quality of the child-environment transaction.

Therefore, surveying both the historically evolved programming efforts for disturbed children as well as emerging ones, we might categorize their intervention strategies as follows.

Exciter-Centered Interventions

In almost all operational patterns and programs that intervene in child disturbance, there has been a bias toward exciter-centered interventions; that is, they aim their change-effects almost exclusively at the exciter, the disturbed child. When they do give consideration to others who are interacting with the child or to the environmental conditions that may be involved in the disturbance, these factors are treated as ancillary or secondary in importance. They are treated as collateral to the disturbance which is perceived as a property or attribute of the child. In general, these interventions make an entry into either the physical or psychological state of the exciter. Typical of this strategy is psychotherapy or psychopharmacology.

Psychotherapy has enjoyed a long period of popularity as a preferred method for alleviating the problem of child disturbance. This method has allowed the community to place major responsibility for disruptive states on deviating children. The psychotherapy conception also allows for the isolation and reduction of complex problems to the simple terms of a disease—a psychological disease. The condition could be localized spatially in the exciter child. All of the scientific orientation toward physical intervention that had been developed by medicine could be carried over into the psychological realm. These conceptions could be applied directly to the exciter and the process of cure could be reenacted within the psychological sphere.

Other interventions into the exciter side of the exciter-respondent disturbance are behavioral intervention, behavioral therapy, behavioral modification, modeling, and so forth. Here we use the behavioral science model to conceptualize and to deal with the problem as a property or attribute of the exciter. Instead of talking about disease, these interventions presuppose that the disturbance arises from "maladapted" behavior which is creating problems for the child and for his environment.

Respondent-Centered Interventions

These interventions concentrate on the other side of the transaction—the responding environment or responding setting of the disturbance. In this case, the setting in which the exciter functions is seen as the antecedent, contemporaneous, or consequent "causes" of the condition is called the disturbance.

Interventions into the setting or environment have taken on increasing importance in recent years. At the macroscopic level, such efforts as neighborhood organization, community development, and urban development have been the strategies employed in this particular orientation.

At the microscopic level, efforts at environmental remodeling include system reorganization, system engineering, milieu-therapy, among others.

In intervening in the exciter-respondent exchange situation, these techniques, like the exciter-centered interventions, are unilateral measures; that is, they deal with only one side of the exchange—namely, the responding environment.

Just as the exciter-centered interventions can reduce the agitation and upset in exchange situations, the concentration on the environment can have the same effect. That is, the reciprocally engendered disturbance is frequently alleviated or abated. Also, by carefully structuring the environment, one can reduce quite markedly the number and frequency of "emotional disturbances."

Exchange-Centered Interventions

More nearly an amalgamation of the other two strategies is one that centers intervention on the threat exciter-respondent exchange patterns themselves. This strategy is relatively new in community-intervention approaches. It has not evolved into an institutionalized system of intervention nor are there yet specific programming efforts derived from its viewpoint. It attempts to influence both sides of the disturbed and disturbing transactions between the child and the responding environment. It attempts to deal with both sets of contingencies (those of the exciter and those of the responding environment) that control the disturbance.

In the long run, this strategy is probably the only one that could enter into and influence the associational dynamics of the community generated by the deviance and response pattern. Perhaps the "Child Advocacy System" recommended by the Joint Commission on the Mental Health of Children (1970) will be an effort in that direction.

Condensation of Cognitive Framework

In the cognitive framework provided in this chapter, we have tried to take a look at the functional ecosystem within which programming takes place. First, there are various scientific models of madness that exist within the scientific fraternity: the behavioral models, the sociological and ecological models, and so forth. Each claims to be a complete, self-contained explanatory and intervention model. The influence of a model depends on (1) the strength of a guild and the power of its operational facilities in a particular community combined with that guild's recognition by and preferred status with the political structures and (2) the prevailing psychological climate and value system of the community with respect to human behavior (deviating behavior is bad, sinful, sick, etc.).

The translation of a model into a public program and community structure is fueled by current and past social threat and recoil crises. In the current crisis, a particular behavioral style and particular behaving groups become the threat-focus of the crisis and produce concerted community recoil and reaction. This threat-recoil cycle is transmitted to power and action-taking sources and the threat-recoil tension is then usually discharged through existing community behavior-regulating structures. These existing structures and facilities are, themselves, products of past social crises in the community. The structures represent community channels created at the height of a historical period of crisis that could not be contained by the then-existing community channels, so that new ones were invented (i.e., the juvenile judicial-correctional structures, the child-guidance structures).

The channel is actually a crisis system translation of a philosophy of human nature, a body of knowledge, a group of specialists, a set of techniques, and a set of facilities through which all these elements are combined and brought to bear on threatening groups.

The concrete structural part of such a crisis system usually becomes an archaeological deposit in communities, whose form can be carried over from crisis to crisis. Even though this form may undergo radical transformations to fit into prevailing community images of the nature of human threat, it tenaciously maintains elements of the old crisis system (i.e., the "new" narcotic hospital, the new "residential" treatment facility, etc.).

Having presented the cognitive framework for programming, let us now turn toward a review of some of the specific techniques and tactics of intervention that are being experimented with by guild groups within various social systems. These natural experiments will offer examples of the vast range and breadth of efforts to deal with child problems in the community.

They might be viewed as the surplus defensive efforts supported and condoned by particular communities or collective bodies to protect against the threat that is either found or imagined to exist in their midst. They also provide a vast library of prototypes from which the community programmer can choose and select, without having to invent additional ones. For convenience, they will be grouped under the headings of social welfare, judicial, medical mental health, and educational so that the programmer can decide which is the most appropriate to fit the particular ecosystem in which he finds himself.

Social-Welfare System

The exciter-centered intervention may be found in the case-worker approach to social work (Perlman, 1957). The social worker acts as counselor or therapist on a one-to-one basis with the client. Although efforts are made in the direction of family counseling and the restructuring of various aspects of the clients' life space, primary emphasis is on the therapeutic role of the professional. The social workers engaged in these processes may utilize psychodynamic techniques such as those employed by clinical psychologists or behavior modification, as in behavior therapy.

Respondent-centered interventions are becoming increasingly important for social workers. In these situations, the social worker does not have direct contact with the child receiving the benefit of his services, but consults with other professionals dealing with the case. Adams and Weinick (1966) describe a program to a school which included both consultation with individual teachers and group seminars in an in-service training effort.

Social work consultation can offer unique advantages in a project reported by Kane (1966) in which a consultant serves priests. The social worker is able to offer individualized guidance for specific problems (case consultation) without supervision of the consultee, dilution of right or responsibility to remain sole judge of action, or betrayal of confidentiality.

Systems reorganization appears to be heavily influencing the roles of social workers. Social work activists have been among the leaders in demanding and attempting change in basic societal structures. Social workers within Head Start programs, Community Action programs, or other antipoverty programs have designed and implemented innovative structures for organizing and educating communities to create a more effective voice for these communities. Levin (1967) describes the establishment of 84 centers in 50 impoverished communities of the Child Development Group of Mississippi. These programs were developed so as to include the poor themselves in the center's functioning, decision making, and resulting consequences.

Community organization with more of a process orientation is found to be effective by Ginsberg (1966). The planning and initiating of new community programs were effected through process-oriented efforts with the total community through committees or councils representing all the small groups including, but not concentrating exclusively on, leadership or power groups. By establishing and maintaining clear and sensitive channels of communication throughout the community, the resources of the community for planning and executing their own programs could be fully tapped.

A Youth Service Project described by Ambrosino (1966) illustrated the effect that a family service agency had on a slum community through its organizational techniques. Efforts to motivate youth and their families to take some form of action concerning the social conditions of their community were successful. Emphasis was placed on methods of enacting social change and community development. After the initial organizational and motivational efforts, the social agency implemented the recreational, educational, vocational, and social work programs evolved from the community action. After four years, significant decreases were found in the rates of vandalism, delinquency, and school dropouts. Ambrosino (1968) stresses the importance of such family agencies in creating long-range planning machinery so as to anticipate the future, in tackling the complex philosophical questions of purpose and in defining priorities. Only then can an agency focus program intervention in order to be effective and preventative in nature.

Perhaps one of the most comprehensive community organization projects that utilizes most models of intervention including some confrontation techniques such as picketing is found in the Mobilization for Youth Program established for the prevention of delinquency in New York City's Lower East Side (Beck, 1966). The avowed purpose of the project is changing the environment instead of the individuals. Small storefront "helping stations" are established for a type of walk-in crisis service. The professional workers try to provide more than a crisis relief, however, by first assuming the role of "social brokerage" agent in mediating between the client and the bureaucracy that is supposed to serve him (i.e., police, welfare, school). An "advocacy role" has evolved in which the worker fights along side the client in order to gain recognition and more appropriate services from the established social agency bureaucracy. The goal, then, is institutional change as well as crisis service. Community development is emphasized in this program as an effort to help residents come to grips with their problems. The evolution of new types of social services such as the organization of consumer cooperatives and voter registration programs have been results of the designing of innovative systems.

Designing or organizing a microenvironment such as that of an institution or agency is also a legitimate role of the social worker. Resnik (1967) sees the social worker as an organizing force in a residential treatment center. It is the function of the worker to use casework and group therapy efforts as well as the coordination of all other social or psychological services in order to effect the cottage treatment milieu.

A confrontation model of intervention in social work may be illustrated by the methods of Alinsky (1965). His primary purpose is to organize and to educate a community to a position of political power. Social workers have been involved in such organizational methods with delinquent gangs in programs of "detached workers" (Spergel, 1966).

Exchange-centered interventions are beginning to emerge from the theory and research of some sociologists. Mercer (1965) deals with the process of how the mentally retarded become labeled as such and highlights the nature of the reciprocal exchange that occurs in order for such labeling to occur. The "interactionist school" of sociology (Becker, 1963, 1964; Goffman, 1961; Scheff, 1966) looks at this exchange process through the sociologist's perspective, though no comprehensive programming efforts have yet emerged from this literature.

Judicial System

The exciter-centered intervention has traditionally been the chief tool of the judicial system. Various methods emphasizing incarceration, counseling (as in probation and parole), and retraining (usually in tandem with incarceration) are all very specifically focused on changing the exciter. New patterns of correction, however, are emerging which may be seen from the respondent-centered viewpoint.

The problems of delinquency seem such that one type of intervention, that of systems reorganization, seems to be most favored. This mode may be used at different levels, however. It is used at a microlevel in which an institution, agency, or even state correctional system is redesigned so as to be more effective in rehabilitation goals and at a macrolevel in which some basic elements of the community are changed in order to prevent delinquency. The

New York City Family Court, Fordham University, the New York City Office of Probation, and the U.S. Office of Juvenile Delinquency and Youth Development are sponsoring a project in which an attempt is made to penetrate, describe, and assess selected neighborhoods in terms of delinquency-producing cultural or organizational patterns. Community action groups are then established with the intention of altering these patterns (Martin, 1966). Evaluation of this project should be very interesting. If this model is effective, it would open a new role for agencies heretofore "correctional" in nature to engage in preventive measures through community organization.

A great deal of work in systems reorganization has been accomplished by the California Youth Authority (Warren, 1969) and more recently by the Federal Bureau of Prisons (Gerard, 1970). Based on the assumption that the same treatment program is beneficial to some types of offenders and detrimental to others, a series of programs have been developed. Some of the findings of these studies would dictate nationwide reorganization of programming for delinquents. These findings may be summarized as:

1. Offenders can be reliably classified in treatment-relevant ways.
2. A large proportion of youthful offenders can be treated in community-based programs instead of in institutions.
3. Grouping of offenders into homogeneous living units by subtypes decreases institutional management problems.
4. Offenders well matched with their treaters may have higher success rates than those not matched.

System reorganization is also advocated by Davitto and Scullion (1967) and by Burdman (1969) in his program to launch a community-based correctional system. Incorporating some of the ideas of differential treatment, Burdman sees a blending of institutional and field programs for those who must initially be placed in confinement, a wide-range application of community services not now utilized, and extensive and enthusiastic free-citizen participation and understanding. Such an innovative step in our correctional system would certainly call for a different role for the correctional agent in the field. Professionals in the field must work to gain organizational, professional, political, and public acquiescence; to promote understanding among the legal system concerning the goals and methods of the correctional system; to define new staff roles and functions; to reorganize institutional structure; and to evaluate and feedback research results (Burdman, 1969). One may visualize the correctional agent much more easily than in terms of the traditional image of probation officer.

Statewide reorganization is advocated by Sheridan (1967) in which departments of services for all children and youth should be established instead of maintaining separate services for delinquents. A specific statewide innovation is described by McNeil (1967) in which a system of half-way house programs was established in Michigan. Along with the systems reorganization involved, new roles were developed for case workers as they lived with the youthful offenders in an "open" or free situation. This system also approaches the problem of delinquency at the community level where preventive supervision, better probation programs, and volunteer work are coordinated.

Medical Mental Health System

Exciter-centered strategies have been the primary source of programming for the mental health professions. Psychotherapy in all of its forms is the prototype of most exciter-centered interventions. However, other strategies may be respondent-oriented and still operate legitimately within this medical system.

Consultation has long been an important function of the medically oriented professions of psychology and psychiatry. Schools, social service agencies, industry, and correctional institutions have used psychiatric or psychological consultants in planning and executing programs that would promote healthier self-concept, role identity, reduction of anxiety, and other factors involved in maintaining mental health. Although the recent Community Mental Health Centers Construction Act adhered to the traditional medical model, a reference to consultation and educational services has given the psychologist numerous opportunities for expanding his role. It has been mentioned that through consultation with general practitioners, teachers, ministers, judges, and police officers, the community mental health professional "can increase the knowledge and ability of those who deal with the public so that they will be able to promote mental health by helping people meet life crises in constructive ways" (Rosenblum, 1968).

Prevention of mental disturbance through consultation is a chief emphasis of Caplan (1964) in which he is concerned with reducing the prevalency of mental illness rather than investing all efforts in analysis of underlying pathology. He approaches the problem of reducing the length and intensity of the disorder through techniques of early detection. Weisman (1965) supports this trend for preventive measures and emphasis on present interaction rather than analysis of pathology. "If a patient can reverse the pattern of failure in interpersonal relations and succeed, he may be more susceptible to an acceptance of insights into how he had operated in the past." This emphasis would seem to allow other professionals concerned with behavioral change a more legitimate role in interventions less concerned with a medical analysis of pathology. Psychiatry can play a larger role in prevention programs through consultation services to other professionals.

Consultation used in a different manner is a key feature of the Dr. H. Philip Dinan Evaluation Center of Bridgeport, Connecticut. This center's orientation stresses immediate, contemporary problems, the social context within which they occur, short-time and time-limited treatment, the utilization of subprofessionals under supervision, and full involvement of school, parent, and other agencies in the treatment program (Tolor & Lane, 1968). The consultation role is utilized to help increase the effectiveness of highly trained professionals. The actual evaluation and treatment of the client is done by the "social counselor," a new role developed by the center in which women with a background in the social sciences such as teachers, nurses, and welfare workers were trained as counselors. These social counselors then have available to them consultation and supervision by two professional consultants—psychologists and psychiatrists. This center also operates several programs patterned on the medical model such as classes for the disturbed and group therapy sessions at the high school.

Most mental health centers intermix programs arising from at least two modes of intervention—consultation and systems reorganization. As psychology and psychiatry become more prevention-oriented, social action or system reorganization techniques in mental health centers proliferate. Dumont (1968) suggests that psychiatry must also concern itself with the "sick society" by joining other behavioral sciences in creating an environment conducive to the mental health of all people in the community. He feels that significant advances in mental health can come about through social change.

The program of the South Shore Mental Health Center in Quincy, Massachusetts has evolved out of such a philosophy of planned social change in which community mental health plays an integral role. The program has five broad functions: (1) prevention and amelioration of mental disorders through consultation and education, (2) emergency and short-term treatment of disturbed and retarded individuals, (3) involvement in key community planned change programs, (4) training at professional and nonprofessional levels, and (5) research in the community laboratory (Rosenblum, 1968). Consultation in this program takes several forms, some of which seem inseparable from system reorganization or planned change agentry. It involves consulting relationships with those who fill major caretaking and planning roles in the community with such services as crisis consultation, self-help consultation, in-service training and educational programs, and administrative consultation.

To fulfill such functions, Rosenblum suggests that two differently trained psychologists are needed: a clinically oriented psychologist and a community psychologist whose concerns are more oriented toward system reorganization.

The activities of community psychologists at the South Shore Center include involvement with community-planned change organizations such as Operation Head Start, Welfare Department Community Action Program, Neighborhood Youth Corps, and other antipoverty programs. The psychologists perform such services as conducting groups so as to motivate and interest individuals in leaving welfare roles and taking jobs. Sarason, Levine, Goldenberg, Cherlin & Bennett (1966) describe many types of community-based social action programs being performed by mental health centers.

The Neighborhood Service Center, an outgrowth of the Lincoln Hospital Mental Health Service in the Bronx, New York, is yet another innovative structure springing from the dual orientation of a preventive approach to mental health problems and community action. Its primary goals are to expedite and integrate services, to develop a community action program directed toward increased social cohesion in the area, and to effect institutional change in the service-providing institutions of the community (Riessman, 1967).

Systems reorganization or environmental manipulation within the realm of clinical psychology may be on a microenvironmental level as well as communitywide intervention. The structuring of the entire milieu for therapeutic effect has been used for some time in psychiatry. The Sonia Shankman Orthogenic School of the University of Chicago under Bettelheim (1950) has been completely structured so as to bring about clinically derived goals. Milieu therapy in many institutions in which all staff members, professional and nonprofessional, as well as the physical environment have been carefully planned as part of the total treatment program. These programs are operated from both a psychoanalytic tradition and a behavior modification orientation. Lovaas, Freitag, Gold & Kassorla (1965) have extinguished self-destructive behavior in institutionalized children through manipulation of the environment to reinforce only appropriate social behavior.

An exchange-oriented strategy might be seen in the work of Proshansky, Ittelson, & Rivlin (1970) in which they show the interaction of psychiatric patients and their physical environment to be a crucial variable in determining their behavior. They conclude that people, policies, and partitions are the three great determinants of behavior on the ward. Therefore, administrative decisions and the physical design of facilities are very viable intervention techniques to alter behavior in a setting in which the intensive exciter-oriented strategy predominates.

Educational System

As a legacy of exciter-oriented interventions, special classes for "disturbed" children are still the major technique utilized by the school in dealing with this particular group (see Chapter Ten). The crisis teacher program (Morse, 1962) is an attempt to deal with the exciter, but in the context of his regular classroom. The child remains in the regular classroom and is referred to the crisis teacher when isolation is deemed necessary. The crisis teacher works closely with the regular teacher in programming for the child.

However, logistical considerations and the trend toward preventive techniques have stimulated efforts to provide consultation attempts to reduce the incidence of behavioral disorder occurring in the classroom through the promotion of more growth-inducing environments and to provide the teacher with skills enabling her to handle more effectively a greater range of behavior. This type of consultation may be given by professionals already operating in the school. The Psycho-Educational Clinic in the public schools of New Haven, Connecticut have operated in such a manner so as to decrease sharply its traditional function as test-giver and concentrate on consulting with teachers to give them information applicable to the learning situation and related to specific problems arising in the classroom (Sarason, 1967). Morse (1962) defines the prime function of the outside consultant as facilitation of a problem-solving process by bringing to the teacher's attention aspects of the problem and possible ways of seeking a solution.

Consultation is the keystone of a program developed by Newman in Washington, D.C. (Newman, 1967). A program of continuous and regular on-the-spot consultation with teachers and small groups of teachers was developed. The consultant helped the teacher by promoting a more objective viewpoint concerning problems, by offering support, by helping the teacher identify specific problems and possible solutions to them, and by sometimes imparting certain skills to the teacher such as Life Space Interviewing (Long, Morse, & Newman, 1965).

A project at the University of Texas has attempted to bring about more effective utilization of resources already in the school to promote communication between mental health workers and the schools in order to deal with factors handicapping the teacher in working effectively with problems (Iscoe, Pierce-Jones, Friedman, & McGehearty, 1967). The role of the child behavior consultant was developed and consultation is performed in San Antonio and Austin public schools. Here again, the emphasis is on developing and expanding the resources of the teacher instead of on specific servicing of the disturbing child. A similar project is underway at the University of Michigan. The Child Development Consultant Project is training experienced teachers to enter the schools as full-time staff consultants whose concern is the mental health of all children.

A more "process-" oriented consultation closely related to what we have termed planned change agentry has been developed in California. The Self-Enhancing Education program (Randolph & Howe, 1966) seeks to train teachers in innovative methods of conducting classrooms so as to promote better pupil self-concept. The emphasis is on bringing to the teacher skills in conducting group problem-solving sessions and helping pupils improve in communication skills.

Techniques of system reorganization in the school have been developed primarily by those in the field of behavior modification. An entire educational program was designed at the National Training School for Boys in Washington, D.C. based on environmental planning concepts and operant learning and design techniques (Cohen et al., 1967). The CASE (Contingencies Applicable to Special Education) project developed a totally individualized program of instruction utilizing a token economy system with negotiable "points" for purchasing entrance into a lounge where snacks and social contact were available. The resulting behavior was much improved and academic procedures employed in CASE are applicable to general public education and the supporting social environment.

A system reorganization in a public school setting was implemented in Santa Monica and Tulare, California, and Palolo School in Oahu, Hawaii (Hewett, 1967). This program attempts translation of behavior modification theory to the classroom and consists of restructuring the classroom so as to implement these principles. Hewett has devised a hierarchy of educational tasks around which the curriculum and physical arrangement of the room are based. A system of meaningful rewards following accomplishment of task has been incorporated into the program using checkmarks which may be exchanged for candy, etc. The entire system is so constructed so as to give the teacher control over the learning environment. A similar system operating in the context of a resource room has been developed by Glavin, Quay, Annesley, & Werry, 1971).

Project ReED (Hobbs, 1966; Lewis, 1967) was developed as two residential centers in Nashville, Tennessee and Durham, North Carolina in conjunction with Peabody College. Emphasis here was on intervention in social systems or the interaction of the exciter and the responding environment instead of concentrating all efforts on the child or on the manipulation of the environment. "Emotional disturbance," as defined by this project, consisted of an accumulation of discrepancies between role performances and role prescriptions as they apply to social interaction. Intervention, from this perspective, must effectively influence this interaction through increasing congruence between the role prescription held by the systems and those held by the child or by increasing the congruence between these prescriptions and the child's role performances. This project developed an intensive short-term residential program to implement this theoretical framework and developed two new professional roles—that of teacher-counselor and of liaison-teacher. Consultation was extensively used for evaluation of the children's records, for crisis consultation with the teacher-counselors, and on a regular basis with the teacher-counselors. Ecological principles of emotional disturbance as illustrated in this project have been formulated by Rhodes (1967) for use in public school programs.

Another approach, which may be viewed from an ecological exchange viewpoint, is that of Hamblin, Buckholt, Bushnell, Ellis, & Ferritor (1969) in St. Louis at the Central Midwestern Regional Laboratories. Their adaptation of social exchange theory utilizing some of the principles of game theory has been effective with extraordinarily aggressive boys, normal two-year-olds, ghetto children, and autistic children. A token economy system is utilized and very specific training is given to the teacher. Manipulation of the environment is not the chief emphasis, however. The exchange between the teacher and the child receives the focus of attention. Manipulation of environmental contingencies is one technique used in influencing this exchange to reward "good" behavior and discourage "bad" behavior. The system of the classroom is modified to change the "name of the game" from "get the teacher" to "learn."

Another approach that may be termed respondent-centered is that of total reorganization of that environment termed "school." This was done by Dennison (1970) in his First Street School in which half of the children came from public schools with severe learning and behavior problems. By restructuring the environment along "free school" lines, Dennison was able to show remarkable success with these "problem children."

Confrontation models of instituting change in schools are becoming more common. The organization of groups of parents, usually in inner cities, whose children are labeled by the school as disadvantaged/disturbed/retarded has become a vehicle for politically confronting a system to demand change. Alinsky and several other social welfare projects previously discussed have had as one of their concerns the improved service of the schools to the disadvantaged. The concern and involvement of the community in the school has become a major issue confronting educators. This would seem to have great import for our present programming for the disturbed since these classifications and their implications are being called into question by these parents. Special classes and the procedures utilized for filling them are under attack in many large cities through the judicial system and lawsuits instigated by parents. These reactions are usually leveled at the exciter-centered programming offered by the schools and the label and concomitant stigma often applied to children simply because of cultural difference.

Summary and Conclusion

In summary, it becomes evident that community programming for the emotionally disturbed child is a complex process of human ecology. Much of the process of rendering of "services" to children is a complex of community dynamics. Service is enveloped in a recurrent collective phenomenon of the threat of individual variation within the community, on one hand, and the collective tendency to project all forms of collective threat on a few vulnerable individuals or groups within the collective, on the other. Both processes are operating in community programming for emotionally disturbed children.

In many ways, the actions of the individual professional who serves deviant children is as much determined by this community process of individual threat and collective recoil, as is the form that individual deviation takes in a particular community. It is very evident that community programming for deviant children involves much more than scientific knowledge, conceptions, and professional practices. It appears also to be a function of a composite of political factors, public threat, historical precedent, and established frameworks for looking at and controlling social behavior.

If we take a longitudinal look at any of the "systems of care" that have come into existence in this country (such as the juvenile corrections system or the child guidance system), we observe a cycle of associational dynamics revolving around behavioral threat and community reactivity to that threat. A pattern of threatening behavior either occurs or is anticipated by community members. The threatening behavior is captured within some public imagery. The community reacts. Spokesmen for defensive action appear. The collective distress over the threat moves outward in the community like ripples in a disturbed pond. Public distress becomes a political and power issue in the society. At this point a public "service" or public action program is instituted against the threat. It is in this latter phase of the cycle that the community "program" specialist can make his input in terms of a specific operational pattern for coming to grips with the threat.

In general, communities within the United States have available to them a limited number of systems of behavioral control and regulation when public concern is aroused. These include the educational, judicial-corrections, social welfare and rehabilitative, and the medical-mental health systems. Each system has its own conceptions and body of knowledge about deviations such as emotional disturbance. Each has its own characteristic guild groups.

The time has come for us to have a better grasp of this total community process and the meaning that it has for our activities. Intervention into the problem of emotional disturbance requires that we understand the deviance dynamics of communities and the purpose that they serve in community life. We can no longer think in terms of small, specialized programs, in individual facilities or settings for children. We must look at the way in which children are caught up in deviance dynamics of communities and the way in which the "service" complex must be altered.

Perhaps we must go even further. Perhaps we have reached a period in history where the accumulation of this vast social paraphernalia for defense against real or imagined child threat, and the accretion of public and professional imagery regarding disturbed or disturbing children has begun to overwhelm us as human communities. Perhaps radical solutions are necessary. It may be that we must quickly discover methods of "treating" collective dynamics so that we can more adequately come to terms with deviation and individual differences in our midst. Perhaps we must carefully scrutinize the massive institutional forms (such as juvenile corrections and child guidance) and determine how well they serve community needs and to what extent they are solutions to the problems of today. Both efforts are probably long overdue. It is very likely that, in this case, human tendency to permanently record its crises and its structural solutions to those crises in its living culture can become a threat to humanistic existence.

References

Adams, R., & Weinick, H. Consultation: An inservice training program for the school. *Journal of the American Academy of Child Psychiatry*, 1966, **5**(3), 479–489.

Alinsky, S. The professional radical. *Harpers*, 1965, **230**(1381), 137–147.

Alt, H. *Residential treatment for the disturbed child.* New York: International Universities Press, 1960.

Ambrosino, S. A family service agency reaches out to a slum ghetto. *Social Work*, 1966, **11**(4), 17–23.

Ambrosino, S. New directions for the family agency. *Social Casework*, 1968, **49**(1), 15–21.

Axline, V. *Play therapy.* Boston: Houghton-Mifflin, 1947.

Barker, R. *Ecological psychology.* Stanford: Stanford University Press, 1968.

Barker, R. (Ed.) *The stream of behavior.* New York: Appleton-Century-Crofts, 1963.

Beck, B. A (new) social work model. *Social Service Review*, 1966, **40**(3), 270–274.

Becker, H. *Outsiders: Studies in the sociology of deviance.* New York: Free Press, 1963.

Becker, H. (Ed.) *The other side: Perspectives on deviance.* New York: Free Press, 1964.

Bender, L. Childhood schizophrenia: A review. *International Journal of Psychiatry*, 1968, **5**, 211–220.

Berkowitz, P., & Rothman, E. *Public education for disturbed children in New York City.* Springfield, Illinois: Charles C. Thomas, 1967.

Bettelheim, B. *Love is not enough.* Glencoe, Illinois: Free Press, 1950.

Block, H., & Niederhoffer, A. *The gang: A study in adolescent behavior.* New York: Philosophical Library, 1958.

Boshes, B., & Myklebust, H. A neurological and behavioral study of children with learning disorders. *Neurology*, 1964, **14**(1), 7–12.

Burdman, M. Realism in community-based correctional services. *Annals of the American Academy of Political and Social Science*, 1969, **381**, 71–80.

Burks, H. The hyperkinetic child. *Exceptional Children*, 1960, **27**, 18–26.

Calhoun, J. Ecological factors in the development of behavioral anomalies. In *Comparative psychopathology.* New York: Grune and Stratton, 1967.

Caplan, G. *Principals of preventative psychiatry.* New York: Basic Books, 1964.

Clausen, J. The ecology of mental disorders. In *Symposium on preventative and social psychiatry*. Washington, D.C.: U.S. Government Printing House, 1959.

Cohen, A. *Delinquent boys: The culture of the gang*. Glencoe, Illinois: The Free Press, 1961.

Cohen, A. *Deviance and control. Englewood Cliffs,* New Jersey: Prentice-Hall, 1966.

Cohen, H., Filipczak, J., & Bis, J. Case I: An initial study of contingencies applicable to special education. Silver Springs, Maryland: Institute for Behavioral Research, 1967.

Conger, J., & Miller, W. *Personality, social class and delinquency*. New York: Wiley, 1966.

Connery, R. (Ed.) *The politics of mental health: Organizing community mental health in metropolitan areas*. New York: Columbia University Press, 1968.

Cruickshank, W. *A teaching method for brain-injured and hyperactive children*. Syracuse: Syracuse University Press, 1961.

Danitto, B., & Scullion, T. An experiment in community treatment of delinquents. *Social Casework*, 1967, **48**(1), 10–16.

Dennison, G. *The lives of children*. New York: Random House, 1969.

Digest of Crisis in child mental health: Challenge for the 1970's. Final report of the Joint Commission on Mental Health of Children, Inc., 1969.

Dreikurs, R., & Dinkmeyer, D. *Encouraging children to learn. Englewood Cliffs,* New Jersey: Prentice-Hall, 1963.

Dubos, R. *Man adapting*. New Haven: Yale University Press, 1965.

Dumont, M. *The absurd healer*. New York: Science House, 1963.

Duncan, O. *Social organization and the ecosystem*. In R. Faris (Ed.) Handbook of modern sociology. Chicago: Rand McNally, 1964.

Empey, L. *Alternatives to incarceration*. U.S. Department of Health, Education, and Welfare, Welfare Administration, Office of Juvenile Delinquency and Youth Development, 1967.

Erikson, E. *Identity and the life cycle: Psychological Issues, Vol. 1, No. 1*. New York: International Universities Press, 1959.

Eysenck, H. *Behavior therapy and the neuroses*. New York: Pergamon Press, 1960.

Faris, R., & Dunham, H. *Mental disorders in urban areas*. Chicago: Phoenix Press, 1965. (University of Chicago Press, 1939).

Fawl, C. Disturbances experienced by children in their natural habitats. In R. Barker, (Ed.) *Stream of behavior*. New York: Appleton-Century-Crofts, 1963.

Franks, C. *Conditioning techniques in clinical practices and research*. New York: Springer, 1964.

Freud, A. *Normality and pathology in childhood*. New York: International Universities Press, 1965.

Freud, S. *The basic writings of Sigmund Freud*. Translated and edited by A. A. Brill. New York: Modern Library, 1938.

Gerard, R. E. *Differential Treatment: A Way to Begin*. Washington, D.C.: Bureau of Prisons, Dept. of Justice, 1970.

Gerard, D., & Houston, L. Family settings and social ecology of schizophrenia. *Psychiatric Quarterly*, 1955, **27**, 90–101.

Ginsberg, L. Mineral city: An experience in process-oriented community organization. *Journal of Jewish Communal Service,* 1966, **42**(3), 234–238.

Glavin, J. P., Quay, H. C., Annesley, F. R., & Werry, J. S. An experimental resource room for classroom behavior problem children. *Exceptional Children,* 1971, **38,** 131–137.

Goffman, E. *Asylums.* Garden City: Anchor Books, 1961.

Hall, C., & Lindzey, G. *Theories of personality.* New York: Wiley, 1965.

Hamblin, R., Buckholt, D., Bushnell, D., Ellis, D., & Ferritor, D. Changing the game from "get the teacher" to "learn." *Transactions,* 1969, **6**(3), 20–31.

Hartmann, H. *Ego psychology and the problem of adaptation.* New York: International Universities Press, 1958.

Hartmann, H., Kris, E., & Lowenstein, R. Comments on the formation of the psychic structure. *Psychoanalytic Study of the Child, Vol. II.* New York: International Universities Press, 1946.

Hawley, A. *Human ecology: A theory of community structure.* New York: Ronald Press, 1950.

Hawley, A. The approach of human ecology to urban research. *Science Monthly,* 1951, **73,** 48–49.

Hewett, F. Educational engineering with emotionally disturbed children. *Exceptional Children,* 1967, **33**(7), 459–467.

Hewett, F. *The emotionally disturbed child in the classroom.* Boston: Allyn and Bacon, 1969.

Hobbs, N. Helping disturbed children: Psychological and ecological strategies. *American Psychologist,* 1966, **21**(12), 1105–1115.

Hooker, E. Sequences in homosexual identification. Paper read at the American Sociological Association, 1960.

Iscoe, I., Pierce-Jones, J., Friedman, S., & McGehearty, L. Some strategies in mental health consultation. In Cowan, E., Gardner, E., & Zax, M. *Emergent approaches to mental health problems.* New York: Appleton-Century-Crofts, 1967.

Joint Commission on Mental Health of Children, Inc. *Crisis in child mental health: Challenge for the 1970's.* New York: Harper and Row, 1970.

Jones, R. *Fantasy and feeling in education.* New York: New York University Press, 1968.

Jordan, N. Some formal characteristics of the behavior of two disturbed boys. In R. Barker (Ed.), *Stream of behavior.* New York: Appleton-Century-Crofts, 1963.

Kane, R. F. Social work consultation to the priest. *Catholic Charities Review,* 1966, **50**(8), 4–10.

Kephart, N. *The slow learner in the classroom.* Columbus: C. Merrill, 1960.

Klein, M. *The psychoanalysis of children.* London: Hogarth, 1932.

Levin, T. The child development group of Mississippi: A hot sector of the quiet front in the war on poverty. *American Journal of Orthopsychiatry,* 1967, **37**(1), 139–145.

Lewis, W. Project RE-ED: Educational intervention in discordant child rearing systems. In Cowen et al., *Emergent approaches to mental health problems.* New York: Appleton-Century-Crofts, 1967.

Long, N., Morse, W., & Newman, R. (Eds.) *Conflict in the classroom*. Belmont, California: Wadsworth Publishing Company, 1965.

Lovaas, I., Freitag, G., Gold, V., & Kassorla, I. Experimental studies in childhood schizophrenia: Analysis of self-destructive behavior. *Journal of Experimental Child Psychology*, 1965, **2**(1), 67–84.

Martin, J. Juvenile court demonstration project. *Crime and Delinquency Abstracts*, **4**(1), National Clearinghouse for Mental Health Information, U.S. Department of Health, Education, and Welfare, Public Health Service, 1966.

McCorkle, L., Elias, A., & Bixby, F. *The Highfields story: A unique experiment in the treatment of juvenile delinquency*. New York: Holt, Rinehart, and Winston, 1958.

McNeil, F. A halfway-house program for delinquents. *Crime and Delinquency*, 1967, **13**(4), 538–544.

Mercer, J. Social system perspective and clinical perspective: Frames of reference for understanding career patterns of persons labeled as mentally retarded. *Social Problems*, 1965, **13**, 18–34.

Miller, W. B. Lower class culture as a generating milieu of gang delinquency. *Journal of Social Issues*, 1958, **14**, 5–19.

Miller, W. B. Preventive work with street corner groups: Boston delinquency project. *Annals of the American Academy of Political and Social Sciences*, 1959, **322**, 97–106.

Millon, T. *Theories of psychopathology*. Philadelphia: W. B. Saunders, 1967.

Morse, W. The crisis teacher public school provision for the disturbed pupil. *School of Education Bulletin*, 1962, **37**, 101–104.

Newman, R. *Psychological consultation in the schools*. New York: Basic Books, 1967.

Perlman, H. *Social case work*. Chicago: University of Chicago Press, 1957.

Phillips, E., & Weiner, D. *Short term psychotherapy and structured behavior change*. New York: McGraw-Hill, 1966.

Platt, A. *The child savers: The invention of delinquency*. Chicago: University of Chicago Press, 1969.

Proshansky, H., Ittelson, W., & Rivlin, L. *Environmental psychology: Man and his physical setting*. New York: Holt, Rinehart, and Winston, 1970.

Randolph, N., & Howe, W. *Self enhancing education*. Palo Alto, California: Stanford Press, 1966.

Raush, H. Naturalistic method and the clinical approach. In E. Willems & H. Raush (Eds.), *Naturalistic viewpoints in psychological research*. New York: Holt, Rinehart, and Winston, 1969.

Raush, H., Dittman, A., & Taylor, T. Person, setting and change in social interaction, II. A normal control study. *Human Relations*, 1960, **13**(4), 305–332.

Redl, F., & Wineman, D. *The aggressive child*. New York: Free Press, 1957.

Reitan, R. Relationships between neurological and psychological variables and their implications for reading instruction. In H. Robinson (Ed.), *Meeting individual differences in reading*. Chicago: University of Chicago Press, 1964.

Resnik, D. The social worker as co-ordinator in residential treatment. *Social Casework*, 1967, **48**(5), 293–297.

Rhodes, W. Psychological techniques and theory applied to behavior modification. *Exceptional Children,* 1962, **28**(6), 333–338.

Rhodes, W. The disturbing child: A problem in ecological management. *Exceptional Children,* 1967, **33**, 449–455.

Rhodes, W. Utilization of mental health professionals in the school. *Review of Educational Research,* 1968, **38**(5), 497–511.

Rhodes, W. A community participation analysis of emotional disturbance. *Exceptional Children,* 1970, **36**(5), 309–314.

Rhodes, W. Ecological model of emotional disturbance. In J. Paul & W. Rhodes, *Models of emotional disturbance.* Englewood Cliffs: Prentice-Hall, in press.

Riessman, F. A neighborhood-based mental health approach. In Cowen, et al., *Emergent approaches to mental health problems.* New York: Appleton-Century-Crofts, 1967.

Rimland, B. *Infantile autism.* New York: Appleton-Century-Crofts, 1964.

Roman, M. Community control and the community mental health center. Presented at National Institute of Mental Health staff meeting on metropolitan topics: Dilemma of Community Control: University and Community Relations, November 21, 1969, Washington, D.C.

Rosenblum, G. The new role of the clinical psychologist in a community mental health center. *Community Mental Health Journal,* 1968, **4**(5), 403–409.

Rubington, E., & Weinberg, M. (Eds.) *Deviance: The interaction perspective.* London: Macmillan, 1968.

Sarason, S. New directions in psychological services for children with mental, emotional, and cultural handicaps. *New York Society for the Experimental Study of Education Yearbook,* 1967, 48–50.

Sarason, S., Levine, M., Goldenberg, I., Cherlin, D., & Bennett, E. *Psychology in community settings.* New York: Wiley, 1966.

Scheff, T. *On being mentally ill: A sociological theory.* Chicago: Aldine 1966.

Sells, S. Ecology and the science of psychology. In E. Willems & H. Raush (Eds.), *Naturalistic viewpoints in psychological research.* New York: Holt, Rinehart, and Winston, 1969.

Sheridan, W. Structuring services for delinquent children and youth. *Federal Probations,* 1967, **31**(3), 51–56.

Siegler, M., & Osmond, H. Models of madness, *British Journal of Psychiatry,* 1966, **112**, 1193–1203.

Spergel, I. *Street gang work: Theory and practice.* Reading, Massachusetts: Adelison-Wesley, 1966.

Staff of Bronx State Hospital, Bronx State Hospital. Chronicle of the strike, November 21–27, 1968.

Stevenson, G. *Child guidance clinics.* New York: The Commonwealth Fund, 1934.

Tolor, A., & Lane, P. An experimental approach to the treatment of disturbed school-aged children. *Journal of School Psychology,* 1968, **6**(2), 97–103.

Ullmann, L., & Krasner, L. *A psychological approach to abnormal behavior.* Englewood Cliffs, New Jersey: Prentice-Hall, 1969.

Warren, M. The case for differential treatment of delinquents. *Annals of the American Academy of Political and Social Science,* 1969, **381**, 47–59.

Weisman, M. The role of psychoanalysis in community mental health. In J. Masserman, *Communication and community.* New York: Grune and Stratton, 1965.

Whyte, W. *Street corner society.* Chicago: University of Chicago Press, 1946.

Wolpe, J. *Psychotherapy by reciprocal inhibition.* Stanford: Stanford University Press, 1958.

Wolpe, J., & Lazarus, A. *Behavior therapy techniques: A guide to the treatment of neuroses.* London: Pergamon Press, 1966.

Chapter Ten

Educational Programs for Children with Behavior Disorders

Frank M. Hewett

The child with a behavior disorder is perhaps never more visible than when he is faced with demands for attention, participation, direction following, control, socially acceptable behavior, and mastery of academic skills in the classroom. The American school as a primary socializing agency for a society emphasizing conformity and achievement sets these expectations as basic to formal educational training. As children arrive in school unable to meet these expectations, concern immediately arises regarding: (1) How many of such children are there? (2) What are their characteristics? (3) How can they be classified so that what they are called has direct relevance to what might be done with them in the classroom?

If children with behavior disorders are viewed as "severely maladjusted," their incidence in the school population has been estimated from four to seven percent (White & Harris, 1961) based on studies done from 1928 to 1958. If they are viewed as "mildly maladjusted" or as belonging to discrete categories (e.g., neurotic) estimates of their actual number are highly unreliable because of the problems of definition and the variability in sampling techniques and instruments used to obtain data.

Medical and psychiatric classification terms have been relied on in special education to describe children with behavior disorders, but the worthlessness of such a practice is becoming increasingly apparent. Labels such as "brain damage behavior syndrome," "hyperkinetic impulse disorder," "Strauss syndrome" (Clements & Peters, 1962) do little to describe children with behavior disorders in educationally meaningful terms. "Habit disturbances," "neurotic traits," and "psychoses" (Watson, 1961) are essentially useless equivalents from psychiatry, as are "adjustment reactions of childhood" or "adolescence." Moving into broader classification areas we find children with behavior disorders considered "emotionally disturbed," "socially maladjusted," "minimally neurologically impaired," "culturally disadvantaged," "educationally handicapped," and afflicted with a "conduct disturbance." In some instances all of these labels can be collectively pinned on a single child who is experiencing difficulty in school. In this respect they are of little value for the planning of specific educational programs. In another respect, as we shall discover later in this chapter, such labels do reflect the differences in orientation that exist among special educators who are confronted with the task of providing educational programs for children with behavior disorders. We shall return to them for a discussion of these orientations and the specific classroom practices with which they are associated.

It should be stated at this point that behavior disorders may occur in combination with any handicapping condition such as mental retardation, blindness, deafness, and physical and severe neurological impairment. In this chapter the children primarily being discussed are those who are free from intellectual and disabling sensory and physical handicaps, although many of the educational approaches to be reviewed have been utilized with children who are afflicted with these handicaps and who also manifest behavior disorders.

Patterson (1964) has questioned medical-psychiatric classifications of children with behavior disorders and suggests that assessing them according to dimensions of hyperactivity, aggressiveness, immaturity, anxiety, and withdrawn behavior will lead to more workable homogeneous groupings. Quay, Morse, and Cutler (1966) have analyzed characteristics of deviant children in the schools and found their behavior to reflect three major dimensions: conduct, inadequacy-immaturity, and personality problems. Since these dimensions have been discussed at length in Chapter One they need not be further described here.

Despite the authoritative ring to the psychiatric labels and the extensive research related to the factorial dimensions, the ultimate test of their educational worth comes when the teacher who is presented with a child described by them says, "Fine. Now just what do I do with him in the classroom?" It is the continuity between diagnosis and classroom practice that is all too often overlooked. Elaborate case studies which include detailed descriptions of personality characteristics, family background, psychological test findings, and one or more diagnostic labels may be compiled and then promptly filed away fulfilling the administrator's and psychologist's responsibility, but leaving the teacher essentially empty-handed.

In an attempt to deal practically with the "translatability gap" between description, diagnosis, classification, and educational programming, a set of behavioral objectives or educational goals necessary for success in learning and school have been formulated (Hewett, 1968). These goals are arranged in a developmental sequence that begins with *attention* and moves through *response, order, exploratory, social, mastery,* and *achievement* levels. Each goal is described in terms of behaviors related to its attainment, and assessment of the child with a behavior disorder is made on the basis of whether he has acquired these behaviors. A profile is then drawn and a school program is planned accordingly. The goals or objectives stated in the developmental sequence have been found to lend themselves to formulation of such programs along with development of curriculum tasks. This approach admittedly defines broad areas of competence needed by all children for success in school and much work is needed to delineate the specific tasks that will aid in their attainment. Its use in a total classroom design for children with behavior disorders will be described later in this chapter.

With this introduction to the description of children with behavior disorders we turn now to a discussion of the types of educational programs that have been provided for them. It will soon be apparent, that what has been offered has been closely related to how the child whose behavior is deviant in the classroom is perceived by the educator. The critical aspects of such perceptions are: (1) *What* is the source of the behavior disorder? (2) *Why* is it occurring in the classroom? In our discussion of these issues we shall refer to the general labels presented earlier—emotionally disturbed, socially maladjusted, minimally neurologically impaired, culturally disadvantaged, educationally handicapped, and conduct disturbance—since any or all of them have been used to describe children with behavior disorders. Following this we shall review and compare educational programs that have been developed for such children.

When a child is given the label "emotionally disturbed," it is often implied that he suffers from an emotional "illness." What is seen in the classroom is a manifestation of this illness and the psychological conflicts, faulty attitudes about self and others, disturbed perception of the environment, fears, and anxieties that may be at the basis of the illness must be understood before we can hope to effectively teach him. Emotional disturbance is expressed through deviant behavior in the classroom when the child is overwhelmed by people— teachers and peers—whom he mistrusts and fears and with demands that he cannot handle.

A child described as "socially maladjusted" is considered out of step with the values of the society and defective in conscience and capacity to empathize with others. Morse (1967) places three types of children in this category. First is the "semi-socialized child" who has a limited capacity to relate to the broader society but whose basic loyalty may be to a subcultural group such as a gang and its delinquent activities. This child is obviously similar to the socialized delinquent child. Second is the child "arrested at a primitive level of socialization." This child lacks any consistent family or gang culture ties, has a generally hedonistic outlook and is impulsive and primitive in his behavior. The third child, viewed as "lacking capacity to socialize," is the most extreme of the three types with an absence of conscience and feelings of guilt. He may be referred to as a "psychopath" who manifests virtually no ability to relate to others. In school the socially maladjusted child may be quickly alienated because of demands for conformity from rigid authority figures such as teachers and principals. They may be frequently truant, sporadic in attention and concentration, easily frustrated, and unable to learn by experience.

The child considered "minimally neurologically impaired" may exhibit some of the same behavior seen in children called "emotionally disturbed" or "socially maladjusted" (e.g., hyperactivity, distractibility). However, instead of a mental illness or faulty socialization an organic dysfunction is considered the underlying cause of the behavior disorder. The actual existence of neurological impairment in a given case of a child with a behavior disorder is far from simple to establish. While Clements (1966) sees a close relationship between hyperactivity and neurological impairment, Werry (1970) challenges such a supposition as "unsubstantiated" (see also Chapter Three). The child given the label is seen as having particular difficulty in school because of the highly stimulating nature of the classroom environment, which may distract and confuse him, and because of problems in spatial orientation and visual, auditory, and motor functioning, which interfere with his learning.

Children considered "culturally disadvantaged" may also exhibit behavior disorders found among children given the previous three labels. In this case, however, the "cause" of the behavior is viewed as the result of an impoverished environment and experiential deprivation such as is seen among children reared in ghetto and underprivileged areas. When these children enter school they do not bring the knowledge of the environment, awareness of appropriate standards of social behavior or understanding of language concepts—which teachers and schools often take for granted will be established in their students. As a result, the students may "misbehave" from ignorance and frustration.

The "educationally handicapped" child is seen as an academic casualty and the causal factors related to his misbehavior are largely viewed as school achievement deficits in such basic tool subject areas as reading, arithmetic, and written language. As this child is given assignments calling for skills he simply has not acquired, continual failure and frustration may lead to deviant behavior in the classroom.

When the child with a behavior disorder in school is given the label of a "conduct disturbance" a sharp contrast emerges between the implication of the term and some of the terms used to describe the children cited above. For in the case of this child it is the behavior he exhibits in the classroom and not its possible extraschool causal factors that receive major focus. The child is considered a candidate for learning more adaptive behavior in school and concern with causation is narrowed to events in the classroom that are under the control of the teacher.

As can be seen, the pinning of a given label on a child with a behavior disorder carries with it a bias with respect to causal factors considered crucial and explanations of why the behavior is occurring in the classroom. These biases have also determined the nature of educational programs provided for these children. We shall briefly discuss such programs and some of the individuals and research studies associated with them.

Educational programs for children called "emotionally disturbed" have been strongly influenced by psychoanalytic theory (S. Freud, 1949) and psychodynamic psychology (A. Freud, 1954, 1965). The hypotheses set forth by Sigmund Freud regarding the mental structures determining human behavior (id, ego, and superego), the instinctually derived energy underlying behavior (libido), the critical phases of human personality development (psychosexual stages), the unconscious determination of behavior (defense mechanisms) and the relationship between events in early childhood (particularly interpersonal relationships) and later behavior have been utilized to varying degrees as the basis for some such programs over the past several decades.

One of the first of these was developed by Aichhorn in the 1920s and described in his book "Wayward Youth" (Viking Press edition, 1965). Aichhorn was concerned with the punitive corrective practices used with institutionalized delinquent boys of his day. His program was designed to establish positive, trusting relationships at the expense of rigid enforcement of limits particularly in the beginning. As a result considerable freedom was given the boys and few restrictions were placed on their deviant behavior.

Bettelheim (1950) has established a residential treatment and educational program for emotionally disturbed children at the Sonia Shankman Orthogenic School at the University of Chicago. His work has emphasized understanding of the child's psychological problems and establishment of a positive teacher-child relationship before introduction of demands for behavior change and formal learning.

Socially maladjusted children such as the delinquent boys worked with by Aichhorn also have been approached as "emotionally disturbed" by other educators influenced by psychoanalytic and psychodynamic psychology. Redl (Redl & Wineman, 1951, 1952) undertook an extensive project with delinquent boys in their Pioneer House project in Detroit which approached the difficulties in control and conformity exhibited by these boys in terms of faulty ego development. Limits were imposed in the group living and educational program but many opportunities were provided for deviant behavior to be expressed as a means of studying the boys' problems.

Newman (1959) has been concerned with the development of public school programs for hyperactive, aggressive children. As in Redl's project, the children are accepted as they are, opportunities are provided for self-expression, and behavior change is emphasized only when the child evidences readiness for such change. In this approach, as in all educational programs that have been influenced by psychoanalytic theory, there is a reliance on the teacher's capacity to communicate acceptance to students, to demonstrate sensitivity to their emotional needs, to utilize considerable flexibility and resourcefulness in planning programs, as well as to build a positive, trusting relationship before making demands for conformity and academic performance.

More recently a psychoeducational approach to problems of children with behavior disorders who are called "emotionally disturbed" has emerged (Morse, 1966). Morse has advocated establishment of a total mental health program in the public school which would bring together the services of a psychoeducational team including special education teachers, psychometrists, social workers, guidance personnel, speech therapists, and psychological and psychiatric consultants. These specialists would observe and discuss problems of children with behavior disorders and would aid the teacher in understanding and dealing more effectively with them. Temporary placement of such children in resource rooms where they would receive individualized supervision and instruction, use of a "crisis" teacher (Morse, 1965) to support classroom teachers when a given child cannot be maintained in a regular program, and "life space" interviewing (Morse, 1963; Redl, 1959; Morse & Small, 1959), a form of immediate reality-oriented therapy in the context in which the problem has occurred, are techniques that have been formulated as a part of the psychoeducational approach.

Thus, the child considered emotionally disturbed may be viewed as needing a kind of psychotherapeutic assistance in the classroom. Provision of this assistance assumes that the educator possesses an understanding of personality dynamics and a clinical judgment and knowledge of interdisciplinary approaches far beyond that normally expected of the average classroom teacher.

School programs for emotionally disturbed children may also rely on a thorough psychodiagnostic evaluation by the psychologist as well as parent counseling and individual or group therapy for the children themselves in an effort to augment assistance provided in the classroom.

When the child with a behavior disorder is viewed as "minimally neurologically impaired" the focus of the educator shifts from concern with psychological conflicts and interpersonal relationships to (1) creating a classroom environment conducive to learning, (2) training the child to accurately perceive visual and auditory stimuli and to become oriented in terms of time and space, and (3) developing efficient and consistent motor patterns of behavior. As the child gains proficiency in these areas, it is assumed he is a better candidate for acquisition of more complex skills such as reading and that he will experience a greater degree of success and less frustration in school and as a result his adjustment will improve.

The sensory-motor training approach in special education was emphasized as far back as the beginning of the nineteenth century with the work of Itard (1962). Itard developed specific exercises to develop sensory discrimination and beginning language abilities in Victor, a feral child discovered living under extremely primitive conditions in a forest. Itard's work was continued by Seguin (Talbot, 1964) who later strongly influenced Montessori (1912) in her efforts to develop a "scientific approach to pedagogy," which included a highly organized program for visual, auditory, and tactile training.

Strauss (Strauss & Lehtinen, 1947; Strauss & Kephart, 1955) conceived of training procedures for children with suspected neurological impairment who were hyperactive and distractible. Control of stimulation in the classroom, separation of children to lessen distraction, and heightening of the stimulus value of teaching materials were educational considerations that he advocated.

Cruickshank, Bentzen, Ratzeburg, and Tannhauser (1961) have also emphasized the value of stimulus control for such children. In addition to recommending the procedures of Strauss, they have explored the use of individual study booths to reduce environmental space and a structured school program with carefully planned routine. In a study that compared four small classes of hyperactive and brain-injured children, two of which rigidly adhered to the methods of Cruickshank et al., and two which served as controls but had knowledge of such methods available, all children made significant gains in achievement, visual perception, and social behavior over a two-year period.

Kephart (1960) has formulated a developmental framework of perceptual-motor behaviors that underlie complex learning. He has also developed specific training procedures for assisting children who are deficient in such behaviors as balance, maintenance of posture, and manipulation and in accurate perception of spatial and directional relationships.

The behavior disorders exhibited by children considered minimally neurologically impaired are seen as related to certain irritability, distractibility, and hyperactivity tendencies associated with such impairment as well as disorientation, confusion, and frustration resulting from inability to function successfully in school. The teacher in an educational program oriented toward this label would be particularly concerned with diagnosis of perceptual-motor deficits and devising specific training procedures for their remediation. The program would be well structured with order and routine emphasized, and every effort would be made to establish basic visual, auditory, and motor competencies before emphasizing academic skills. In addition to extensive diagnostic testing, a neurological examination, including an electroencephalogram (EEG) may be recommended by the school. Medication may be prescribed by a physician in an effort to control the child's distractibility and hyperactivity, and the school nurse might be given the responsibility for administering it during the day.

Children considered "culturally disadvantaged" and who often display behavior disorders in school, have become of increasing national concern. Community action programs such as Operation Headstart have been underwritten by the federal government in an attempt to attack problems of early deprivation and pseudoretardation, which are commonly found among children of the poor. Although research and development of specific educational programs for these children are relatively new, Frost and Hawkes (1966) advocate thorough assessment of developmental levels, achievement motivation, experiential background, and special strengths and weaknesses of the disadvantaged as an essential first step. Preschool enrichment programs, smaller pupil-teacher ratios, in-service training for teachers, nongraded and individualized teaching strategies, revamped curriculum materials focused on the language and interest level of the child, and parent counseling in an effort to narrow the differences in values between home and school are all seen as important in providing a more effective education for the disadvantaged child.

An innovative approach to preschool preparation of the disadvantaged has been presented by Bereiter and Engelmann (1966). They define cultural deprivation as "a lack of those particular kinds of learning that are important for success in school." Their highly specific academic objectives include teaching the child to handle polar responses (e.g., big versus little) to correctly use such prepositions as "on, in, under, over, between" in describing arrangements of objects, to name basic colors, to count to 20 aloud without help, to distinguish printed words from pictures, to rhyme, and to develop a sight reading vocabulary of at least four words. Two methods suggested for attainment of these objectives are "verbal bombardment" by the teacher and "direct instruction" consisting of carefully planned lessons, demonstrations, drills, and exercises.

Fifteen severely deprived four-year-olds were subjected to a program of such "direct instruction." Although they were over a year retarded in language abilities, they tested within the normal range after the nine-month program and also had made substantial gains in IQ, arithmetic, and reading. While the assumptions Bereiter and Engelmann make about language deficits in the disadvantaged are open to question, their approach has attested to a way of increasing the behavioral repertoire of deprived children.

The task-oriented approach of Bereiter and Engelmann is in marked contrast to the exploratory, self-expressive, and interpersonal approach often taken in traditional preschool programs. The emphasis of the former is on readying the child for the realities of learning in school and putting him on an equal footing with his peers on entrance to kindergarten, thereby eliminating certain stresses, frustration, and failure, which may lead to later behavior problems.

The term "educational handicap" has been used to describe any child who is not clearly a candidate for labels relating to intellectual, sensory, neurological, or physical deficits and who is having trouble learning in school. This is particularly true in California where "educationally handicapped" is applied to many children who are emotionally disturbed, minimally neurologically impaired, socially maladjusted, and culturally disadvantaged and who are functioning below capacity in school subjects. In this discussion we shall consider the approach that views the academic deficiencies of a child with a behavior disorder as a major cause of his problems in school.

Coleman (1953) has described a remedial education approach taken during a six-week study with ten boys and ten girls, eight to sixteen years of age, who had serious school problems but who were generally free from "disabling emotional handicaps" in the Fernald School (formerly Psychology Clinic School), a center for assessment and treatment of school learning problems on the campus of the University of California, Los Angeles. Despite an initial psychological screening examination, which included projective personality testing and sought to eliminate severely maladjusted children, the children in the program had various behavior problems and one child eventually manifested a "serious personality maladjustment of a deep-seated nature" that had not been picked up during the screening.

According to Coleman, eight of the students in the study had been subjected to unsuitable teaching methods in the past and this was central to their school problem. Factors such as beginning reading instruction before an appropriate readiness level was attained and exclusive use of visual and verbal methods of instruction were related to the child falling behind in learning from the start and then becoming "hopelessly lost." Three of the students had such frequent absences from school or had changed schools so often that the normal course of their education had been seriously disrupted. Parental rejection, overpermissiveness, unreasonable expectations, and other home problems were seen as central to the school problem of seven of the students.

In the remedial program undertaken, there were seven distinguishing features.

1. *Creation of a favorable learning atmosphere,* which included establishment of good pupil-teacher and pupil-group rapport, removal of competition between students, and provision of success experience through use of teaching materials and techniques geared to each child's level.
2. *Creation of a need to learn* through making learning situations and materials as meaningful as possible.
3. *Filling in weaknesses and gaps in the pupil's educational background* by means of task assignments based on a thorough individual achievement evaluation with each child.
4. *Remedial work as an approach to the whole person* with emphasis on "reestablishing shattered self-confidence," social interaction, creative self-expression, and helping the child learn ways of communicating with others and coping with his problems.
5. *Integration of home environment with school program* via parent conferences and discussions designed to alleviate home conditions that were interfering with the child's learning.
6. *Specific remedial techniques* based on methods outlined by Fernald (1943) such as the experiential approach to reading (the child writes stories on topics that are meaningful to him) and kinesthetic tracing of words. For all subject matter an attempt was made to follow this sequence: (a) create a need, (b) offer concrete experience, (c) emphasize concept development, and (d) offer application in a meaningful problem situation.
7. *Keeping the child up with his classes* was attempted by giving work which paralleled that of the public school and which aimed at getting the child up to expected grade level as quickly as possible.

The students in Coleman's study attended a half-day summer school program for six weeks. Following this period, all but one child made appreciable academic gains (mean achievement gain was 0.8 of a grade in all subject areas, five times the improvement to be expected had the students remained in their regular schools for the same period). In addition, the majority expressed a positive attitude toward the school experience (as compared to none before the program) and teachers reported increased self-confidence among the students as reflected in decreasing dependence and an increase in ability to tolerate mild competition and failure "without feeling unduly devaluated." There was also a reduction in hostility and deviant behavior, with blowups and fights that occurred in the early phases of the remedial program lessening over the six-week period and a more friendly and relaxed class atmosphere developing. Finally, increased self-expression was observed and the children became active participants in regular school subjects, projects, and social activities.

Coleman describes the program as utilizing a "total push" approach in all areas felt to be related to the children's school problems, but it is apparent that major emphasis was on creation of a unique educational experience in the classroom designed to alter previously established negative attitudes about school and learning and to help the child achieve academic success.

We turn now to consideration of the child with a "behavior disorder" in school as a child with a "behavior disorder" in school instead of as a victim of emotional, social, neurological, cultural, or primarily academic handicaps. As was stated earlier, this focus on observed behavior in the classroom and its relation to events under the control of the teacher contrasts to approaches stressing concern with causal factors outside such control. Despite this contrast, it is still possible to keep many of the major tenets associated with these other approaches in mind while fully mobilizing and utilizing the resources unique to the teacher and school in an effort to help the child learn more adaptive behavior.

Mobilization and utilization of teaching resources to directly assist the child in changing his behavior requires a strategy. Such a strategy has emerged in the field of special education from experimental work with behavior modification (see Chapter Seven). The behavior modification strategy directs the teacher to discern those behaviors which the child exhibits in the classroom that interfere with his learning or getting along. Next, it emphasizes the importance of determining why these behaviors are being maintained in the classroom. Such a determination involves studying the total classroom environment in an effort to find either the stimuli (e.g., demands that the child cannot handle) which provoke such behavior or the rewarding consequences which follow such behavior and reinforce it. Finally, it urges the teacher to carefully review the classroom environment and manipulate stimuli and consequences so that the total learning situation supports the child in the development of more adaptive behavior. A thorough discussion of the learning theory principles and concepts underlying the behavior modification strategy may be found in Chapter Seven.

A brief example will be useful in illustrating the behavior modification strategy in action in the classroom. Mark is a nine-year-old boy seated in a reading group with the teacher and four classmates. The teacher opens a page in a book, points to a line and hands the book to Mark with the instruction that he is to read it aloud to the group. Mark takes the book from the teacher without a word, but in the next instant he throws it down on the floor making a loud noise. This results in all the other children in the room looking up from their work and directly at him, the uncontrolled giggling of the members of the reading group and the teacher's face assuming a gradually reddening color from mounting anger.

The teacher wishing to utilize the behavior modification strategy in such a situation would have no trouble identifying the maladaptive behavior interfering with learning (e.g., Mark's throwing the book down). A more difficult problem would arise in assessing the classroom events—stimuli and consequences that were related to its occurrence. Was it the presence of the book and the demand to read it aloud and perhaps fail in front of his classmates that triggered off the behavior or was it because the full attention of the class, the giggling delight of those in the reading group, and the fuming frustration of the teacher had made similar acts so rewarding in the past that Mark deliberately took advantage of the situation to obtain further gratification? Being in a classroom for a short time with Mark would undoubtedly reveal the classroom events that most likely determined the outburst. Once these were obvious, the teacher might alter the type of reading assignment given Mark or the manner in which it was given (e.g., within an oral reading group) or she might set firm limits with the other children regarding their not responding to Mark's bid for attention. In addition the teacher would need to control her own behavior and perhaps ignore Mark's outbursts, therefore eliminating one more possible source of reinforcement. Of course, both classroom events—the book that he wished to avoid and the promise of a rewarding classroom disruption—might be related to Mark's problem behavior and the teacher would have to act accordingly. Another possible approach would be to punish Mark, that is, make his outburst nonrewarding by sending him from the room, giving him an "F," writing an unsatisfactory note home to his parents, keeping him after school, and so forth. In general, however, use of negative consequences or punishment may not be as effective as planning ahead and anticipating such problems in the future, attempting to eliminate rewarding consequences when they did occur, and consistently providing these consequences when Mark exhibited appropriate behavior.

Birnbrauer, Bijou, Kidder, and Wolf (1965) utilized behavior modification principles in an educational program for institutionalized retardates, many of whom had behavior disorders at the Rainier School in Buckley, Washington. Careful control of stimuli and consequences in the program resulted in behavioral and academic gains not ordinarily expected of children with such limited intellectual abilities.

Haring and Phillips (1962) found that use of a structured classroom with clear-cut expectations and rewarding consequences for appropriate behavior and academic accomplishment resulted in definite academic gains for children with behavior disorders.

Hewett (1964, 1965) undertook reading and speech training programs with two autistic boys who were highly distractible, inattentive, and uncooperative. The programs were based on the behavior modification strategy and in both cases substantial progress was made.

Quay, Sprague, Werry, and McQueen (1967) successfully increased the "attention" behavior of aggressive, unsocialized boys in the classroom by flashing a light on their desks if they were attending to the teacher during a group listening period. These light flashes could later be converted into pieces of candy and served as positive consequences.

Use of primary or tangible rewards is often relied on as a part of the behavior modification strategy because of the lack of demonstrated effectiveness of more typical rewards in the classroom such as a verbal praise with children who have conduct disorders (Levin & Simmons, 1962).

One type of social reinforcement that has been found to have an effect on the study behavior of disruptive and dawdling students is teacher attention. Hall, Lund, and Jackson (1968) systematically varied this reinforcement with one first-grade and five third-grade students with study behavior problems. The children were given teacher attention only when working appropriately and were ignored when they were inattentive. Under such conditions the study rates of the children increased sharply. A reversal procedure during which time the teacher paid attention to nonstudy behavior brought about an immediate decline in study rates. Once the initial approach was reinstated, study rates again markedly increased and these were maintained even after the experimental program terminated.

The loudness of teacher reprimands was shown to have an effect on the behavior of disruptive children in a study by O'Leary, Kaufman, Kass, and Drabman (1970). Initial observations revealed that most teacher reprimands were loud in nature and could be heard by many other children in the classroom. When the teachers were asked to use a soft voice audible only to the child being reprimanded, the frequency of disruptive behavior declined in most of the children. As in the study cited above, reversal of procedures increased disruptive behavior which decreased again when the "soft voice" condition was reinstated.

Control of disruptive behavior in elementary classrooms was achieved by a "game approach" (Wolf, Hanley, King, Lachowicz, & Giles, 1970). A bell rang every twenty minutes and students earned token reinforcers exchangeable for later privileges if they were in their seats at that time. Barrish, Saunders, and Wolf (1969) engaged a regular fourth-grade class in which there were several behavior problem children in another type of game based on a behavioral approach. The class was divided into two teams. Whenever a child on either team left his seat or talked out, a mark was placed on the chalkboard which meant possible loss of privileges by all members of his team. This approach was successful in improvising the problem student's behavior during arithmetic and reading periods.

Whelan (1966) and Nolen, Kunzelmann, and Haring (1967) have described the use of high interest activities as rewarding consequences in school programs for children with learning and behavior problems. The children are expected to maintain appropriate behavior and undertake academic tasks in order to obtain points, which they can later exchange for free time pursuing activities (e.g., arts and crafts) they select on the basis of their interests. Whelan has also summarized the implications of the total behavior modification strategy for education of children with behavior disorders.

Special educators who view the child with a behavior disorder as a candidate for learning within the classroom setting and who avoid preoccupation with causal events outside this setting have been increasingly effective in creating successful school programs for these children. Haring and Lovitt (1967) have utilized a classroom approach called "precision teaching" based on the work of Lindsley (1966). This approach involves selecting a specific behavior (e.g., number of arithmetic problems done correctly), recording the occurrence of the behavior, and charting it on a graph, recording changes in the teaching program, analyzing the child's performance to determine the relationship between program and behavior, and systematically changing the program variable and reevaluating its effect on performance. Walker, Mattson, and Buckley (1969) have also utilized this approach.

Quay and Glavin (1970) undertook a four-year investigation of self-contained special classes and resource rooms that utilized principles of behavior modification with behaviorally disordered children in the public school. The results of their study indicated that social behavior and academic achievement definitely improved in these experimental classes and suggested that the resource room concept in which the child participates part time in the regular class program is the most cost-effective method for the education of children with behavior problems currently available in the public school.

Over a period of several years, Hewett has explored the development of an engineered classroom design for children with learning behavior problems (Hewett, 1966, 1967, 1968) and the remainder of this chapter will be devoted to describing this design in terms of its goals and methods and summarizing the data obtained from evaluation of its use in the public school.

The use of the term "engineered" in describing a school program immediately suggests, as does "behavior modification," an emphasis on methodology and teacher manipulation of the classroom environment instead of educational goals and strictly child-centered considerations. That such methodological emphasis not readily accepted in education was recognized by Charters in

1945 when he wrote concerning "Is There a Field of Educational Engineering?" Skinner (1965) has also commented on the "extraordinary neglect of method" reflected in current efforts to improve education.

The behavior modification strategy, which was previously discussed, is essentially an engineering strategy concerned more with methods than goals. Its recommendation to the teacher to identify maladaptive behavior and then to set out to modify the classroom environment in order to change that behavior leaves some questions unanswered: What maladaptive behavior? Which behaviors are more important to modify than others? What are the critical behaviors associated with success in learning and school?

In an effort to incorporate the powerful methodological features of the behavior modification strategy yet compensate for its neglect of specific educational objectives, the engineered classroom design first directs its attention to the establishment of goals. These goals were introduced in the opening section of the chapter and are conceived as a developmental sequence of behavioral objectives—attention, response, order, exploratory, social, mastery, and achievement.

It is the child and his demonstrated capacity in relation to each of these goals that will influence the teacher in planning an educational program for him. More specifically, the teacher is interested in answers to the following questions in connection with each goal:

1. *Attention*
   (a) Does the child pay attention to visual, auditory, and tactual stimuli associated with learning tasks given him?
   (b) Does the child attend to reality events instead of fantasy?
   (c) Does the child pay attention to behavior associated with assignments in the classroom or is he preoccupied with compulsive, ritualistic acts such as excessive handwashing or pencil sharpening?
   (d) Has the child developed accurate beliefs about himself and the environment and does he manifest interests that are appropriate for his age and sex?
   (e) Does the child pay attention to the teacher?
   (f) Does the child retain directions and information given him and profit from such instruction?

2. *Response*
   (a) Will the child freely undertake an assignment given him?
   (b) Is the child constricted in his performance in the classroom and unwilling to do more than a limited amount in relation to an assignment?

(c) Does the child display a broad range of interests in subject matter and activities in the classroom?

(d) Does the child withdraw from contact with teacher and peers?

(e) Can the child function in a regular class setting or does he need a special class placement or individual tutoring?

3. *Order*

    (a) Does the child follow directions and start, follow through, and complete assignments in the manner prescribed?

    (b) Is the child impulsive and uncritical in his attempts to do assignments given him?

    (c) Does the child respect the working rights of others or is he disruptive in a class group?

4. *Exploratory*

    (a) Does the child have accurate knowledge about his environment and does he freely and thoroughly engage in multisensory exploration of it?

    (b) Is the child overly dependent on the directions and choices of others in selecting interests and activities?

    (c) Is there any evidence of motor, physical, sensory, perceptual, or intellectual deficits that limit the child's capacity to freely and accurately explore the environment?

5. *Social*

    (a) In general, does the child's behavior gain the approval of others and avoid their disapproval?

    (b) Is the child overly dependent on obtaining attention and praise from others?

6. *Mastery*

    (a) Has the child acquired the ability to take care of himself and has he mastered cognitive and academic skills commensurate with his intellectual capacity?

7. *Achievement*

    (a) Is the child self-motivated in learning and does he give evidence of being rewarded by acquisition of knowledge and skill?

By means of a planned assessment procedure (Hewett, 1968), the teacher describes the child with a behavior disorder within the guidelines provided by the developmental sequence. Thus, the "behavior disorder" is approached as a failure to achieve one or more of the stated educational goals.

Such an assessment assists the teacher in answering such questions as "Who is the child with a behavior disorder?" and "What does he need in order to achieve success in learning and school?" But it fails to answer a most critical and often neglected question: "How can I do something about his problem in the classroom?" It is at this point that the behavior modification strategy is extremely useful. The teacher must select some objective or goal most basic to the child's problem in school (e.g., on the lowest level of the developmental sequence where he is having difficulty), relate it to a specific curriculum task or class assignment, present it to the child making clear what is expected, and then guarantee a meaningful reward will be provided if the child successfully accomplishes it. When the child is not successful the teacher reflects on the nature of the task assigned (stimuli) and the available rewards (consequences) as well as demands made in association with the task and as "when," "where," "how," and "how well" it was to be done. Such reflections are based on the teacher's assuming responsibility for the child's inability to be successful. This is in contrast to the approach implicit in some of the other educational programs for children with behavior disorders cited earlier where child failure may be attributed to emotional, medical, and extraschool factors that make it possible for the teacher to more readily view the problem as "outside my control."

Despite the grimmest of extraschool factors that relate to children's behavior disorders in the classroom, the teacher utilizing the behavior modification strategy takes him as he is when he walks through the classroom door and accepts full responsibility for assisting him in taking at least a small step in the direction of positively modifying his attention, response, order, exploratory, social, or mastery behavior. This is done by constant manipulation of the stimuli and consequences within the classroom environment and although this approach does not specify that a "positive teacher-child relationship" and "more adequate self-image" on the part of the child are major goals, the guarantee of success implicit in it seldom fails to produce such results over time.

The engineered classroom design formulates a practical and workable room environment and a class schedule and set of operations that will enable the teacher to help children with behavior disorders acquire the essential competencies for learning specified on the developmental sequence. In addition, it attempts translation of the behavior modification strategy for realistic use in the classroom.

Starting with the room and composition of the class, there are nine double desks for each of nine students who are under the supervision of a teacher and teacher-aide. The room is divided into three major centers paralleling levels on the developmental sequence. The *mastery-achievement* center includes the student desk area and two study booths where work may be undertaken free from visual distraction.

The *exploratory-social* center is in one corner of the room and consists of three distinct areas. One features science equipment necessary for simple experiments as well as a fish tank and various animals in cages. Another is used for arts and crafts projects and the third for communication tasks—games and social activities for two or more students.

The *attention-response-order* center is in the opposite corner. Here puzzles, discrimination and matching exercises, and intriguing tasks emphasizing attention, participation, and direction-following are undertaken.

The class schedule covers four hours and includes a ten-minute order period, an hour reading period, a ten-minute recess, an hour period devoted to arithmetic, a nutrition period, physical education, and a final hour of exploratory activities in the science, art, and communications areas described earlier. Thus it can be seen that emphasis is given to building of basic academic skills as well as involving the child in order and exploratory experiences. These activities are the basis for the "stimuli" that the teacher manipulates in an effort to assist the child in learning.

The "consequences" in the engineered classroom are largely provided at first by the check-mark system. When each child enters the room in the morning, he picks up his individual Work Record Card near the door. This is a 4x6 card with 200 ruled squares.

As he moves through the class day, the child's efforts are acknowledged by check marks given on the card by both teacher and aide. First thing in the morning, the child gets five check marks if he is on time, has remembered to pick up his card as he entered, and is seated and ready to go to work at his desk. Following the ten-minute order period (a short visual-motor, hand-eye coordination exercise to get him paying attention, responding and following directions) a possible ten check marks are given—two if he started, three if he tried and followed through, and a possible five bonus. The "bonus" check marks are administered by teacher and aides on a wholly individual basis. They reflect the child's accomplishment on the levels of the developmental sequence most basic to his problem. Therefore some children get the five bonus for just trying (response level), others for following directions (order level), and finally others for doing the assignment correctly (mastery level).

Throughout the day, ten check marks are given as described above, every fifteen minutes to let the child know where he stands. In giving these check marks, the teacher verbalizes the reason the child does or does not get the ten which are possible. At other times the teacher does not engage in a great deal of verbal interaction with students. An attempt is made to establish her as a "shop foreman" carefully assigning tasks on the basis of the child's learning needs and fairly and predictably acknowledging his accomplishments by giving him what he has "earned." Completely filled check-mark cards can be exchanged weekly for tangible rewards such as candy and prizes or for 15 minutes of privilege time at the arts and crafts area.

Central to the engineered classroom design is constant manipulation of assignments or "stimuli" in the class to assure a given child's continued success. These manipulations are referred to as "interventions" and involve locating an assignment on the developmental sequence where the child has a maximum probability of success. Therefore, if the child is experiencing difficulty during the reading or arithmetic period, the teacher has a possible nine interventions to consider: (1) send him to the study booth with the original assignment (mastery), (2) change the assignment and have him continue at his desk or go to the study booth (mastery), (3) verbally restructure demands that he do the assignment (social), (4) send him to exploratory center for science or art task (order), (6) take him outside the room and get him to agree on some task (e.g., swinging on swings) for which he can earn check marks (response), (7) place him in one-to-one tutoring with teacher and increase number of check marks given (attention).

Each of the above seven interventions involve the child continuing to earn check marks with no penalty is extracted because he changes activity. The change is considered necessary to maintain appropriate behavior and keep the child learning successfully. If none of these work, however, the teacher may try intervention (8) send the child outside the room where he must wait quietly for 5, 10, or 15 minutes without earning check marks. If this fails to assist the child in bringing his behavior under control, the teacher may consider sending him home. When this is done it is with the understanding that the child was unable to "be a student" and since "only students stay in school" it will be necessary for him to leave. There is no lecturing or admonishing regarding his behavior and when he returns the next day there are no grudges held and he is welcomed back into the classroom by the teacher who uses every resource in the room to prevent a recurrence of difficulties and to successfully maintain him in school. An attempt is also made to enlist the support of the school principal, clerks, and parents with respect to treating the child's removal from the classroom during a "time out" or when he is sent home in a matter-of-fact manner. All are concerned he is unable to remain, but they approach such removal as a necessary consequence at a particular time, not an indictment of the child as "sick" or "incorrigible." In summary, the engineered classroom design (1) provides an educational program for the child based on his developmental learning deficits instead of his extraeducational descriptions, (2) provides a system of consequences (check marks) that continuously (every 15 minutes) and predictably lets the child know where he stands and rewards him for demonstration of desired behavior, nonrewards him for failure to meet demands which according to everything known about him are reasonable to expect, and (3) manipulates the total classroom environment through a series of planned interventions so that at all times the child is assigned tasks at developmental levels where he needs to work, is ready to work, and can be successful working.

A study was undertaken in the Santa Monica Schools in California to demonstrate and evaluate the engineered classroom design with children with behavior disorders. Included in the Santa Monica Project (Hewett, Taylor, Artuso, 1967) were six classrooms, each with nine students and a teacher and aide. The children in the classroom met the criteria for inclusion in a state-supported program for the educationally handicapped:

> Educationally handicapped minors are minors other than physically handicapped minors . . . or mentally retarded minors . . . who, by reason of marked learning or behavioral problems or a combination thereof, cannot receive the reasonable benefit of ordinary education facilities (State of California Education Code, Chapter 7.1, Section 6150).

Each child was given an individual intelligence test, a physical examination, and portions of the California Achievement Test (Elementary level) and the Wide Range Achievement Test. Mean IQ for all classes was 94 (individual range 85–113), mean age 10 years, 3 months (individual range 8–0 to 11–11), mean reading achievement level 2.8 (individual range 0 to grade 6.2) and mean arithmetic fundamental achievement level 3.3 (individual range 0 to grade 5.2). Six teachers were selected from applicants to the Santa Monica district and all were trained in the operation of the engineered classroom and use of the developmental sequence for describing students. Following this the six teachers were randomly assigned to experimental or control classrooms.

The independent variable or experimental classroom condition was rigid adherence to the engineered classroom design including the giving of tangible rewards and check marks. The control classroom condition was use of any teaching strategy (including aspects of the engineered approach) *except* the giving of check marks or any tangible reward. One class (Class E) used the experimental condition over the entire school year and one (Class C) used the control condition over the entire school year. Two classes (Classes EC) began the year with the experimental condition and abruptly withdrew from it at midyear when they became control classes. The two other classes (Classes CE) started using the control condition and abruptly introduced the experimental condition at midyear. These rotations permitted consideration of three questions:

1. What will be the effect of rigid adherence to the engineered classroom

design on children with behavior disorders who have previously been in a regular class?

2. What will be the effect of rigid adherance to the engineered classroom design on children with behavioral disorders who have previously been in a small individualized class that did not use the reward system of the engineered design?

3. What will be the effect of abruptly withdrawing the reward system of the engineered design from a class of children with behavior disorders who have become accustomed to it?

The major dependent variable in the study that attempted to shed light on answers to these questions was *task attention*. Task attention was defined as the time spent by a student maintaining eye contact with a task or assignment given him by the teacher. In situations where eye contact was irrelevant to the task (e.g., listening to a record) appropriate head or body orientation was credited. Two observers sat in the front of each of the six project classrooms for two and one-half hours every morning during the entire year. Each held a stopwatch and was assigned either four or five children to regularly observe. The children were observed for five-minute segments in random order so that at least five separate samples of task attention were obtained on each student each day. Reliability was established beyond the 85 percent agreement level for all observers.

The individual task attention measures were recorded as percentages and daily class task attention percentage means were computed for each project class. These were later averaged for four-week intervals.

Figure 1 depicts these four-week means graphed over the project year. In the discussion which follows, "significant" difference refers to the .05 level of confidence. A complete statistical analysis of all data was done to arrive at the findings discussed but is not presented here.

As can be seen, Class C started out with a superior task attention percentage level than Class E but by interval 2 this was reversed in favor of Class E, which maintained a task attention advantage over the remainder of the year. With respect to question 1 the engineered design produced a significantly higher task attention percentage among students than the control condition during intervals 3 to 8. The teacher in Class C relied on mastery, and social and exploratory rewards and initially was more successful than the teacher in Class E. But within a short period of time, Class E's provision for more basic rewards using the check-mark system sustained students at a higher task attention level for the entire year.

Classes CE, which started the year using the control condition and then introduced the engineered design at midyear, showed a significant increase in task attention when this design was implemented as shown in Figure 1. This

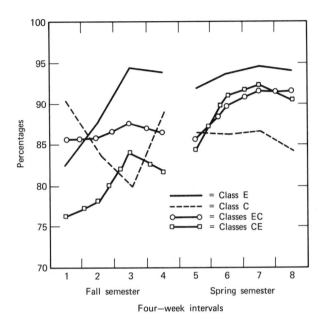

100
95
90
Percentages
85
80
75
70

——— = Class E
----- = Class C
○——○ = Classes EC
□——□ = Classes CE

1   2   3   4   5   6   7   8

Fall semester   Spring semester

Four—week intervals

Graph of Class E, Class C, Classes EC, and
Classes CE mean task attention percentages
averaged for four-week intervals during the
fall and spring semesters.

provides evidence concerning question 2 and the effect of adding the design to a small class with a teacher and aide which is already established.

Classes EC used the design for the first half of the year and then abruptly withdrew it at midyear when they introduced the control condition. As can be seen from Figure 1 these classes actually made significant gains in task attention percentages on removal of the check-mark system and rigid adherence to the engineered design. This seemed to result from the fact that during the first half of the year a consistent structure was firmly established in the classrooms through use of the check-mark system and on removal of this system reliance on social and mastery rewards actually enhanced the effectiveness of the program. This finding offers evidence regarding question 3 in the study.

The other dependent variable used in the study was achievement level of students. While reading and spelling gains were not significantly different among students enrolled in the two classroom conditions, significant gains in arithmetic fundamentals were positively correlated with presence of the engineered classroom design. Class E made a gain of .2 years in this area while Class C gained only .4 of a year. Classes CE did not differ significantly from Class C in gain in arithmetic fundamentals during the first half of the year when all classes were using the control condition but gained .8 of a year during the second half as compared to .1 year gain made by Class C. The correlation between gain in arithmetic fundamentals and the presence of the engineered design is seen as reflecting the value of the strong emphasis on building attention, response, and order behaviors in the engineered design. These behaviors are probably more directly linked to functioning in arithmetic than in language arts areas where no significant differences were observed.

In a follow-up study (Hewett, Taylor, Artuso, & Stillwell, 1969), 30 classes of elementary students matched on the basis of age, sex, and IQ were tested for achievement gains over a one-year period. One group was made up of educationally handicapped children in an engineered classroom, one group educationally handicapped children left in regular classrooms, and one group of normal children. Reading and arithmetic gains for the engineered classroom were significantly greater than those for the educationally handicapped children remaining in the regular classroom.

In summary, the engineered classroom design appears to be particularly effective in "launching" children with behavior disorders into learning and more actively involving them in attention, responding, and direction-following. Once an investment is made in establishing these basic competencies, the child actually moves on to higher levels of the developmental sequence where he is more susceptible to approaches using exploratory, social, and mastery emphases.

In this chapter a review of educational programs with children with behavior disorders has been presented. What has been done educationally with these children has related to how their problems were perceived. While all special educators share a concern for helping such children achieve greater success in school, they have approached that goal from emotional, neurological, cultural, academic, and behavioral points of view. Sidetracking the teacher with ominous labels that may have nothing to do with educational practices and that may lead the teacher to consider the child largely a psychiatric, medical, or social problem is seen as detrimental. The implication that teachers must acquire expertise associated with the psychotherapist or diagnostician or that they should approach educational problems of children with behavior disorders as strictly academic is also seriously questioned. A developmental behavioral approach to the education of the child with behavior disorders has been introduced. Evaluation of this approach in the public school suggests that systematic control of stimuli and consequences in the classroom and focus on building attention, response, and order skills can successfully launch such a child into learning.

References

Aichhorn, A. *Wayward youth.* New York: The Viking Press, 1965.

Barrish, H. H., Saunders, M., & Wolf, M. M. Good behavior game: Effects of individual contingencies for group consequences on disruptive behavior in a classroom. *Journal of Applied Behavior Analysis,* 1969, **2**, 119–124.

Bereiter, C., & Engelmann, S. *Teaching disadvantaged children in the pre-school.* Englewood Cliffs: Prentice-Hall, 1966.

Bettelheim, Bruno. *Love is not enough.* Glencoe, Illinois: Free Press, 1950.

Birnbrauer, J., Bijou, S., Wolf, M., & Kidder, J. Programmed instruction in the classroom. In L. Ullmann & L. Krasner (Eds.), *Case studies in behavior modification.* New York: Holt, Rinehart, and Winston, 1965.

Charters, W. Is there a field of educational engineering? *The Educational Research Bulletin,* **24**, 1945, 29–37.

Clements, S. Minimal brain dysfunction in children, in *NINDB Monographs,* No. 3, United States Public Health Service. Washington, 1966.

Clements, S., & Peters, J. Minimal brain dysfunctions in the school age child. *Archives of General Psychiatry,* 1962, **6**, 185–197.

Coleman, J. Results of a program of remedial instruction, *Elementary School Journal,* **54**, 1953, 454–458.

Cruickshank, W., Bentzen, F., Ratzeburg, F., & Tannhauser, M. *A teaching methodology for brain-injured and hyperactive children.* New York: Syracuse University Press, 1961.

Fernald, G. *Remedial techniques in basic school subjects.* New York: McGraw-Hill, 1943.

Freud, A. The relation between psychoanalysis and pedagogy, *Psychoanalysis for Teachers and Parents* (translated by B. Low). New York: Emerson, 1954.

Freud, A. *Normality and pathology in childhood.* New York: International Universities Press, 1965.

Freud, S. *An outline of psychoanalysis.* New York: W. W. Norton, 1949.

Frost, J., & Hawkes, E. *The disadvantaged child.* Boston: Houghton Mifflin, 1966.

Hall, R. V., Lund, D., & Jackson, D. Effects of teacher attention on study behavior. *Journal of Applied Behavior Analysis,* 1968, **1**, 1–2.

411

Haring, N., & Lovitt, T. Operant methodology and educational technology in special education. In N. Haring & R. Schiefelbusch (Eds.), *Methods in Special Education.* New York: McGraw-Hill, 1967.

Haring, N., & Phillips, E. *Educating emotionally disturbed children.* New York: McGraw-Hill, 1962.

Hewett, F. Teaching reading to an autistic boy through operant conditioning, *The Reading Teacher,* 1964, **17**, 613–618.

Hewett, F. Teaching speech to an autistic child through operant conditioning, *American Journal of Orthopsychiatry,* **35**, 1965, 927–936.

Hewett, F. The Tulare experimental class for educationally handicapped children, *California Education,* 1966, **3**, 6–8.

Hewett, F. Educational engineering with emotionally disturbed children. *Exceptional Children,* 1967, **33**, 459–467.

Hewett, F. *The emotionally disturbed child in the classroom: A developmental strategy for educating children with maladaptive behavior.* Boston: Allyn and Bacon, Inc., 1968.

Hewett, F., Taylor, F., & Artuso, A. The Santa Monica project: Demonstration and evaluation of an engineered classroom design for emotionally disturbed children in the public school: Phase I: Elementary level. *Final Report. Project No. 62893, Demonstration Grant No. OEG-4-7-062893-0377, Office of Education, Bureau of Research, U.S. Department of Health, Education and Welfare,* 1967.

Hewett, F., Taylor, F. D., Artuso, A. A., & Stillwell, R. The Santa Monica engineered classroom: Progress Report I. Unpublished manuscript, 1969.

Itard, J. M. G. *The wild boy of Aveyron.* New York: Appleton-Century-Crofts, 1962.

Kephart, N. *The slow learner in the classroom.* Columbus, Ohio: Charles E. Merrill, 1960.

Levin, G., & Simmons, J. Response to food and praise by emotionally disturbed boys, *Psychological Reports,* 1962, **11**, 539–546.

Lindsley, O. Personal communication, 1966.

Montessori, M. *The Montessori method.* Philadelphia: F. A. Stokes, 1912.

Morse, W. Working paper; Training teachers in life space interviewing. *American Journal of Orthopsychiatry,* 1963, **33**, 727–730.

Morse, W. The crisis teacher. In N. Long, W. Morse, & R. Newman (Eds.), *Conflict in the classroom: The education of emotionally disturbed children,* Belmont: Wadsworth, 1965.

Morse, W. Public schools and the disturbed child. In P. Knoblock (Ed.), *Intervention approaches in educating emotionally disturbed children,* Syracuse: Syracuse University Press, 1966, 113–128.

Morse, W. The education of socially maladjusted and emotionally disturbed children. In W. Cruickshank & G. Johnson (Eds.), *Education of exceptional children and youth* (Second Edition), Englewood Cliffs, N.J.: Prentice-Hall, 1967.

Morse, W., & Small, E. Group life space interviewing in a therapeutic camp. *American Journal of Orthopsychiatry,* 1959, **29**, 27–44.

Newman, R. G. The assessment of progress in the treatment of hyperaggressive children with learning disturbances within a school setting. *American Journal of Orthopsychiatry,* 1959, **29**, 641–642.

Nolen, P., Kunzelmann, H., & Haring, N. Behavioral modification in a junior learning disabilities classroom. *Exceptional Children*, 34, 1967, 163–169.

O'Leary, K. D., Kaufman, K. F., Kass, R. E., & Drabman, R. S. Effects of loud and soft reprimands on the behavior of disruptive students. *Exceptional Children*, 1970, 37, 145–155.

Patterson, G. R. An empirical approach to the classification of disturbed children. *Journal of Clinical Psychology*, 1964, 20, 326–337.

Quay, H. Dimensions of problem behavior and educational programming. In P. Graubard (Ed.), *Children against schools*, New York: Follett, 1969.

Quay, H. C., & Glavin, J. The education of behaviorally disordered children in the public school setting. *Final Report Project No. 482207*, Department of Health, Education, and Welfare, U.S. Office of Education, Bureau of Education for Handicapped, 1970.

Quay, H., Morse, W., & Cutler, R. Personality patterns of pupils in special classes for the emotionally disturbed. *Exceptional Children*, 1966, 32, 297–301.

Quay, H. C., Sprague, R. L., Werry, J. S., & McQueen, M. M. Conditioning visual orientation of conduct problem children in the classroom. *Journal of Experimental Child Psychology*, 1967, 5, 512–517.

Redl, F. Strategy and techniques of the life space interview. *American Journal of Orthopsychiatry*, 1959, 29, 1–18.

Redl, F., & Wineman, D. *Children who hate*. Glencoe, Ill.: The Free Press, 1951.

Redl, F., & Wineman, D. *Controls from within*. Glencoe, Ill.: The Free Press, 1952.

Skinner, B. Why teachers fail, *Saturday Review*, 1965, 48, 80–102.

Strauss, A., & Kephart, N. *Psychopathology and education of the brain-injured child*, Volume II. New York: Grune and Stratton, 1955.

Strauss, A. A., & Lehtinen, L. E. *Psychopathology and education of the brain-injured child*, Volume I. New York: Grune and Stratton, 1947.

Talbot, M. E. *Edouard Seguin: A study of the educational approach to the treatment of mentally defective children*. New York: Bureau of Publication, Teachers College, Columbia University, 1964.

Walker, H., Mattson, R., & Buckley, N. Special class placement as a treatment alternative for deviant behavior in children. In F. A. M. Benson (Ed.), *Modifying deviant social behavior in various classroom settings*. Eugene: University of Oregon Press, 1969.

Watson, R. *Psychology of the child*. New York: John Wiley, 1961.

Werry, J. The diagnosis, etiology and treatment of hyperactivity in children. In J. Hellmuth (Ed.), *Learning disorders*. Seattle: Special Child Publications, 1970.

Whelan, R. J. The relevance of behavior modification procedures for teachers of emotionally disturbed children. In P. Knoblock (Ed.), *Intervention approaches in educating emotionally disturbed children*. Syracuse: Syracuse University Press, 1966.

White, M., & Harris, M. *The school psychologist*. New York: Harper and Row, 1961.

Wolf, M., Hanley, E. L., King, L. A., Lachowicz, J., & Giles, D. K. The timer-game: A variable interval contingency for the management of out-of-seat behavior. *Exceptional Children*, 1970, 37, 113–117.

Chapter Eleven

Follow-up Studies of Behavior Disorders in Children

Lee N. Robins

Kinds of Problems Amenable to Investigation Through Follow-up Studies

The State Commissioner of Mental Health asks himself, "If 50,000 babies are born this year, how many child psychiatrists, school social workers, and psychologists are we likely to need to care for them in the next two decades?"

The mother of a new born baby asks herself, "Is there anything I must do or avoid doing if I want to prevent the appearance of behavior problems? My husband drinks too much, will my baby be affected? If my baby is colicky and fussy at three months does this mean he is going to be a problem child? If we live in a bad neighborhood, will my son become a delinquent?"

The parent or doctor of a child who already has behavior problems wants to know answers to a different set of questions: "How long are these problems likely to continue? Are there any treatments likely to shorten their natural course? Do they presage some serious illness in adult life?"

Follow-up studies have addressed themselves to all these problems: The risk of the appearance of pathological behavior in populations of children; the different rates of risk in children with different kinds of heredity, social settings, early behavior, and maternal practices; the duration of problem behavior; the evaluation of treatment; and the predictive value of problem behavior in childhood for adult adjustment. This chapter will discuss what special advantages the follow-up study brings to the solution of these problems and it will illustrate the contribution of follow-up studies by presenting findings from some of the more interesting ones that have been done.

What Is a Follow-up Study?

The word "follow-up" has been used in many ways. The only concept common to all the uses is that some measure has been taken at two or more points in time. The time interval may be short or long. Measures may be taken only at the beginning and end or recurrently throughout the time interval. The *kinds* of things measured at the beginning and end may be the same or different. If we study how many children aggressive at Time I are still aggressive at Time II, we are studying the *same* behavior measured twice. But if we study how many children with sleep disturbance at school entry are failing school at age 12, different behaviors are measured. Even the *people* studied at Time I may or may not be the same as the people at Time II, although there must be a stated relationship between them. In our previous examples, the *children's* behavior is studied at both times, but if we investigate whether children from broken or impoverished *homes* at Time I will have behavior disorders at Time II, we are studying connections between the behavior of their *parents* and their own behavior.

Follow-up studies can be very much like laboratory experiments if during the elapsed time some planned intervention has taken place (for instance, treatment). But they may also treat elapsed time as a period of spontaneous change and development only—and thus become explorations of natural histories.

In this chapter, two restrictions will be added to the broadest use of the term "follow-up." First, the time interval must be of sufficient length so that there has been an opportunity for an important amount of change to occur. Second, the measurements at either end of a time interval must be independent of each other. These strictures rule studies comparing the diagnoses of children on entering and leaving a treatment facility, since changes in diagnosis over such a short interval probably more often reflect changes in the *amount of knowledge* about the child acquired by his physician than changes in the state of the child himself. They also rule out studies in which a teacher's evaluation at the beginning of the school term is found to correlate with the child's grades at the end of the term, since the fact that the same person (the teacher) has provided both the initial rating and the final grade makes the two measures fail the test for independence.

Why Use Follow-up Studies?

Granted that questions about risks of pathological behavior, the evaluation of treatment, and the predictive value of childhood behavior are important, why use follow-up studies to answer them? What can follow-up studies do that other studies cannot?

Follow-up studies are uniquely adapted to learning which children are most likely to develop behavior disorders, the outcome of behavior disorders, or the results of therapy. To study which children develop behavior disorders, at Time I family and social backgrounds are evaluated, and then a number of years later the children themselves are studied to identify those who have developed behavior disorders. One can thus learn from which backgrounds problem children are most likely to come. To study the *outcome* of behavior disorders, one selects children known to have a disorder and a matched group of normal children, and then reexamines them after a number of years to see what proportion of each group is then having difficulties. The normal children serve as the control group, so that one can estimate to what extent the difficulties found in the disturbed children at follow-up can be attributed to their earlier disorder and to what extent their difficulties could have been expected to emerge independently of the history of childhood disorder. To study the effects of *therapy*, the design is similar except that the control group is not made up of normal children, but is rather an untreated group *with* behavior disorders, whose outcome can be compared with the outcome of children who received therapy.

One reason the follow-up study is preferable to a cross-sectional study for these purposes is that it is not subject to retrospective falsification or selective recall. If in a cross-sectional study, the mother of a disturbed child is asked about family variables present before the child showed symptoms, her account is likely to be distorted in at least some of the following ways: (1) It will revise the past so as to "make sense" of the relationship between past events and the child's behavior. For instance, the mother may report that the grandmother's death occurred before the child began having nightmares, when in fact the nightmares had started months earlier. (2) She will remember things that mothers of normal children would not because she is seeking explanations for her child's problems. For instance, she may recall that the child was frightened by a dog, or that a distant relative had a somewhat similar kind of problem. The researcher may be persuaded that a particular event or a genetic factor is relevant to the child's problems, even though such events and affected relatives occur just as frequently in the history of normal children, but are too trivial to be recalled by a mother who is not concerned over her child's behavior. (3) She may try to assume blame for the child's problems by exaggerating her own inadequacies as a parent, or to avoid blame by painting a blacker picture of the father's drunkenness and a more whitewashed version of her own behavior than she would if she did not have a problem child. (4) Like the mother of the normal child, she may simply misremember important events or confuse the age at walking and talking of one of her other children with that of the patient. In follow-up studies, the information about the past was *collected* in the past. It is, therefore, more likely to be accurate because it deals with recent events and because it cannot be altered to explain or to justify what happened later.

One advantage that has been claimed for the follow-up study is that it can discover the *causes* of behavior disorders. In fact, the follow-up study contributes to the understanding of cause in only a limited way. *No* nonexperimental study, whether cross-sectional or longitudinal, can *demonstrate* cause. The only way to do so is by manipulating experimentally a variable that you think produces behavior disorders and then looking to see whether you have in fact changed the rate. But nonexperimental studies *can* help one decide which factors are *probable* causes. To argue that some particular circumstance is a probable cause of a behavior disorder, you have to be able to show that when it occurs in a child *without* behavior disorder, the risk of a behavior disorder's appearing later is increased. The hard part is to show that the circumstance or event that you think caused the disorder actually was present *before* the disorder got started. For instance, parents are often hostile and unloving toward delinquent children, but this does not necessarily mean that the parents' attitude influenced the children's behavior. What we want to know is whether the parent was hostile *before* the child showed any kind of abnormal behavior or whether the hostility was simply the parents' response to the child's provocative acts. It is obvious that a retrospective study that starts with delinquent children, who may have been discipline problems at home long before they were known to the courts, has trouble in deciding whether the parent was already rejecting and disapproving before the child *ever* did anything to provoke the parent. But can follow-up studies do better? If the follow-up study is following children who were already delinquent when selected for the study and finds they have hostile parents, there is still no way to be sure whether the hostility or the problems came first. On the other hand, if a study starts with normal children, some of whom have hostile parents, and follows them to see which ones develop problems, and if the children with hostile parents *do* develop behavior problems, it appears probable that the hostility of the parent has played a part. But it is difficult to find such children for a study. One has to identify the children at that critical period when they have *already* been exposed to the factor that we think causes difficulties, but *before* they have reacted to that exposure by showing problem behavior. It must be obvious, then, that we can use follow-up studies to test causal hypotheses in quite limited circumstances. Although follow-up studies solve *some* of the dilemmas of research into the causes of behavior problems, they are by no means the panacea that some researchers believe them to be.

A final area in which follow-up studies are particularly valuable is in estimating what proportion of the population of children ever develop behavior disorders. A cross-sectional study is much more likely to miss the most seriously disturbed cases than is a follow-up study. Suppose we decided to find out how many children develop behavior problems before puberty by doing a cross-sectional study of seventh graders. We would miss all the children whose behavior problems were severe enough so that they never entered seventh grade—children in hospitals, correctional institutions, special schools, and un-graded rooms—as well as the small group whose behavior had been so reckless that it led to fatal accidents. On the other hand, if we were to select a representative sample of very young children, chosen before behavior problems can make them less accessible to us, and *follow* them to the age of 12, we would be forced to account for all our cases and our figures for the rate of development of behavior disorders before puberty would include children dead, out of school, or retarded in school. Consequently, our estimates of rates would be much more nearly correct.

The main advantages of follow-up studies, in short, are (1) that information about early life is more accurate; (2) the temporal order between environmental factors and the development of behavior disorders can sometimes be ascertained; (3) a more complete sampling of the population can be achieved.

These advantages, however, do not accrue automatically. Many of the follow-up studies we shall discuss have not taken full advantage of the potentials of the follow-up design. Nonetheless, some important results have been achieved that could not have been achieved with cross-sectional studies.

Some Follow-up Studies and What They Find

How Many Children Ever Develop Behavior Disorders?

The proportion of children who will ever develop behavior disorders can be estimated in two different ways. The most direct method is to choose children at birth, follow them until the age designated as the end of "childhood," and see how many developed problems at any time in the interval. A second way is to select well children of various ages (or children born at different periods), follow them for a fixed period of time, a period long enough so that *some* of them will have reached the age designated as the end of childhood, and see how many new cases of behavior disorders emerged at each age level. With proper statistical treatment the risk of the development of a disorder within the whole age span of childhood can then be calculated.

We have an example of the first method in the Berkeley Growth Study. Every third child born in Berkeley, California, over an 18-month period was followed at yearly intervals until he reached age 14 (Macfarlane, Allen, & Honzik, 1954). The behavioral status of the children at each age was evaluated according to the presence or absence of 39 symptoms. Although this study does not attempt to label children as having or not having behavior disorders, the proportion of children having each symptom has been reported by sex and age and the average number of symptoms present at various ages was computed. This kind of information enables us to say, for instance, that less than 5% of children have more than 10 of the 39 symptoms at age 11. We also know what symptoms tend to occur together, and what symptoms are rare at what ages. For instance, poor appetite is a very rare complaint at age 14, but occurs so frequently in little girls of 6 (40%), that it probably has no psychiatric significance at that age. Running away from home, on the other hand, occurs in fewer than 10% of children at every age, and presumably then should always be considered a possible indicator of serious problems. Similar findings *could* have been obtained with a cross-sectional instead of a longitudinal design by sampling children of all ages and comparing the proportions at each age showing each symptom. But then we would have had to *infer* that the reason fewer 11-year-old boys steal than do 6-year-olds is because stealing drops out of the repertoire of behaviors with aging. In a follow-up study, using the *same* boys at different ages, we *know* that this happens. We do not have to wonder whether our 11-year-olds, by some fluke of the selection process, just happened to be drawn from less antisocial children than were our 6-year-olds.

Two Swedish studies have collected data appropriate for the second kind of study. Unfortunately both present only the raw figures for the number of new cases found without calculating how many new cases would have been found if all children had reached the upper age limit.

One of these studies (Jonsson & Kälvesten, 1964) selected over a 9-year period one-sixth of all birth records of boys born on the 15th of the month in Stockholm (0.5% of all boys born during this 9-year period), and then located these boys when they were aged 7 to 16. The rate of problem behavior was then calculated from information obtained from school records; interviews with teachers, mothers, and fathers; examination by a psychiatrist; and psychological tests. One-fourth of the boys were found to have serious enough problems to warrant referring them for treatment and 2% were found to be institutionalized. It is interesting to note the frequency with which various types of problems occurred. Excess activity was found in 6%; 5–10% were defiant and aggressive; 20–25% were oversensitive; and 18% had reading or writing difficulties. Serious delinquent behavior (truancy, vagrancy, stealing) was reported for 2–3%.

The second Swedish study followed the whole population of one community after a 10-year interval (Hagnell, 1966). Although this study was not interested in children alone, by presenting results separately for each age group, it provides us with information about children. Of the children under 10 who were free of psychiatric disease in 1947, 7% of both boys and girls developed psychiatric illnesses by 1957, as assessed in interview. This incidence was less than half the incidence of new cases of psychiatric illness among adults well in 1947 (17.6%). The most common diagnosis for children was what the author called "childhood neurosis," which apparently corresponds to antisocial behavior in this country. Boys (6%) developed this pattern more frequently than girls (1%). Girls' problems were more commonly what we think of as neurotic in this country: fatigue, depression, anxiety, and mixed neurosis. None of the children developed a psychosis. During the 10-year period, only 2% of the children had consulted a psychiatrist, and only 0.5% had been in a psychiatric hospital. The proportion of those becoming ill who were hospitalized was lower for children than for adults (7% versus 12.5%). Apparently, then, <u>children less often develop psychiatric illness than do adults,</u> <u>and their illnesses may be less severe,</u> since when sick, they less often require hospitalization.

Which Children Develop Behavior Disorders?

Predictors of behavior disorders in children can be sought in characteristics of the social environment or in early characteristics of the child himself. The kinds of behavior disorders with which these early environmental and personal characteristics have been shown to be associated include delinquency, coming to psychiatric attention, and poor school performance. (We omit here what is probably the most common measure of abnormality sought in children, low IQ, since low IQ does not properly belong under the "behavior disorders" umbrella.)

Socioeconomic Factors and Parental Performance. By far the most ambitious study ever undertaken concerning the effect of socioeconomic and family factors on the life chances of children is the follow-up study of a sample of 5362 children born in a single week of 1946 in England and Wales (Douglas, 1964, 1966; Mulligan et al., 1963). These children have been repeatedly restudied from birth to age 20. Findings published thus far report family and social status factors affecting the child's risk of delinquency, of passing examinations for entrance into "grammar schools," and of neurotic symptoms.

<u>Low social status, as indicated by the father's having a manual instead of</u> <u>a white-collar job, was found to be related to official delinquency and to the</u> <u>appearance of aggressive behavior in school, to low scores on school achieve</u> <u>ment tests,</u> to *declining* scores on school achievement tests when scores at ages 8 and 11 are compared, to critical comments by teachers such as "poor worker" or "lazy," and to failure to enter schools for the intellectually able even when achievement scores warranted admission. That is, lower class children have more antisocial behavior, *achieve* less, and do not even reap the rewards of what they do achieve. No class differences were found in the number of

neurotic symptoms reported (bedwetting, nightmares, nailbiting, thumbsucking, abdominal pain, or vomiting).

This study sheds light on *why* lower class status is associated with behavior problems. When the families of delinquents were compared with other working class families of *nondelinquents,* the delinquents were found to come from families in which the parents were inadequate. That is, the parents were less educated; they had made less use of health services available; they had more often quarreled and separated. If such inadequate parents are more common in the lower class than in the middle class, this would explain why the lower class produces a higher proportion of children with behavior disorders. It is reasonable that inadequate parents *should* be more common in the lower classes, because inadequacy would show itself in an inability to hold a job or to obtain jobs other than those at the lowest level, as well as in poor performance as a parent.

The observation that the adequacy of the parents matters more than their class status in predicting children's problems has been affirmed in a number of studies. To demonstrate that class status is not the crucial factor, it must be shown that (1) an improvement in social status does *not* lead to a decrease in children's behavior problems unless there is comparable improvement in family performance, and (2) that inadequate parents produce children with behavior problems even in middle class homes.

The first question—does improvement in standard of living lead to improved behavior—was answered negatively by a study of Negro slum children whose families were moved to a spacious, clean, new housing project (Wilner, 1962). The children who moved into the project showed no greater gains in school achievement than did a matched group of children who stayed in the slum, although there was a slight decline in school absences among the project children. There is a question, of course, as to whether improved housing is enough to constitute a rise in social status. It is hard to imagine another *kind* of improvement in social status, however, that can occur without the parents' showing especially good work performance.

The second question, does inadequacy in the family produce equally severe behavior problems in children in middle class families as in lower class families was answered affirmatively by a study of the behavior of three generations (Robins & Lewis, 1966). It was found that having antisocial parents or grandparents (i.e., parents or grandparents who as adults had been arrested, drank excessively, failed to work regularly, deserted or neglected the children, beat the children or spouse, or had extramarital sexual relations) considerably increased the chances of a son's dropping out of high school and appearing in police or juvenile court records. This relationship between problem behavior in a boy and his relatives appeared in *both* white-collar and blue-collar families. Indeed, when both had antisocial relatives, boys in white-collar families had no advantage over boys in blue-collar homes with respect to graduation or arrests. At both class levels, the effect on the son was greater the *more* antisocial relatives he had.

Psychiatric Illness in Parents. The studies cited above suggest that parental behavior is probably a more important predictor of behavior problems in children than in social class. We might expect that parents *treated* for psychiatric illness would show extreme behavior problems and should thus be especially likely to have children with behavior disorders. Unfortunately, most studies reporting on psychiatric illness in the offspring of psychiatrically ill parents have been conducted after the offspring are already adult. It is not possible to tell from these reports whether the disorders reported for the offspring began *in childhood* or later. Some problems found *must* have been visible in childhood, especially mental deficiency and antisocial behavior, since we know that these rarely, if ever, first appear in adulthood.

Most studies investigating disorders in the offspring of psychiatrically ill parents have been interested in finding evidence for a genetic factor in psychiatric illness. These studies have considered it evidence for such a genetic factor when children develop the same disorder that their parents had. By contrasting the offspring of parents with differing diagnoses, they show that psychiatric disorders tend to run "true to type" within families. One study presenting such evidence sought hospital records for the offspring of parents both of whom had been hospitalized with either schizophrenia or a depressive illness (Lewis, 1957). When both parents were schizophrenic, 23% of their offspring had been hospitalized for schizophrenia and none had been hospitalized for depressive illness. When both of the parents had had an affective (depressive) illness, only 8% of their offspring had been hospitalized for schizophrenia, and 19% had had a depressive illness. When one parent was schizophrenic and the other depressed, the rates of the two diseases in their children were almost equal—10% schizophrenic and 13% depressed.

But disorders *other* than those of their parents also appear in the children of the psychiatrically ill. Are such disorders more common in the children of the psychiatrically ill than in the general population? If so, does this indicate that genetic inheritance is not specific with respect to diagnosis? Or does the excess of disorders unlike the parents' show the environmental effects of living with a psychotic parent or of suffering separation from the parent when he or she is hospitalized?

Two studies have shown that disorders unlike the parents' do occur more frequently in the children of schizophrenics than in the children of parents not known to be psychiatrically ill. One study compared the children of patients diagnosed "dementia praecox" (schizophrenia) with the children of patients seen in a medical clinic (Canavan & Clark, 1923a, 1923b). Since most of these children were still young at follow-up, the number developing behavior disorders was not a final figure. However, a comparison of the *kinds* of disorders shows not only more cases of schizophrenia among the children of schizophrenic parents (6% of the children over 16 with a schizophrenic parent versus less than 1% of the control children over 16 years) but more cases of conduct disorder as well (11% versus 2% for school-aged children). A study of adult children separated from their mothers in early life and placed in foster homes or institutions (Heston, 1966) similarly showed not only an excess of schizophrenia in the children of schizophrenic mothers (11% versus none in the control children) but also an excess of antisocial behavior (15% convicted of a felony versus 4% of the control children) and mental deficiency (8.5% versus none of the control children). This second study indicates that the excess of disorders other than schizophrenia in the children of schizophrenic parents cannot be attributed to living with the psychotic parent nor to the experience of separation from the parent, since in this study *all* children had been early separated from the mother, whether or not she was psychotic. While this study might then seem to suggest that a *genetic* component may be reflected in diverse kinds of pathology, this inference cannot safely be made because no information is available about the father of the child. It is possible that schizophrenic women more often have children by antisocial or mentally defective men than do other women whose children are removed from them. If so, the high rate of nonschizophrenic pathology in the children may well reflect the genetic contribution of the father.

Children's Early Behavior as a Predictor of Later Problems.   Most studies following the behavior patterns of children have been concerned only with normal development, not with the appearance of behavior disorders. This was a wise choice, since the small samples used made the chances of turning up many children with behavior disorders slim. There are, however, a few studies that do relate early behavior to the development of problems.

The Berkeley Growth Study, which we discussed earlier as contributing to our knowledge of the frequency of various kinds of symptoms found in children of various ages, has also exploited its repeated assessment of symptoms in the same children to learn at what age high symptom levels tend to persist and to learn which symptoms are transient and which are lasting (Macfarlane et al, 1954).

Most children's problems do seem to be age-specific. That is, a problem present at one age will not be found later. The symptoms that were found to be exceptions to this rule were destructiveness, demanding attention, somberness, jealousy, shyness, and excess reserve. When these were present at age 6 or 7, they were also likely to be present at 13 or 14. But while most other specific symptoms change from one age to another, children with *many symptoms* at one age tend to have *many* symptoms later as well. This consistency in the overall level of disturbance does not appear, however, until age 6 or 7. Before then, symptoms have little predictive value for later adjustment.

The fact that early symptom levels are not good prognosticators seems consistent with the findings of a study of 136 normal babies first observed shortly after birth and followed by observation and parent interviews regularly thereafter. These babies were evaluated along 9 behavior scales. Before the age of 7, 29 of these children were referred and accepted for psychiatric help (Rutter et al., 1964). By age 9, 42 were given psychiatric care (Thomas, Chess, & Birch, 1968). This unusually high rate of psychiatric referrals apparently occurred for two reasons. First, the children came from New York Jewish professional families, a group which every study of the utilization of psychiatric facilities finds unusually interested in and accepting of psychiatric intervention. Second, the psychiatrist doing the research freely offered services as a recompense for the family's cooperation. Although it is unlikely that the children seen had behavior disorders of the severity ordinarily seen in psychiatric practice, they were children whose behavior caused enough concern to their parents that a consultation was sought. And the psychiatrist agreed that the problems were not simply normal behavior for their ages. When an attempt was made to correlate psychiatric treatment with the 9 behavioral attributes scored in infancy, little could be found in the observations of early behavior of patients to distinguish them from the less troubled children. Only 1 of the 9 attributes (high activity level) scored in the first year of life was significantly related to pathology; none of the variables scored in the second year; and only 1 score (high intensity) in the third year. Grouping of attributes (negative mood, high intensity, withdrawing, and nonadaptivity) during the first 2 years still showed no significant correlation with later behavior problems.

However, another study using data collected before school-age (Westman, Rice, & Bermann, 1967) indicates that behavior at age 3 or 4 may have predictive value. Immaturity, getting along poorly with other children, and eccentric behavior noted in the nursery school teacher's records were related to receiving mental health services before completing high school. Failure to get along with peers in nursery school was related to trouble with peers and teachers later on and to childhood neurotic symptoms. Eccentric behavior in nursery school was also related to neurotic symptoms later.

Three studies of school-aged children confirm the Berkeley Study's observation that behavior after age 6 is indeed a very good predictor of later adjustment problems. These studies sought predictors of delinquency and school achievement in teacher's comments and evaluations by other students. All three studies (Mulligan, Douglas, Hammond, & Tizard, 1963; Conger & Miller, 1966; Havighurst, Bowman, Liddle, Matthews, & Pierce, 1962) agree in showing that delinquents-to-be do poor school work, challenge the teacher's authority, and are unpopular with their schoolmates. In the British study (Mulligan), predelinquents were "underachievers" by age 8. Later they disobeyed teachers, quarreled and fought, cheated, and played truant. In Denver (Conger), by fourth grade, predelinquents were resentful of authority, getting along badly with classmates, daydreaming, and doing poor work. In "River City" (Havighurst), children chosen as most aggressive by teachers and classmates in the sixth and seventh grades later became delinquent, particularly if they also had school failures. Two of the studies agree as well that neurotic symptoms ("nervousness" in Denver, stammering, nailbiting, vomiting, bedwetting, thumbsucking in England) are unrelated to later delinquency. (Comparable data are not presented in the River City study.) Such neurotic symptoms neither predict delinquency *nor* predict that a child will *not* be delinquent. Delinquency and nervousness are unrelated but not incompatible (see also Chapter One).

School achievement, unlike delinquency, was predicted by *both* neurotic symptoms and aggressive behavior. In England the achievement test scores of children with neurotic symptoms were found to deteriorate between the ages of 8 and 11. Since achievement scores are important determinants of which children the teachers will nominate for admission to schools for the academically talented ("grammar schools"), having symptoms in early childhood does predict that a child will not be admitted to the "grammar schools," and consequently will end his schooling early. In River City, more than half (57%) of the children among the most aggressive in the sixth and seventh grades failed to finish high school, compared with only 17% of the least aggressive.

Traumatic Experience and Later Problems. Much literature has been devoted to the discussion of whether maternal deprivation is followed by behavior disorders in childhood (World Health Organization, 1962). The belief that maternal deprivation was important was fostered by the observation that children in orphanages often seemed to be suffering from a lack of spontaneity, low intelligence, and rather constricted ability to make relationships with others. The interpretation that this kind of behavior problem in institutionalized children is a result of experiencing separation from the mother is no longer so widely accepted. Such behavior might be simply a consequence of inadequate care in the institution. Or it might be a continuation of behavior problems present *before* separation from the mother or caused by the mother's neglect or maltreatment prior to the child's removal. Separation from the mother is so severely disapproved in our society that it rarely occurs in the absence of serious pathology in either the mother or the child. When Bowlby studied separations from the mother because of tuberculosis in the child, a cause not related to behavior problems in either the child or his mother, little or no difference could be demonstrated between the children who had been in a sanatorium and control children in their school class, after they had returned to school (Bowlby, Ainsworth, Boston, & Rosenbluth, 1956).

One kind of traumatic experience—abuse at the hands of the parents—
has been found to be associated not only with very serious psychiatric problems for children, but with serious medical problems as well (Elmer & Gregg,
1967). Among 50 abused children, defined by their being found to have
multiple bone injuries at various stages of healing at admission to a hospital,
who were followed a year and 5 months to 10 years later, 8 were found to have
died and 5 to have been permanently institutionalized in hospitals for the
mentally defective. Among those 20 available for interview, half had IQs below
80, half had speech problems, and 40% had "emotional disturbance" (undefined). Children who had been moved out of their homes showed better
physical and intellectual development than those remaining, suggesting that
when maternal handling is sufficiently abnormal, being deprived of the mother
is an advantage. If this study had *not* found that removal from the mother was
associated with a better outcome, we would have had to consider the possibility
that the gross defects found in the children might have been what *incited* the
mother to abuse them rather than being the result of maltreatment. Even *with*
improvement after removal, it is possible that some of the children had mental
defect or brain damage prior to being abused, defects which may have made
them particularly demanding or irritable babies. But the parental abuse, along
with the neglect and poor nutrition that often accompanied it, must also have
contributed its share to the disastrous findings at follow-up. Indeed, in the
case of such an extreme experience as parental abuse, the very life of the child
is threatened if he is not removed from the home.

Can Behavior Disorders Be Prevented?

Beginning with Cyril Burt's study of the delinquent in 1925 and continuing with the studies by Healy and Bronner a few years later, it became
obvious that the social situations of delinquents differed from that of nondelinquents. These early reports, plus the Gluecks' history-making *Unraveling
Juvenile Delinquency* in 1950, underscored the fact that the families and
social environment of delinquents were unfortunate. The boys who became
delinquent had few "good influences" in their lives. It was an easy step from
this observation to experiments in delinquency-prevention by offering good
influences and attempting to counterbalance the influence of "bad companions"
and of parents who were uninterested or rejecting. The efforts at prevention
centered on children thought to be "predelinquent" as judged by criteria
developed from the studies comparing delinquents and nondelinquents.

The results of these efforts have been consistent if disheartening. No
experiment in delinquency-prevention has succeeded. The techniques used
have been those of counseling of children and their parents, psychotherapy,
encouragement to participate in wholesome recreation, offering of friendship,

good examples, and understanding. The treatment has been applied at various ages—to boys around age 11 (Powers & Witmer, 1951; McCord & McCord, 1959), to adolescent girls (Meyer, Borgatta, & Jones, 1965), to children from kindergarten through sixth grade (Tait & Hodges, 1962), and to boys just entering elementary school (Craig & Glick, 1963). Since each of these studies provided a carefully selected control group to allow comparisons between children for whom prevention was attempted and children for whom it was not, there is every reason to have confidence in the negative results.

Although none was able to prevent delinquency, all the studies demonstrated that the *predictors* of delinquency were correct. Those children expected to become delinquent did in fact do so more often than children for whom delinquency was not anticipated, although prediction was far from perfect. (In most prediction of deviant behavior, professionals tend to be excessively pessimistic—they *overpredict* later difficulties.) The predictions were much better than chance whether the predictors used were family type, the parents' assessment of the child's behavior, home visitors' judgment of the family, or teacher's assessments and school records. And they were accurate whether what was being predicted was juvenile delinquency, graduation from school, or discipline problems in school. The failure of these studies was not in prediction but in prevention.

Efforts to prevent children's problems other than delinquency are common, but have seldom been evaluated carefully. Prenatal clinics hold parents' meetings to help prepare parents psychologically for handling their prospective baby. Many PTAs have psychiatrists in to answer parents' questions and show "mental health" films followed by discussion groups. But there have been few attempts to learn whether these efforts do in fact reduce the incidence of problems in children. One such study has been done in St. Louis, contrasting over a 3-year period classrooms in which the mothers have been offered group therapy sessions and mental health films followed by discussion programs with classrooms in the same school not exposed to the program (Gildea, Glidewell, & Kantor, 1967). Likes the efforts to prevent delinquency, these efforts to prevent other kinds of symptoms in school children could not be demonstrated to have had any beneficial effect. Teachers' ratings of the children's behavior and mothers' reports of symptoms in the children both proved resistant to these preventive efforts.

Can Behavior Problems Be Successfully Treated?

If our current techniques for preventing behavior disorders in childhood are inadequate, it is still possible that we might be able to treat them once they occur.

To decide whether a treatment has helped, one thinks first of evaluating the child before and after treatment to see if there has been an improvement. But it is not so simple to decide whether the improvement that has occurred should be attributed to the treatment experience. Many cases of behavior disorder have a fluctuating course. Children usually come to professional attention because of the sudden onset of a new symptom or the worsening of existing symptoms. If the seeking of treatment results from a temporary exacerbation of symptoms, it is not surprising that a few weeks or months later the level of symptoms will have receded—*whether or not* treatment was obtained. The questions to which we need an answer are not whether children have improved after a course of treatment, but whether *more* of them have improved and whether they have improved *more permanently* than could have been expected if they had not been treated. To decide whether treatment has "worked," then, we need to know how much improvement over the same time interval would have occurred in untreated children with similar complaints, and we need to know how many are still improved some years later.

There has been considerable argument about how to obtain the necessary base-line figures for how much improvement can be expected without treatment. One method used is to assess the improvement of children assigned to the waiting lists of clinics. A careful review of the studies that compared treated and untreated cases referred to child guidance clinics (Lewis, 1965) finds little support for the idea that treatment makes much difference. Improvement rates of two-thirds to three-quarters are regularly reported for both treated and untreated populations studied immediately after treatment, and rather high relapse rates are reported in treated children followed a number of years later.

Questions have been raised about whether these negative findings do not result from hidden differences between the initial degree of illness in the treated and untreated groups. For instance, emergency cases may be accepted for treatment and less severe cases may be assigned to waiting lists. Or perhaps the children assigned to the waiting lists were not really untreated—they may have sought help elsewhere.

Perhaps an even more basic problem than whether waiting lists constitute proper control groups is whether it is reasonable to evaluate treatment by studying improvement rates in a total clinic population in the first place. No one would think of evaluating the effectiveness of medical treatment by seeing how many attenders of a general medical clinic are well or improved a year or two later, while comparing them with people who approached the clinic for treatment but were not seen. We know that some patients of a medical clinic will have a self-limited illness, such as influenza, from which *all* will have recovered. For them the revelant question is not whether they are improved a year later, but whether the course of the disease was milder as a result of treatment. Other patients, those with arthritis, for instance, have presently incurable illnesses with spontaneously occurring remissions and exacerbations. The relevant question for such patients at follow-up is neither cure nor improvement as measured by current symptom level, but rather whether treatment has increased the proportion of the follow-up interval during which the patient has been able to function effectively. For other syndromes, the goal for therapy is to prevent progress of the illness. Indeed, at the present level of medical knowledge, the medical syndromes for which the relevant measure of treatment is whether the patient is cured at follow-up or even much improved is a small minority of the total.

Yet many of the studies reviewed by Lewis have failed to specify the disorders being treated or what the goals of treatment were, as well as failing to ascertain whether the control group was really comparable. But these failings do not seem to account for the poor showing made by treatment. Studies dealing with specified problems, using clearly defined goals (for example, preventing recidivism), or carefully matching controls with treated cases on the basis of the nature and the severity of their disturbance have not been able to demonstrate greater effectiveness of therapy.

Although the total population of child guidance clinics shows a *high* rate of improvement whether or not they are treated, among one subgroup of that population, the psychotic children, we find just the opposite. Children diagnosed as psychotic have grossly abnormal behavior, usually including the absence of relationships with their peers, an absence of speech or abnormal speech characterized by repeating questions verbatim and reversing pronouns (referring to themselves as "you"), preoccupation with their own activities and failure to respond to interruptions, dislike for and resistance to changes in routine, stereotyped repetitive movements, failure to achieve toilet training, and temper tantrums. Such children *rarely* improve, whether or not they receive treatment. The psychotics form so small a proportion of most clinic populations that their poor prognosis does not much influence the overall improvement rates. Among 15 psychotic children given very intensive therapy, first in the hospital and subsequently as outpatients, only two children showed a little improvement, and even these two children were still grossly abnormal 5 years after initial diagnosis (Eaton & Menascolino, 1967). These children had had almost all current therapeutic maneuvers attempted—play therapy, milieu therapy, special education, speech therapy, drugs, as well as therapy with the parents, but all to no avail.

The California Youth Authority forestry camps have a modern treatment program for delinquency, including counseling, work experience, and planned recreation. Early reports showed less recidivism for delinquents assigned to these camps than to traditional reformatories or to a prison. In a recent study (Molof, 1967), judges were asked to select boys they would ordinarily send to forestry camps. The boys selected were then randomly assigned to the camps or to reformatories or prison. No differences were found in rates of later offenses between boys sent to camps as compared with boys sent to prisons or reformatories. This study of delinquents points out the great importance of making certain that experimental and control groups are truly comparable. The previously reported success of the forestry camps apparently had resulted from judges' selecting only good-risk delinquents for them. The high rate of improvement reported for child guidance cases may have a similar explanation. Treatment may be recommended disproportionately for patients with the best prognosis. *These* patients may do well no matter how treated, or even if not treated at all. The recommendation of the least sick patients to treatment is not so irrational as it may at first sound. Patients who recover quickly make way for new patients in overcrowded facilities, and doctors may interpret their rapid recovery as evidence that they derive the greatest benefit from treatment.

Some studies have claimed success for modern facilities for delinquents based on the way attitude test questions are answered at the end of the period of incarceration. Such indirect methods of assessing "delinquency-proneness" are not very satisfactory. One wants to prevent delinquent acts, not change questionnaire answers. It is still an unanswered question as to whether there is any correlation between such answers and later behavior.

The effect of treatment in a child guidance clinic on *nondelinquent* and *nonpsychotic* children was studied by comparing the proportion improved over a two-year period with the proportion improved among untreated school children carefully matched with the clinic sample with respect to the nature and severity of their symptoms (Shepherd, Oppenheim, & Mitchell, 1966). This match for presenting symptoms was achieved by first screening the school population for children showing symptoms similar to those in the clinic, as ascertained by questionnaires administered to the parents of both groups, and then personally interviewing the parents of both groups until a good match for severity was located. At follow-up two years later improvement rates for treated and untreated children were indistinguishable. As in less rigorously controlled studies, approximately two-thirds of both clinic and school problem groups had improved.

The Duration of Childhood Disorders

We noted in the last section that childhood disorders seen in clinics, whether treated or untreated, usually improved with time. We also noted that delinquents and psychotic children, both treated and untreated, had much lower rates of improvement than the usual run of clinic children. Some studies have been interested in these spontaneous rates of improvement and in how much they differ between types of problem behavior or disorders of differing degrees of severity. Follow-up studies interested in spontaneous changes in symptom pictures over time are called natural history studies. Since treatment was found not to be an important modifier of the course of childhood disorders, it will be no surprise to you that natural history studies also find that most childhood disorders improve or disappear with time, but that the psychotic disorders and extreme antisocial behavior tend to persist.

Obviously, treated clinic cases cannot be used to study the natural history of childhood disorders if one thinks treatment makes a difference. Consequently, natural history studies of total populations of disturbed children have been based on school populations.

When teachers were asked to identify children who were "problems" or emotionally disturbed, they selected 7.6% of their classes, and twice as high a proportion of boys as of girls (Cumming & McCaffrey, 1964). When teachers were again asked to so designate children two years later, half of the group originally designated were renominated. Boys were somewhat more likely to be renominated than girls. We cannot optimistically report, however, that 50% of all disturbed children recover within 2 years, since no attempt was made to locate children who had not remained in the school system or who had not been promoted both years. Almost certainly those not promoted and transferred to special schools had higher rates of problems than those progressing normally.

A similar study of second through fifth grades (Glavin, 1967) reported only 30% of those originally identified as still "emotionally disturbed" four years later. This figure may be spuriously low because of the methods used to specify who was "emotionally disturbed." Instead of being asked to nominate any children they considered problems, as in the preceding study, teachers were asked to pick the 5 most poorly adjusted children in their classes and fellow-pupils were asked to nominate the 3 children they liked least. These nominations were combined with scores on a personality test to decide who was maladjusted. In classes with fewer than 5 children with serious problems, teachers had to nominate children with trivial difficulties, which might be expected to disappear. Even when children with serious problems were selected, their failure to be renominated later need not indicate a disappearance of problems. Perhaps enough children not previously nominated became seriously maladjusted during the interval to displace the child originally selected from among the teacher's "worst" 5 or their classmates' most disliked 3.

Follow-up studies of young offenders generally attempt to find out how many again commit a crime after an arrest. The Gluecks (1940) followed 1000 juvenile delinquents in 3 5-year periods. During the initial 5-year period, at the end of which their average age was 19, all but 20% had been rearrested. Similarly, among juvenile drug offenders in California (Roberts, 1967), all but

18% had another arrest in the next 4 or 5 years. When the drug arrest was not their *first* juvenile offense, only 9% failed to be rearrested. These studies emphasize the fact that serious antisocial behavior, as reflected in a juvenile police record, is much more persistent than is the general run of childhood disorders noted by teachers or by child guidance clinics.

When child guidance populations are divided into diagnostic groups, it becomes clear that the one-third who do *not* quickly improve are predominantly the antisocial and psychotic children, rather than the ones with neurotic diagnoses. In a Detroit children's clinic (Cunningham, Westerman, & Fischoff, 1956), cases were divided into those with personality disorders (antisocial behavior), psychosomatic disorders, and neurotic disorders (fears, eating, and sleeping problems, etc.). The children were followed a year or two after referral, through telephone interviews with their mothers. The mothers reported most improvement for children originally classified as neurotic.

Similarly, in a follow-up study from the Worcester Clinic (Shirley, Baum, & Polsky, 1940–1941), neurotic symptoms were found to be associated with good outcome, while restlessness and inattention, symptoms commonly described in antisocial children, were associated with poor outcome.

A 5-year follow-up of 72 adolescents in an outpatient clinic again found a good prognosis for neurotics (91% unimpaired at follow-up) and a poor prognosis for antisocial adolescents who were diagnosed "sociopathy" (Masterson, 1967). All the sociopaths were moderately or severely impaired at follow-up. Similarly, none of the schizophrenics was unimpaired 5 years later.

The same pattern is found for adolescents disturbed enough to require hospitalization. Two to five years after admission, the schizophrenics have the poorest outcome (19% recovered and 23% improved), the antisocial behavior disorders (sociopathy) are next (38% recovered and 22% improved), while the neurotics do well (40–55% well and 24–50% improved) (Annesley, 1961). For the antisocial behavior disorders the most important prognostic variable for continued problems was the presence of *multiple* antisocial symptoms (stealing, violence, *and* truancy). With only an isolated antisocial symptom, no matter what its nature, adolescents had good prognoses.

Warren classified his adolescent psychiatric inpatients as "neurotic," "conduct disorders," "mixed neurotic and conduct disorders," and "psychotic" (Warren, 1965). We can assume his psychotics include patients Annesley and Masterson would have called schizophrenics and that his conduct disorders are similar to Annesley and Masterson's behavior disorders and sociopathy. If so, the findings of all 3 studies agree well. Among children younger than 15 at admission, Warren found at follow-up 6 or more years later that most (74%) of the neurotics were well, while only a third of the conduct disorders had recovered. More than half of the children who had been delinquent before referral had further arrests, while children with some antisocial behavior but no official delinquency prior to referral became delinquent in one-third of the cases. Almost all of the psychotic children were still sick at follow-up.

How Should Childhood Disorders Be Classified?

One reason for doing follow-up studies of childhood disorders is to learn how to recognize early forms of an adult disorder. Lacking laboratory tests for psychiatric illness, the psychiatrist relies heavily on the past history of the illness in order to make a diagnosis. When the patient is a child, there is very little past history available. One does not yet know whether his illness has a remitting or deteriorating course nor what the full spectrum of symptoms will be when the disorder had been present for some time. By following children with disorders over a period of years it is possible to learn whether they do turn out to have an illness that fits into the adult diagnostic system. Such follow-up studies are the only way to settle arguments as to whether illnesses seen in adults do or do not occur in children.

One adult psychiatric disorder about which this question has been asked is hysteria (also called "conversion reaction"). Hysteria in adults is a disorder characterized by a great profusion of symptoms typically including menstrual problems, anxiety symptoms, frigidity, pain with no known physical basis, and multiple surgical operations. It occurs primarily if not exclusively, in women and almost always begins before the age of 25. To learn whether it can occur in children, a follow-up study was done of all the children in a children's hospital who had been diagnosed hysteria and hypochondriasis, as well as those diagnosed mixed neurosis if their symptoms included any of the classical "hysterical" symptoms: pain, vomiting, paralysis, amnesia, fits, urinary retention, blindness, trances, or aphonia (Robins & O'Neal, 1953). Of 23 children examined a number of years later, only 4 were found to be diagnosable as hysterics. The 4 for whom the original diagnosis was valid were all girls who had presented more than 5 symptoms. They averaged 8.25. Children later found *not* to have hysteria averaged only 3.53 symptoms. The diagnosis for children who did *not* have hysteria as adults was most frequently anxiety neurosis (8 cases). Four children were found to have no psychiatric disease. This study indicates that hysteria *can* begin before puberty, but that most children who show a combination of nervousness and unexplained physical complaints will as adults still be nervous, but their physical complaints will either have been discovered to have some physical basis or will have dissipated without ever having been diagnosed.

Another diagnosis about which a question has been raised as to whether it occurs in children is schizophrenia. Although some psychiatrists make a diagnosis of childhood schizophrenia in withdrawn children who show little or inappropriate emotion, others feel that this syndrome is quite distinguishable from true schizophrenia and is, in fact, associated with brain damage. (Schizophrenia is a so-called "functional" psychosis, which means that it is not possible to demonstrate any structural or physiological abnormality of the central nervous system.)

Support for the occurrence of schizophrenia in childhood was claimed by a study in which a series of 120 prepubertal children diagnosed "childhood schizophrenia" at Bellevue Hospital, between the ages of 4 and 13, were located again when they were aged 11 to 20 (Bender, 1953). Fifty-seven percent had received a diagnosis of "schizophrenia" in another hospital after leaving Bellevue, and an even higher proportion were diagnosed schizophrenic at follow-up by the Bellevue staff themselves. Other diagnoses received while hospitalized included mental defect, psychoses other than schizophrenia, and personality disorder. While the author argues that the high rate of diagnosis of schizophrenia both by the Bellevue staff and by other hospital staffs shows that true schizophrenia does occur in children, this is not necessarily an appropriate inference. The Bellevue staff was interested in confirming its original diagnosis. And the other hospitals' staffs presumably had the Bellevue diagnosis in hand while making *their* diagnosis. No objective criteria for the diagnosis of schizophrenia were applied at either intake or follow-up. At intake, the only requirement appeared to be that the symptomatology invade every area of the child's functioning. The specific symptoms could be not only varied but at opposite ends of a continuum—from anxiety and withdrawal to "over-adapted and relating to others too well." It is difficult to decide the meaning of a follow-up study in which the original diagnostic criteria are unspecified and where no provision has been made to avoid contamination between the original diagnosis and the follow-up diagnoses.

More recent studies (Rutter, 1965; Rutter & Lockyer, 1967; Rutter, Greenfeld, & Lockyer, 1967; Eaton & Menolascino, 1967) throw considerable doubt on the idea that children who are psychotic before puberty are really schizophrenic. Among 63 children first seen between the ages of 2 years and 9 months and 10 years and 8 months and then followed 10 years later by Rutter, none was found at follow-up to have the cardinal symptoms of schizophrenia, that is, delusions, hallucinations or paranoid ideas. This same failure to develop delusions or definite hallucinations had been reported in an earlier study of autistic children (Kanner & Eisenberg, 1955). Eaton and Menolascino found children originally diagnosed childhood schizophrenia indistinguishable clinically at follow-up 5 years later from children with known neurological defects at intake, and much more severely damaged than would be expected in ordinary "simple schizophrenia" of adult life. In addition, the families of Rutter's psychotic children did not contain an excess number of schizophrenics, as families of adult schizophrenics do. The childhood psychotics were very predominantly male, while there is no excess of males among adult schizophrenics. On three grounds, then, symptomatology, family history, and sex distribution, the childhood psychotics did not resemble schizophrenics when they grew older. An alternative hypothesis to the theory that psychosis in early childhood is schizophrenia was suggested by the frequency with which these children developed fits and other neurological signs during the follow-up interval. The delayed appearance of neurological signs shows that there must have been brain damage present even in some children who showed no neurological abnormality early in their illness. The brain damage could simultaneously explain the low IQ, the odd behavior, and the failure to develop normal speech. These follow-up studies, therefore, strongly suggest that childhood psychosis is not simply an early form of schizophrenia.

Another contribution that follow-up studies can make is to distinguish between *primary* and *secondary* symptoms. Many child psychiatrists, noting that an absence of speech and a total withdrawal from social interaction were characteristic of psychotic children, had inferred that psychotic (autistic) children *could* speak, but did not do so because they had no interest in communicating with others. However, in some of the nonspeaking autistic children Rutter followed, the extreme social withdrawal *disappeared* as they got older, but speech did *not* appear. This finding suggested to him that the absence of speech was *not* simply an expression of social withdrawal. Indeed, he wondered whether the social withdrawal was not instead a consequence of the child's inability to understand the communication of others and to communicate with them.

While disagreeing with Bender about whether psychotic children are schizophrenic, the Rutter, Eaton, and Menolascino, and Kanner and Eisenberg studies all agree with her that the prognosis is very poor. In all studies, about half the children were institutionalized at follow-up. An evaluation of those out of institutions show a poor level of adjustment with almost none employed. These studies, then, add to the studies of psychotic adolescents mentioned in the previous section, to show that when psychosis occurs in very young children, the prognosis is also very poor.

Do Childhood Disorders Portend Adult Problems?

One of the common folk feelings about disliked childhood behavior is that children "grow out of it" before they reach adulthood. Many a grandmother has comforted a distraught mother whose child embarrasses her by sucking his thumb in public with the observation that "after all, you don't see any adults sucking their thumbs. He'll quit when he is ready." Much of this advice is sound—certainly many children *do* give up inappropriate behavior before adulthood. But if the mother thinks beyond the thumb-sucking itself, she may be worried not that the child will be a thumb-sucking adult, but that his childhood behavior may portend disturbed adult behavior of some other kind—perhaps he will substitute alcohol for thumb-sucking.

Research investigating the likelihood that the behavior disorders of childhood will be carried over into adulthood have been of two types: (1) investigations that start with *children* known to have had behavior disorders and then locate information about their adult adjustment and (2) investigations that start with persons known to have psychiatric problems as *adults* and then search childhood records to learn whether they had problem behavior as children. The second type of study may not at first appear to belong under the heading of follow-up studies, since the index reference point is the *later* period of time, just as it is in cross-sectional studies that ask the patient about his early history in an attempt to elucidate the causes of his present difficulties. But it differs from such retrospective studies in that the data about childhood were collected *independently* of the ascertainment of adult problems. The childhood information, whether obtained from juvenile court records, school records, or child guidance clinic records was written down when the subject was a *child*, and could not therefore be contaminated by the knowledge that he would be an adult with psychiatric problems. Such studies do, indeed, therefore, meet the criteria for follow-up studies we delineated earlier: Measures were taken at two different points in time, the time interval was long enough for significant change to have occurred, and the measures were independent of each other.

Studies that begin with children as the point of reference are only extensions in time of the studies of the duration of childhood symptoms which we described in an earlier section. The children are merely followed beyond adolescence into adulthood. In some of the studies reported in the last section, at least some of the sample were over 20 years old at follow-up. In this section, we shall discuss only those studies in which the children are old enough at follow-up so that we have some assurance that stable adult patterns can be discerned. We shall report only on studies in which at least some subjects were 25 years of age or older at follow-up. Our criteria for having had childhood behavior problems include being known to psychiatrists, being known to the police or courts, and having evidence for learning or disciplinary problems in elementary school.

Children Known to Psychiatrists. Two studies have investigated outcomes of children hospitalized in psychiatric facilities. Masterson followed 153 adolescents hospitalized in the Payne Whitney Hospital 5 to 19 years after discharge (1958). His findings are very similar to the results of follow-up studies of hospitalized adults. That is, adolescents diagnosed schizophrenia had a better prognosis when onset was late, when there were symptoms of depressed mood or confusion, when the personality prior to the illness was good, and when there was marked improvement while in the hospital. (In the opinion of some researchers, these results, in both adolescent and adult studies might best be interpreted to mean "when the patients were *mis*diagnosed schizophrenia.") Psychoneurotics almost all had good outcomes. About half the sociopaths had good outcomes, and those sociopaths who improved had *not* had difficulties in school and had improved markedly while in the hospital. (Might these also be examples of misdiagnosis?)

Morris also followed hospitalized children, but his group was younger (aged 4 to 15) when initially hospitalized (Morris, Escoll, & Wexler, 1956). Instead of studying *all* children hospitalized during a given period, as Masterson had, he confined himself to nonpsychotic, nonbrain-damaged, antisocial children of normal intelligence. This group is probably most comparable to the group in Masterson's study who were diagnosed sociopathic. Out of a group of 90, 47 were followed at least to age 26. Although nonpsychotic as children, one-fourth of these antisocial children were diagnosed schizophrenic as adults and one-third (including the schizophrenics) had been chronically hospitalized. Only one-fourth had a good adult social adjustment. Those who were well adults had shown least symptomatology prior to hospitalization. This study suggests that while childhood *psychosis* may not be an early form of schizophrenia, antisocial behavior serious enough to lead to hospitalization may sometimes forebode schizophrenia.

Studies of child guidance clinic populations have shown the same striking patterns found in the more seriously ill hospitalized populations. Both in Dallas (Michael, Morris, & Soroker, 1957; Michael, 1957) and in St. Louis (Robins, 1966) poor outcomes were largely confined to *antisocial* children. Indeed, in St. Louis, children seen for neurotic disturbances had almost as good adult adjustment as had normal school children selected for freedom from school problems and matched with the clinic children with respect to IQ, neighborhood, age, and race. (The Dallas study did not include a control group.) Antisocial children had not only more psychiatric hospitalization as adults but also more difficulties with the law, with their jobs, with their families, and with social relationships of all kinds than either neurotic or control children.

The Dallas study found a later hospital diagnosis of schizophrenia most common in the "ambiverts"—boys judged to be neither introverts nor extroverts. In the St. Louis study, schizophrenia was somewhat more common as the number of childhood neurotic symptoms increased (4% of children with 2 or fewer, 6% of those with 3 to 5, and 9% of children with 6 or more) while the presence of antisocial symptoms did not change the risk. In a sense these findings agree, since patients in the St. Louis study with a high degree of *both* antisocial and neurotic symptoms (more than 6 of each) produced a higher proportion of schizophrenics than did any other group (11%). Both studies agree that the shy, withdrawn personality, often thought to be predictive of schizophrenia, predicts *neither* schizophrenia nor other psychiatric illness, and that some antisocial children are schiopzhrenic adults.

⭐ The St. Louis study found that having a *father* whose behavior was antisocial increased the risk that antisocial behavior would persist into adulthood. Social class, broken homes, gang membership, on the other hand, had little predictive value. One important finding was that *no* childhood variables, neither the child's behavior problem nor his family type, predicted adult neurosis. Indeed, many of the symptoms for which children are commonly referred to psychiatrists, tics, speech difficulties, shyness, fears, oversensitiveness, "nervousness," irritability, tantrums, and insomnia, occurred as often in children *well* as adults as they did in those who were later neurotic. These findings suggest that while adult antisocial behavior has its roots in childhood behavior disorders, adult neurosis for the most part does not. (An exception was the neurotic diagnosis "hysteria," which could be predicted by both family patterns and behavior.)

The later military history of boys seen in child guidance clinics of several cities (Roff, 1956) was contrasted with the military history of a control group of randomly selected school boys. Child guidance clinic patients were found to have obtained more rejections from Service for behavior problems and criminal records and fewer deferments because of dependency and essential jobs during World War II. Among boys inducted, the clinic cases received more dishonorable discharges and more honorable discharges for psychiatric illness or "unsuitability," indicating that they had adjusted less well to life in Service. Despite their higher rate of problems, most clinic patients (74%) had uneventful military careers. It was found possible to predict from the clinic records *which* patients would fail in Service with considerable accuracy. One of the best prognostic clues was poor relationships with other children, as reported by teachers, supplemented by evaluations by family members and clinic personnel (Roff, 1961a).

Children Known to Legal Authorities. There is much literature on the prediction of recidivism among juvenile delinquents, a literature which has grown out of the needs of judges and probation officers to decide on the proper disposition of children in their custody. But there have been few studies which followed juvenile delinquents long enough to judge their long-range risk of arrests as adults or of problem adjustment in other areas. Nor have there been many studies which compared their adult adjustment with that of nondelinquent boys.

The Gluecks followed 1000 boys referred to the Judge Baker Clinic by the juvenile court until they reached an average age of 29 (Glueck & Glueck, 1940). Of the 1000, arrest records were studied for the 848 who had survived the whole period and on whom follow-up data were available throughout. Only 13% of these delinquents were found to have been entirely free of delinquency throughout the 15 years since their initial referral, and 58% had been arrested in the last 5 years (between the ages of 24 and 29, approximately).

While this study does not provide a control group, the number arrested seems extremely high. That it *is* very high is validated by studies in St. Louis. Two-thirds of the male white child guidance clinic cases and normal controls had been known either to the police or juvenile court before the age of 17 (Robins, 1966). More than half (58%) of those subjects known to the police as juveniles had a significant adult police record (sentenced for a nontraffic offense, or if not sentenced, arrested at least three times for nontraffic offenses). When the subjects had had *no* police contacts as juveniles, only 14% ever had a significant adult police record. A similar strong relationship between delinquency and adult arrest records has been found in a follow-up study of normal Negro school boys in St. Louis (Robins, unpublished). Two-thirds of the Negro men with a juvenile police record had a significant adult record, but of those free of juvenile offenses only one-fourth had. It will be noted that while the relationship between juvenile and adult arrests holds for both races, Negro men have more adult arrests and incarceration than whites, both with and without a juvenile police record.

Juvenile arrest history was a more powerful predictor of adult arrest records for both whites and Negroes than was any measure of family stability or social class. However, for whites, but not for Negroes, family pathology and lower class status in childhood did *add* to the risk of later arrests for delinquents. More than 4 out of 5 (84%) of the white delinquents from lower class, problem families had significant adult arrest records.

A comparison of the military careers of juvenile delinquents with the careers of a random sample of school boys (Roff, 1961b, 1963) found that about a quarter of juvenile delinquents were rejected by the services on "moral" grounds, as compared with only 7% of a random sample of boys. When delinquents were inducted, more than half had unsatisfactory service records, compared with only 13% of the control group of school boys. This study shows that the bad adult prognosis for juvenile offenders is by no means limited to their criminal histories.

The widespread predictive power of juvenile delinquency appears also in a study of delinquent and nondelinquent children known to a Child Welfare Board in Sweden (Otterstrom, 1946). Children were referred to the Board because of bad homes, delinquent behavior, or both. Children referred for *delinquency* had worse adult outcome than children from bad homes, not only in terms of their police records, but also in terms of marital disruptions, poor occupational success, and high rate of alcoholism. Like the St. Louis study, Otterstrom's study emphasizes that the presence of childhood behavior problems is a more powerful predictor of adult outcome than is family pathology.

Both studies also show that antisocial behavior in childhood predicts a wide variety of adult difficulties.

Children Identified in School as Showing Problem Behavior.   In the St. Louis study, the very high level of adult success in the slum-dwelling control group, chosen for an absence of elementary school retardation and serious truancy, was in marked contrast to the outcome of the child guidance clinic patients (Robins, 1966). Most of these control children, although from impoverished families, as adults had little crime, stable family lives, steady employment, and rising social status. Finding that an absence of elementary school problems predicted such good adult adjustment suggested to us that the *presence* of retardation and truancy in elementary school should predict the kind of adult *mal*adjustment associated with poverty and slum living. This prediction is being tested in a sample of Negro men. Although analysis of the data is not complete, the combination of being held back at least one semester in elementary school plus being absent more than 20% of the time in 5 or more school quarters has already been shown to predict death before the age of 33 (11% versus 2% for the remainder of the sample) (Robins, 1968a), problem drinking among those surviving to age 33 (32% versus 20% of the remainder of the population) (Robins, 1968b), and a serious adult criminal record (57% versus 34% for the remainder of the sample).

We counted as "solid citizens" those adult Negro men who met all of the following criteria: employed at follow-up, not unemployed as much as 6 months within the last 5 years, currently married, not divorced more than once previously, continuously supporting legitimate children, no current drug use, no alcohol problems in the last 3 years, and no dependence on crime or gambling for support in the last 5 years. Only 17% of Negro men achieved this level of conformity to middle class standards when they had been held back and truanted in elementary school, as compared with twice that proportion (33%) when the elementary school record showed fewer problems.

A comparison of these findings for Negroes with findings for whites in the earlier study indicates that the direction of the relationships is the same, but that the risk of adult problems is so much greater for Negroes that problems *do* occur at an appreciable rate even in children with innocuous school records. (Among white boys, an absence of elementary school problems was almost a *guarantee* of later successful adjustment.) But with *poor* school records, there is almost a certainty that the Negro men will fail to conform to adult middle class standards of behavior.

The Childhood Histories of Sick Adults.   When childhood predictors of *rare* adult psychiatric disorders are the topic of interest, it is wasteful of research time and funds to start with a random sample of children. One would follow them into adulthood only to discover that too few have developed the disorder to allow statistical comparisons between their childhoods and the childhoods of subjects *without* the disorder. One solution is to select children thought to have a high rate of *predisposition* to the disorder (as the St. Louis clinic population had to adult antisocial behavior), but when the disorder is as rare as schizophrenia, for instance, a population of deviant children still will not produce enough cases. If one chooses a still more highly predisposed sample, as for instance the offspring of schizophrenic mothers, the schizophrenics one discovers at follow-up will not be a *representative* sample of schizophrenics. Most schizophrenics, after all, do not have a mother so diagnosed.

A solution to this problem is to select a representative sample of *adult* schizophrenics and then locate appropriate records dating from their childhoods. A control group can be chosen from the same childhood records—for instance, the next name in the list of classmates or clinic attenders—or from the adult records, depending on the question one seeks to answer.

This technique of following cases "backwards" has been used in a number of studies of patients identified in mental hospital records. In one study (Huffman & Wenig, 1954), the names of State Hospital patients admitted from one metropolitan area were checked against the records of a child guidance clinic operated during their childhoods by the Board of Education. Patients *not* located in the clinic records were assumed to have been free of significant maladjustment in childhood. Very impressive differences in the frequency of appearing in the childhood records were found among different diagnostic groups. Almost all of the patients with an adult diagnosis of schizophrenia (dementia praecox type), sociopathy, or mental deficiency had been known to the clinic as children, but none of those with depressions, and few of those with situational reactions or acute organic psychoses.

A somewhat similar study in England, starting with adult patients and locating psychiatric records made for them as children (Pritchard and Graham, 1966), again found that adults with conduct disorders (sociopathy) more often had been seen as children than had the depressions. (Rates of schizophrenia were not discussed, probably because this diagnosis was much less common in the acute psychiatric hospitals studied than in the State Hospital population.) This study also attempted to relate childhood symptoms to the adult diagnoses. Among patients seen as children, depression and anxiety in adulthood had been prefigured by neurotic symptoms in childhood (predominantly anxiety, depression, and somatic complaints). Adults with conduct disorders (sociopathy) came predominantly from those children referred for antisocial behavior (stealing, truanting, lying, fighting). This part of the study confirmed the St. Louis study's findings that antisocial behavior in childhood was strongly related to the diagnosis of sociopathy in adults.

Male patients diagnosed schizophrenic in one hospital were searched for in the records of a child guidance clinic in the same city (Frazee, 1953). When a name was located, the next boy of the same age seen by the clinic was selected as a control subject. The purpose of this study was to see whether child guidance clinic patients destined to be schizophrenic had a different pattern of symptoms from other clinic patients. The preschizophrenics were found to have lower IQ scores, to be generally sicker, as measured by the number of symptoms, and to have had a gradual onset of symptoms. They had more school failures and came from more disturbed families. Particularly striking symptoms were their inability to make normal social relationships, their frequent temper tantrums, and their description as listless. They did *not* show symptoms of psychosis in childhood.

Two studies sought school records of persons hospitalized with a diagnosis of schizophrenia and compared their records with records of matched controls in the same school. In one study (Bower, Shellhamer, & Daily, 1960), school personnel were interviewed about patients and control subjects using "double blind" methods (i.e., neither the interviewer nor the school personnel knew which boy was hospitalized and which was well). Patients differed from controls in having lower IQ scores, in being poorer students, in more often showing deteriorating grades, and in more frequently dropping out of school. The patients also more often were described as careless, apathetic, depressed, fewer social contracts, and less athletic. Despite their having more indicators of poor adjustment in high school, about one-fifth of the patients had been extremely well-adjusted students.

This study shows that some schizophrenics have poor prepsychotic personalities, but it fails to answer some important questions. Many studies have reported an association between lower class status and schizophrenia. While some recent work suggests that this association is a *consequence* of the poor prepsychotic personality (Goldberg and Morrison, 1963), one still wonders whether the poor grades and deficient social interaction may not simply be evidence of the lower class status of the preschizophrenics. One study has overcome this limitation by comparing IQ scores on elementary school records of adult schizophrenics with the scores of their *own* siblings (Lane & Albee, 1965). Since siblings share both class status and family environment, differences in IQ could not be environmental. When compared with their *own* brothers and sisters, the future schizophrenics were found to have lower IQ scores. Correlations between their IQ scores and their siblings' were much lower than the correlation between siblings in the general population. These findings suggest a disease process already started in elementary school which depresses IQ and wipes out the correlations attributable to genetic factors and family environment found in normal siblings. Since similar findings did *not* occur between siblings when one had been diagnosed neurotic in a child guidance clinic, this finding does not appear to apply to *all* psychiatrically ill persons. Schizophrenics were also found to have lower birth weights recorded on their birth certificates than had their siblings (Lane and

Albee, 1966). From this, we may infer that the pre-schizophrenic child is different at birth. Either whatever produces schizophrenia also influences birth weight, or perhaps babies in less robust health at birth are more vulnerable to schizophrenia-producing variables.

Conclusions

This chapter has discussed studies in English principally published prior to 1969 which meet the following criteria: The studies have dealt with children's behavior disorders, broadly defined as reported symptoms, difficulties at school or with the law, or referral to a psychiatrist before the age of 18; measures have been taken at two or more points in time, at least one measure having been taken before the age of 18; the measures have been made independently of each other; and more than a year has elapsed between the initial measure and the follow-up measure. An effort has been made to select examples of studies meeting these criteria from each major area in which follow-up studies have made a contribution. In areas in which several studies have been published, quality of the research has been the guiding factor in choosing which studies to present. Judgment as to quality was based on the size and representativeness of the sample, the clarity with which methods were reported, and the use of adequate control samples.

Although some of the less rigorous studies have thus been eliminated, the scientific qualities of the studies presented vary widely. It is perhaps a tribute to the contribution that follow-up studies can make that concordant findings appear despite major differences in the orientations of the researchers to one school of psychological thought or another and in the scientific rigor with which the studies have been pursued. We would argue that this concordance stems at least in part from the fact that follow-up studies require independent measures at two points in time, a requirement which reduces the possible bias of results in the direction of the researcher's preconceptions.

As of the writing of this chapter, there are many questions about childhood disorders which could be answered by follow-up studies but to which satisfactory answers have not yet been found. Among these questions for which we have sought answers in existing studies, the least well covered are the incidence of behavior disorders among children, the duration of childhood disorders, and proper classification of childhood disorders. A major difficulty in answering these questions stems from researchers' failure to agree on criteria for what constitutes a behavior disorder of childhood. Without such criteria, they can agree on neither rates of *appearance* nor rates of *disappearance* of disorders. As the studies presented indicate, being seen by a psychiatrist cannot be a satisfactory measure of the number of children with behavior disorders, since that figure can vary between 2% of Swedish children seen in a 10-year period to more than 10 times that rate, 21%, referred to a psychiatrist before the age of 7, when parents are particularly accepting of psychiatric intervention. Nor can the presence of at least one symptom be a satisfactory measure, since all children would qualify at one age or another (Macfarlane et al., 1954). At the present time, we can say only that difficulties severe enough to cause concern to teachers and psychiatrists occur in at least 7% of children (the proportion diagnosed as psychiatrically ill in a 10-year period in one Swedish study). But the figure may be considerably greater than 7%, since another Swedish study found 25% in need of treatment. We do not yet have a reliable figure for the occurrence of behavior disorders at some time during childhood.

We do know that most children identified as having behavior problems in clinics and in schools are considered as well or improved a year or two later, but no study has yet attempted to ascertain the length of time between onset and disappearance either for individual symptoms or for syndromes. Consequently, we cannot yet prognosticate with any assurance how long a child's disturbance is likely to last. We know only that neurotic symptoms are much more likely to dissipate or improve in a short time than are symptoms of psychosis or antisocial behavior.

Nor have follow-up studies yet produced a comprehensive classificatory system for childhood behavior disorders. To develop a comprehensive classification will require both more "backward" follow-ups of representative samples of adults with well-defined syndromes and more prospective follow-up studies into adulthood of children identified by symptom clusters and family histories. Only when the whole spectrum of adult disorders has been identified as beginning or not beginning in childhood, and when these early appearing adult disorders can be separated from disorders limited to children, can we begin to develop a coherent classification scheme for childhood disorders. The studies presented here have made only a small beginning in this enterprise. They have shown that psychosis appearing before puberty is never or almost never an early form of adult schizophrenia, but that the psychotic child does have an illness that continues into adulthood, where it accounts for only a small proportion of hospitalized adults. They have shown that hysteria can, but rarely does, begin in childhood, while the common adult neuroses seem *not* to begin in childhood. Finally, they have shown that the widespread adult antisocial behavior called sociopathy begins almost exclusively in childhood. We as yet do not know what proportion of childhood disorders these early forms of adult disorders account for, nor can we readily distinguish by symptom pattern childhood disorders which will and which will not be continued into adulthood. Indeed, our best clue at the present time as to whether a disorder will be transient seems to be the severity of incapacitation and number of symptoms rather than its classification by syndrome.

We are on firmer ground at the present time when it comes to predicting *which* children will develop a behavior disorder, however we define the disorder. We know that psychiatric illness in the parents is reflected in an elevated rate of behavior problems in their children, and that antisocial parents have antisocial children. When the parents' antisocial behavior takes the form of physical abuse of the child, the child shows very severe disability. We also know that childhood behavior problems are more common in the lower classes, and that this relationship may be largely accounted for by the higher prevalence of antisocial and psychiatrically ill parents in the lower classes. To what extent the influence of the parent's disturbance on the child's behavior is genetic and to what extent it is environmental is still an unanswered question.

We can also predict certain behavior disorders of later childhood from behavior first observable around the age of starting school. A combination of poor relationships with schoolmates, working below intellectual capacity, and failing to accept the teacher's authority predict delinquency. A high level of neurotic symptoms predict poor school success. Early behavioral predictors of other kinds of childhood disorders are not yet clearly identified.

We also know a good deal about the adult prognosis for disturbed children. The weight of evidence at the present time is that two kinds of childhood disorders, psychosis and serious antisocial behavior, have gloomy prognoses for adult life. Psychosis in children, whether it begins before puberty or whether it is schizophrenia beginning in adolescence, almost always persists into adulthood. Most psychotic children will spend much of their lives in institutions. Serious antisocial behavior in childhood is not so uniformly disastrous, but in a large minority of cases it presages life-long problems with the law, inability to earn a living, defective interpersonal relationships, and severe personal distress. In fact, if one could successfully treat the antisocial behavior of childhood, the problems of adult crime, alcoholism, divorce, and chronic unemployment might be vastly diminished. These two disorders, psychosis and antisocial behavior, along with severe mental retardation, which we have not discussed here, are the childhood psychiatric categories for which serious adult difficulties can be predicted. Neurotic disorders of childhood, quite to the contrary, have very good long term prognoses, no matter how disturbing they may be to the family and child while they exist.

At the present time, unfortunately, there is no substantive evidence that childhood psychosis or antisocial behavior can be either prevented or treated successfully. All carefully controlled studies have agreed in showing poor results no matter what techniques have been attempted. It is, however, encouraging that follow-up methods provide us with a technique for evaluating our attempts at prevention and treatment that produces clear and consistent answers. When we do find successful techniques for preventing or modifying childhood disorders, we can expect follow-up studies to demonstrate their *effectiveness* as dramatically and consistently as they now demonstrate our present failures in prevention and cure.

References

Annesley, P. T. Psychiatric illness in adolescence: Presentation and prognosis. *Journal of Mental Science,* 1961, **107**, 268–278.

Bender, L. Childhood schizophrenia. *The Psychiatric Quarterly,* 1953, **27**, 1–19.

Bower, E. M., Shellhamer, T. A., & Daily, J. M. School characteristics of male adolescents who later became schizophrenic. *American Journal of Orthopsychiatry,* 1960, **30**, 712–729.

Bowlby, J., Ainsworth, M., Boston, M., & Rosenbluth, D. The effects of mother-child separation: A follow-up study. *British Journal of Medical Psychology,* 1956, **29**, 211–244.

Burt, C. *The young delinquent,* New York: D. Appleton and Company, 1925.

Canavan, M. M., & Clark, R. The mental health of 463 children from dementia praecox stock, 1. *Mental Hygiene,* 1923a, **7**, 137–148.

Canavan, M. M., & Clark, R. The mental health of 581 offspring of non-psychotic parents. *Mental Hygiene,* 1923b, **7**, 770–778.

Conger, J. J., & Miller, W. C. *Personality, social class, and delinquency,* New York: Wiley, 1966.

Craig, M. M., & Glick, S. J. Ten years' experience with the Glueck social prediction table. *Crime and Delinquency,* 1963, **9**, 249–261.

Cumming, J., & McCaffrey, I. Onondaga County school studies. Interim Report No. 1. Persistence of Emotional Disturbances Reported Among Second and Fourth Grade Children, Mental Health Research Unit, New York State Department of Mental Hygiene, Syracuse, New York, 1964.

Cunningham, J., Westerman, H. H., & Fischoff, J. A follow-up study of patients seen in a psychiatric clinic for children. *Amer. J. Orthopsychiat.,* 1956, **26**, 602–612.

Douglas, J. W. B. *The home and the school.* London: Macgibbon & Kee, 1964.

Douglas, J. W. B. The school progress of nervous and troublesome children. *The Brit. J. of Psychiat.,* 1966, **112**, 1115–1116.

Eaton, L., & Menolascino, F. L. Psychotic reactions of childhood: A follow-up study. *Amer. J. Orthopsychiat.,* 1967, **37**, 521–529.

Elmer, E., & Gregg, G. S. Developmental characteristics of abused children. *Pediatrics,* 1967, **40**, Part I, 596–602.

Frazee, H. E. Children who later became schizophrenic. *Smith Coll. Studies in Social Work*, 1953, **23**, 125–149.

Gildea, M. C.-L., Glidewell, J. C., & Kantor, M. B. The St. Louis school mental health project: History and evaluation. In E. L. Cowen, E. A. Gardner, & M. Zax (Eds.), *Emergent Approaches to Mental Health Problems*, New York: Meredith Publishing Company, 1967.

Glavin, J. P. "Spontaneous" improvement in emotionally disturbed children. George Peabody College for Teachers, Doctoral Dissertation, August 1967.

Glueck, S., & Glueck, E. *Juvenile delinquents grown up*. New York: The Commonwealth Fund, 1940.

Glueck, S., & Glueck, E. *Unraveling juvenile delinquency*. New York: The Commonwealth Fund, 1950.

Goldberg, E. M., & Morrison, S. L. Schizophrenia and social class. *Brit. J. of Psychiat.*, 1963, **109**, 758–802.

Hagnell, O. *A prospective study of the incidence of mental disorder*, Stockholm: Svenska Bokförlaget, 1966.

Havighurst, R. J., Bowman, P. H., Liddle, G. P., Matthews, C. V., & Pierce, J. V. *Growing up in River City*. New York: John Wiley, 1962.

Healy, W., & Bronner, A. F. *New light on delinquency and its treatment*. New Haven: Yale University Press, 1936.

Heston, L. L. Psychiatric disorders in foster home reared children of schizophrenic mothers. *Brit. J. of Psychiat.*, 1966, **112**, 819–825.

Huffman, P. W., & Wenig, P. W. Prodromal behavior patterns in mental illness, Department of Public Welfare, State of Illinois. Mimeo., 1954.

Jonsson, G., & Kälvesten, A.-L. *222 Stockholmspojkar*, Uppsala, 1964. A summary in English appears in G. Jonsson, Delinquent boys, their parents and grandparents, *Acta Psychiatrica Scandinavica*, 1967, Suppl. 195, Appendix I, 227–256.

Kanner, L., & Eisenberg, L. Notes on the follow-up studies of autistic children. *Psychopathology of Children*, New York: Grune & Stratton, Inc., 1955, pp. 227–239.

Lane, E. A., & Albee, G. W. Childhood intellectual differences between schizophrenic adults and their siblings. *Amer. J. Orthopsychiat.*, 1965, **35**, 747–753.

Lane, E. A., & Albee, G. W. Comparative birth weights of schizophrenics and their siblings. *The Journal of Psychology*, 1966, **64**, 227–231.

Lewis, A. J. The offspring of parents both mentally ill. *Acta Genetica*, 1957, **7**, 349–365.

Lewis, W. W. Continuity and intervention in emotional disturbance: A review. *Exceptional Children*, 1965, **31**, 465–475.

Macfarlane, J. W., Allen, L., & Honzik, M. P. *A developmental study of the behavior problems of normal children between twenty-one months and fourteen years*. Berkeley and Los Angeles: University of California Press, 1954.

Masterson, J. F., Jr. Prognosis in adolescent disorders. *Am. J. Psychiat.*, 1958, **114**: 1097–1103.

Masterson, J. F., Jr. The symptomatic adolescent five years later: He didn't grow out of it. *Am. J. Psychiat.*, 1967, **123**, 1338–1345.

McCord, W., & McCord, J. *Origins of crime.* New York: Columbia University Press, 1959.

Meyer, H. J., Borgatta, E. F., & Jones, W. C. *Girls at vocational high.* New York: Russell Sage Foundation, 1965.

Michael, C. M. Relative incidence of criminal behavior in long term follow-up studies of shy children. *Dallas Medical Journal,* January 1957.

Michael, C. M., Morris, D. P., & Soroker, E. Follow-up studies of shy, withdrawn children II: Relative incidence of schizophrenia. *The Amer. J. of Orthopsychiat.,* 1957, **27**, 331–337.

Molof, M. J. Forestry camp study: Comparison of recidivism rates of camp-eligible boys randomly assigned to camp and to institutional programs, Research Report No. 53, State of California, Department of the Youth Authority, 1967.

Morris, H. H., Jr., Escoll, P. J., & Wexler, R. Aggressive behavior disorders of childhood: A follow-up study. *Am. J. of Psych.,* 1956, **112**, 991–997.

Mulligan, G., Douglas, J. W. B., Hammond, W. A., & Tizard, J. Delinquency and symptoms of maladjustment: The findings of a longitudinal study. *Proceedings of the Royal Society of Medicine,* 1963, **56**, 1083–1086.

Otterström, E. Delinquency and children from bad homes. *Acta Paediatrica,* 1946, **33**, Suppl. 5.

Powers, E., & Witmer, H. *An experiment in the prevention of delinquency.* New York: Columbia University Press, 1951.

Pritchard, M., & Graham, P. An investigation of a group of patients who have attended both the child and adult departments of the same psychiatric hospital. *Brit. J. of Psychiat.,* 1966, **112**, 603–612.

Roberts, C. F., Jr. A follow-up study of the juvenile drug offender. Institute for the Study of Crime and Delinquency, Sacramento, California, October 1967.

Robins, E., & O'Neal, P. Clinical features of hysteria in children, with a note on prognosis. *The Nervous Child,* 1953, **10**, 246–271.

Robins, L. N. *Deviant children grown up.* Baltimore: The Williams & Wilkins Co., 1966.

Robins, L. N. Behavior patterns and the high Negro death rate. *Trans-action,* 1968.

Robins, L. N., & Lewis, R. G. The role of the antisocial family in school completion and delinquency: A three-generation study. *Sociological Quarterly,* 1966, **7**, 500–514.

Robins, L. N., Murphy, G. E., & Breckenridge, M. B. Drinking behavior in young urban Negro men, *Quart. J. Stud. Alc.,* 1968.

Roff, M. Preservice personality problems and subsequent adjustments to military service; Gross outcome in relation to acceptance-rejection at induction and military service. School of Aviation Medicine, USAF Randolf AFB, Texas, Report 55-138, 1956.

Roff, M. The service-related experience of a sample of juvenile delinquents. U.S. Army Medical Research and Development Command, Report No. 61-1, 1961a.

Roff, M. Childhood social interactions and young adult bad conduct. *J. Abnorm. Soc. Psychol.,* 1961b, **63**, 333–337.

Roff, M. The service-related experience of a sample of juvenile delinquents. II. A replication on a larger sample in another state. U.S. Army Medical Research and Development Command, Report No. 63-2, 1963.

Rutter, M., Birch, H. G., Thomas, A., & Chess, S. Temperamental characteristics in infancy and the later development of behavioural disorders. *Brit. J. of Psychiat.*, 1964, **110**, 651–661.

Rutter, M. The influence of organic and emotional factors on the origins, nature and outcome of childhood psychosis. *Developmental Medicine and Child Neurology*, 1965, **7**, 518–527.

Rutter, M., & Lockyer, L. A five to fifteen year follow-up study of infantile psychosis I. Description of sample. *Brit. J. of Psychiat.*, 1967a, **113**, 1169–1182.

Rutter, M., Greenfeld, D., & Lockyer, L. A five to fifteen year follow-up study of infantile psychosis II. Social and behavioural outcome. *Brit. J. Psychiat.*, 1967b, **113**, 1183–1199.

Shepherd, M., Oppenheim, A. N., & Mitchell, S. Childhood behaviour disorders and the child-guidance clinic: An epidemiological study. *Journal of Child Psychology Psychiatry*, 1966, **7**, 39–52.

Shirley, M., Baum, B., & Polsky, S. Outgrowing childhood's problems: A follow-up study of child guidance patients. *Smith College Studies in Social Work*, 1940–41, **11**, 31–60.

Tait, C. D., Jr., & Hodges, E. F., Jr. *Delinquents, their families, and the community*. Springfield, Ill.: Charles C. Thomas, 1962.

Thomas, A., Chess, S., & Birch, H. G. *Temperament and behavior disorders in children*. New York: New York University Press, 1968.

Warren, W. A study of adolescent psychiatric in-patients and the outcome six or more years later II. The follow-up study. *J. Child Psychol. Psychiat.*, 1965, **6**, 141–160.

Westman, J. C., Rice, D. L., & Bermann, E. Nursery school behavior and later school adjustment. *Amer. J. Orthopsychiat.*, 1967, **37**, 725–731.

Wilner, D. M., Walkley, R. P., Pinkerton, T. C., & Tayback, M. *The housing environment and family life*. Baltimore: The Johns Hopkins Press, 1962.

World Health Organization. Deprivation of maternal care: A reassessment of its effects. *Public Health Papers*, No. 14, 7-165, 1962.

Name Index

Subject Index